Essential Otolaryngology

Essential Otolaryngology

Edited by **Chad Downs**

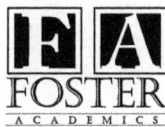

FA
FOSTER
ACADEMICS

New Jersey

Published by Foster Academics,
61 Van Reypen Street,
Jersey City, NJ 07306, USA
www.fosteracademics.com

Essential Otolaryngology
Edited by Chad Downs

International Standard Book Number: 978-1-63242-432-7 (Hardback)

Contents

Preface   IX

Chapter 1 **Correlation of Lateral Cephalogram and Flexible Laryngoscopy with Sleep Study in Obstructive Sleep Apnea**   **1**
Anila Narayanan and Bini Faizal

Chapter 2 **Subclinical Hearing Loss, Longer Sleep Duration, and Cardiometabolic Risk Factors in Japanese General Population**   **8**
Kei Nakajima, Eiichiro Kanda, Ami Hosobuchi and Kaname Suwa

Chapter 3 **From Inpatient Notes to Outpatient Followup: Enhancing the Rhinology Service in a Tertiary Centre through Student Led Projects**   **19**
M. Sayma, R. Hyne,M. Sharma, L. Kyle, M. Abo Khatwa, I. MacKay-Davies, A. Poulios and H. S. Khalil

Chapter 4 **Effect of Preoperative Mastoid Ventilation on Tympanoplasty Success**   **24**
Mehmet Metin, Zeynep Kizilkaya Kaptan, Sedat Dogan, Hasmet Yazici, Cem Bayraktar, Hakan Gocmen and Etem Erdal Samim

Chapter 5 **Evaluation of the Nasal Surgical Questionnaire for Monitoring Results of Septoplasty**   **28**
Rolf Haye, Magnus Tarangen, Olga Shiryaeva and Liv Kari Døsen

Chapter 6 **Effects of Sacrificing Tensor Tympani Muscle Tendon When Manubrium of Malleus is Foreshortened in Type I Tympanoplasty**   **35**
Sohil Vadiya

Chapter 7 **Aerodigestive Foreign Bodies in Adult Ethiopian Patients: A Prospective Study at Tikur Anbessa Hospital, Ethiopia**   **38**
Abebe Bekele

Chapter 8 **Evaluation of Etiology and Treatment Methods for Epistaxis: A Review at a Tertiary Care Hospital in Central Nepal**   **43**
Ramesh Parajuli

Chapter 9 **Impact of Educational Program on the Management of Chronic Suppurative Otitis Media Among Children**   **48**
Yousseria Elsayed Yousef, Essam A. Abo El-Magd, Osama M. El-Asheer and Safaa Kotb

Chapter 10 **Elicitation of the Acoustic Change Complex to Long-Duration Speech Stimuli in Four-Month-Old Infants**   **56**
Ke Heng Chen and Susan A. Small

Chapter 11   **Gastric Decompression Decreases Postoperative Nausea and Vomiting in**
              ENT Surgery   68
              Kerem Erkalp, Nuran Kalekoglu Erkalp, M. Salih Sevdi, A. Yasemin Korkut,
              Hacer Yeter, SertuL Sinan Ege, Aysin Alagol and Veysel Erden

Chapter 12   **Pressure Flow Analysis in the Assessment of Preswallow Pharyngeal Bolus**
              Presence in Dysphagia   73
              Lara Ferris, Taher Omari, Margot Selleslagh, Eddy Dejaeger, Jan Tack,
              Dirk Vanbeckevoort and Nathalie Rommel

Chapter 13   **Individual Optimization of the Insertion of a Preformed Cochlear Implant**
              Electrode Array   79
              Thomas S. Rau, Thomas Lenarz and Omid Majdani

Chapter 14   **The Relationship of the Facial Nerve to the Condylar Process:**
              A Cadaveric Study with Implications for Open Reduction Internal Fixation   101
              H. P. Barham, P. Collister, V. D. Eusterman and A. M. Terella

Chapter 15   **What Are the Trends in Tonsillectomy Techniques in Wales? A Prospective**
              Observational Study of 19,195 Tonsillectomies over a 10-Year Period   104
              Hussein Walijee, Ali Al-Hussaini, Andrew Harris and David Owens

Chapter 16   **Importance of "Process Evaluation" in Audiological Rehabilitation: Examples**
              from Studies on Hearing Impairment   111
              Vinaya Manchaiah, Berth Danermark, Jerker Rönnberg and Thomas Lunner

Chapter 17   **Branchial Anomalies: Diagnosis and Management**   118
              Sampath Chandra Prasad, Arun Azeez, Nikhil Dinaker Thada, Pallavi Rao,
              Andrea Bacciu and Kishore Chandra Prasad

Chapter 18   **Mucin Gene Expression in Reflux Laryngeal Mucosa: Histological and**
              ***In Situ* Hybridization Observations**   127
              Mahmoud El-Sayed Ali, David M. Bulmer, Peter W. Dettmar and Jeffrey P. Pearson

Chapter 19   **Chronic Maxillary Rhinosinusitis of Dental Origin: A Systematic Review of**
              674 Patient Cases   133
              Jerome R. Lechien, Olivier Filleul, Pedro Costa de Araujo, Julien W. Hsieh,
              Gilbert Chantrain and Sven Saussez

Chapter 20   **Changing Trends in the Management of Epistaxis**   142
              Henri Traboulsi, Elie Alam and Usamah Hadi

Chapter 21   **More Than One Disease Process in Chronic Sinusitis Based on Mucin**
              Fragmentation Patterns and Amino Acid Analysis   149
              Mahmoud El-Sayed Ali and Jeffrey P. Pearson

Chapter 22   **Prediction of Short-Term Outcome in Acute Superior Vestibular Nerve Failure:**
              Three-Dimensional Video-Head-Impulse Test and Caloric Irrigation   157
              Holger A. Rambold

Chapter 23   **Efficacy of Epley's Maneuver in Treating BPPV Patients: A Prospective**
              Observational Study   163
              Sushil Gaur, Sanjeev Kumar Awasthi, Sunil Kumar Singh Bhadouriya,
              Rohit Saxena, Vivek Kumar Pathak and Mamta Bisht

Chapter 24 **Hearing Preservation in Cochlear Implant Surgery**   168
Priscila Carvalho Miranda, André Luiz Lopes Sampaio, Rafaela Aquino
Fernandes Lopes, Alessandra Ramos Venosa and Carlos Augusto Costa Pires de
Oliveira

Chapter 25 **The Complications of Sinusitis in a Tertiary Care Hospital: Types, Patient
Characteristics, and Outcomes**   174
Saisawat Chaiyasate, Supranee Fooanant, Niramon Navacharoen,
Kannika Roongrotwattanasiri, Pongsakorn Tantilipikorn and Jayanton Patumanond

Chapter 26 **The Correlation of the Tinnitus Handicap Inventory with Depression and
Anxiety in Veterans with Tinnitus**   179
Jinwei Hu, Jane Xu, Matthew Streelman Helen Xu and O'neil Guthrie

Chapter 27 **The Epworth Sleepiness Scale in the Assessment of Sleep Disturbance in
Veterans with Tinnitus**   187
Yuan F. Liu, Jinwei Hu, Matthew Streelman and O'neil W. Guthrie

Chapter 28 **Inferior Turbinate Size and CPAP Titration Based Treatment Pressures:
No Association Found among Patients Who Have Not Had Nasal Surgery**   196
Macario Camacho, Soroush Zaghi, Daniel Tran, Sungjin A. Song, Edward T. Chang
and Victor Certal

Chapter 29 **Patient Satisfaction with Postaural Incision Site**   203
George Barrett, Susanne Koecher, Natalie Ronan and David Whinney

Chapter 30 **Bolus Residue Scale: An Easy-to-Use and Reliable Videofluoroscopic Analysis
Tool to Score Bolus Residue in Patients with Dysphagia**   207
Nathalie Rommel, Charlotte Borgers, Dirk Van Beckevoort, Ann Goeleven,
Eddy Dejaeger and Taher I. Omari

Chapter 31 **The Importance of the Neutrophil-Lymphocyte Ratio in Patients with Idiopathic
Peripheral Facial Palsy**   214
M. Mustafa Kiliçkaya, Mustafa Tuz, Murat Yariktaş, Hasan Yasan, Giray Aynalı
and Özkan Bagci

Chapter 32 **Antrochoanal Polyps: How Long Should Follow-Up Be after Surgery?**   218
Saisawat Chaiyasate, Kannika Roongrotwattanasiri, Jayanton Patumanond and
Supranee Fooanant

Chapter 33 **Vestibular Disorders After Stapedial Surgery in Patients with Otosclerosis**   223
Ditza de Vilhena, Inês Gambôa, Delfim Duarte and Gustavo Lopes

Permissions

List of Contributors

Preface

It is often said that books are a boon to mankind. They document every progress and pass on the knowledge from one generation to the other. They play a crucial role in our lives. Thus I was both excited and nervous while editing this book. I was pleased by the thought of being able to make a mark but I was also nervous to do it right because the future of students depends upon it. Hence, I took a few months to research further into the discipline, revise my knowledge and also explore some more aspects. Post this process, I began with the editing of this book.

This book on otolaryngology is a collective contribution of a renowned group of international experts. It is a vital tool for all researching or studying this field as it gives incredible insights into emerging trends and concepts. Otolaryngology is commonly referred to as ENT (ear, nose, and throat). It is the area of medicine that deals with the diseases of these body parts. It includes sub-specialties such as otology, laryngology and voice disorders, rhinology and sinus surgery, head and neck oncologic surgery, pediatric otorhinolaryngology, etc. As this field is emerging at a fast pace, this book will help the students to better understand the concepts and essentials of otolaryngology. A number of latest researches have been included to keep the readers up-to-date with the global concepts in this area of study. This book attempts to understand the multiple branches that fall under the discipline of otolaryngology. It is a beneficial read for otolaryngologists, head and neck surgeons, ENT specialists, professionals and students engaged in this field.

I thank my publisher with all my heart for considering me worthy of this unparalleled opportunity and for showing unwavering faith in my skills. I would also like to thank the editorial team who worked closely with me at every step and contributed immensely towards the successful completion of this book. Last but not the least, I wish to thank my friends and colleagues for their support.

Editor

Correlation of Lateral Cephalogram and Flexible Laryngoscopy with Sleep Study in Obstructive Sleep Apnea

Anila Narayanan and Bini Faizal

Department of ENT, Amrita Institute of Medical Sciences, Amrita Vishwa Vidyapeetham, Kochi, Kerala 682041, India

Correspondence should be addressed to Bini Faizal; binifaizal@aims.amrita.edu

Academic Editor: Jeffrey P. Pearson

Objective. To study the correlation between lateral cephalogram, flexible laryngoscopy, and sleep study in patients diagnosed with obstructive sleep apnea (OSA). *Background.* Screening tools should be devised for predicting OSA which could be performed on an outpatient basis. With this aim we studied the skeletal and soft tissue characteristics of proven OSA patients. *Methods.* A prospective study was performed in patients diagnosed with obstructive sleep apnea by sleep study. They were evaluated clinically and subjected to lateral cephalometry and nasopharyngolaryngoscopy. The findings were matched to see if they corresponded to AHI of sleep study in severity. An attempt was made to see whether the data predicted the patients who would benefit from oral appliance or surgery as the definitive treatment in indicated cases. *Results.* A retropalatal collapse seen on endoscopy could be equated to the distance from mandibular plane to hyoid (MP-H) of lateral cephalometry and both corresponded to severity of AHI. At the retroglossal region, there was a significant correlation with MP-H, length of the soft palate, and AHI. *Conclusion.* There is significant correlation of lateral cephalogram and awake flexible nasopharyngolaryngoscopy with AHI in OSA. In unison they form an excellent screening tool for snorers.

1. Introduction

OSA has received significant attention in sleep medicine. It is considered to be a significant cause of morbidity alerting us to the need of evaluating all snorers. Though polysomnogram is irreplaceable in diagnosing OSA, it makes sense to have simple clinical tools to evaluate OSA patients in the outpatient setting. All patients may not have the time and resources for cone beam CT [1, 2] or drug induced sleep endoscopy, the latest in the management of OSA.

Routine assessment of the patients with OSA includes body mass index, tonsillar grading, thyromental distance, and Modified Mallampati grading. Lateral cephalogram and flexible nasopharyngolaryngoscopy provide multisegmental assessment of airway. Former provides anteroposterior assessment of craniofacial morphology at the level of soft palate and base of tongue. It may not be effective for lateral diametric measurements. Studies have been conducted on cephalometric variables in nonapneic and apneic snorers which can be based as guidelines for recognizing potential candidates.

Flexible nasopharyngolaryngoscopy with Muller's maneuver (awake endoscopy) [3–6] gives a three-dimensional soft tissue assessment of airway. Both the above procedures can be easily done in an outpatient setting. There is no denying that both procedures have better options in the form of cone beam CT and drug induced sleep endoscopy (DISE).

Despite our knowledge that apneic individuals have a collapsing airway, we still have great difficulty in assessing the exact point of collapse during sleep. A combination of lateral cephalometry and awake endoscopy can be a preliminary screening tool to rule out any bony or soft tissue compromise on the airway. DISE and cone beam CT could be the next line of investigation in case of any surgical intervention. This decreases the economic burden on the patient as well as radiation exposure. The level of obstruction in endoscopy may correlate with an altered reading at the corresponding level in lateral cephalometry. It may suggest the efficacy of surgical procedure or suitability of oral appliance in some cases. Conversely, application of these variables in a snorer may provide insights into the probability of OSA in him. However, as suggested by Cavaliere et al. [7] 22.7% of patients with epiglottis related obstruction may go undetected in awake endoscopy. In our study, we analyzed the parameters from lateral cephalometry and awake nasopharyngolaryngoscopy and compared them with AHI of patients with mild, moderate, and severe OSA.

2. Materials and Methods

2.1. Objectives. To study the correlation of lateral cephalometry and awake flexible nasopharyngolaryngoscopy with Apnea Hypopnea Index of sleep study in patients diagnosed with obstructive sleep apnea.

2.1.1. Study Design. This was a prospective cross-sectional study on patients diagnosed with OSA in a tertiary care centre.

2.1.2. Sample Size and Method of Recruitment. For this study, 70 patients diagnosed with OSA following sleep study, with an AHI of 5 or greater, were included. Patients less than 18 years, who underwent upper airway surgeries, with syndromic anomalies and craniofacial abnormalities like retrognathia, prognathism, and mandibular hypoplasia were excluded. The patients were subsequently divided into 2 groups. group I showed less than 50% of airway collapse on endoscopy and group II had more than 50% collapse.

2.1.3. Data Collection. Patients with symptoms suggestive of OSA underwent sleep study from the Pulmonology Department of our Institute whereby AHI and other parameters like RDI, oxygen saturation, number of apneas, and number of hypopneas were recorded by Apnea Link. OSA is classified as mild (AHI- 5–15), moderate (AHI- 15–30), and severe (AHI-more than 30) depending on the AHI (American Academy of Sleep Medicine).

After routine ENT evaluation, patients underwent flexible nasopharyngolaryngoscopy with Muller's maneuver after adequate nasal preparation with 0.1% Oxymetazoline nasal drops and topical Lignocaine 4%. The following four areas were studied for end expiratory collapse, retropalatal region, retroglossal region, lateral pharyngeal walls, and supraglottic region. Patients were classified into Groups I and II depending on the collapse of airway at these levels.

Digitalized lateral cephalometry was taken from the Dental Department of the institute (Sirona; Orthophos XG5). Before the radiograph was taken, a thin layer of barium sulfate paste was applied on the dorsum of the tongue to enhance soft tissue identification. To standardize hyoid position, radiographs were exposed at the end of expiration, in the natural head position with the teeth in light occlusion. The cephalometric variables included in this study were Angle SNA (skull base angle of maxilla), Angle SNB (skull

TABLE 1: Showing the normal values of the variables studied.

Lateral cephalogram	Normal values (mm)
SNA	81.1 ± 0.66
SNB	78.3 ± 0.65
MPH	22.5 ± 0.88
PAS	10.4 ± 0.55
PNS-P	39.8 ± 0.57

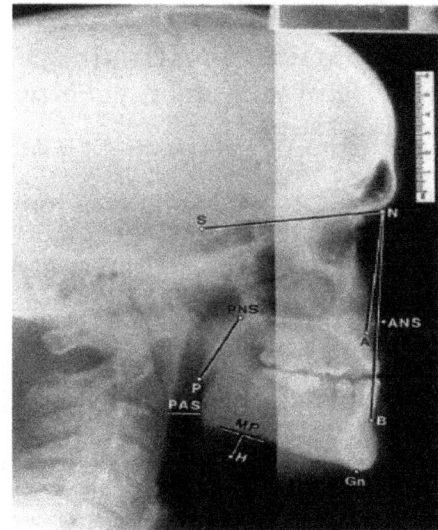

FIGURE 1: Standard lateral cephalogram with markings for SNA, SNB, PAS, MP-H, and PNS-P. Angle SNA: the angle from sella at the centre of pituitary fossa of sphenoid bone to nasion and the most posterior point on the curve between anterior nasal spine and supradentale of the maxilla. Angle SNB: the angle from sella, nasion, and the point of greatest concavity on the anterior surface of mandibular symphysis. PAS (posterior airway space): the distance from base of tongue to the posterior pharyngeal wall at the level of C2 vertebra. PNS-P (length of the soft palate): the distance from the most posterior point on the sagittal plane of hard palate (PNS) to the tip of the soft palate (P). MP-H (mandibular plane to hyoid bone): measured at the mentum (Me) as the line joining MP (mandibular plane) to H (the most anterosuperior point of the hyoid bone). MP: the line joining (Me) and Go (Gonion, most lateral external point at the junction of the horizontal and ascending ramus of the mandible).

base angle of mandible), PAS (posterior airway space), PNS-P (length of the soft palate), and MP-H (mandibular plane to hyoid bone) (Table 1; Figure 1). These areas were plotted after manual tracing of the lateral cephalograms. The corresponding normal values standardized in our cephalogram are shown in Table 1.

2.2. Statistical Analysis. To test the statistical significance of the differences between the two groups, Student's *t*-test was applied. To test the statistical significance of the association of the group with categorical variables Chi square test was done.

TABLE 2: Association of retropalatal region on flexible nasopharyngolaryngoscopy with lateral cephalometric variables.

	Retropalatal				
Lateral cephalogram indices	Group I <50% obstruction ($n = 28$)		Group II >50% obstruction ($n = 42$)		p value
	Mean	SD	Mean	SD	
SNA	82	0.7	82	0.7	0.947
SNB	79.5	1.3	79.4	1	0.653
PNSP	30.3	3.7	31	2.3	0.379
PAS	16	4.3	14.1	6.3	0.152
MPH	18.2	2.6	21	3.6	<0.001
AHI	19.9	10.2	38	18.6	<0.001

TABLE 3: Association of retroglossal region on flexible nasopharyngolaryngoscopy with lateral cephalometric variables.

	Retroglossal				
Lateral cephalogram indices	Group I <50% obstruction ($n = 43$)		Group II >50% obstruction ($n = 27$)		p value
	Mean	SD	Mean	SD	
SNA	82.1	0.7	81.8	0.6	0.097
SNB	79.6	1.2	79.2	0.9	0.157
PNSP	30.1	3.3	31.7	1.8	0.011
PAS	14.9	4.2	14.8	7.4	0.934
MPH	18	2.4	22.7	3.1	<0.001
AHI	21.7	10.3	45.2	18.5	<0.001

3. Observations, Results, and Discussion

Our study compared the lateral cephalogram and awake endoscopy with AHI. We could find several significant associations between these investigations.

3.1. Correlation of Lateral Cephalometric Variables and Flexible Nasopharyngolaryngoscopy (Awake Endoscopy). The measurements were taken at the usual sites of collapse, namely, the retropalatal, retroglossal, posterior pharyngeal wall, and supraglottic areas.

3.1.1. Correlation at the Retropalatal Region. In group 1 (less than 50% collapse) there were 28 patients and in group 2 (more than 50% collapse) there were 42 patients. MP-H in group 1 was 18.2 mm and in group 2 was 21.1 mm. This value is much less than the normal range of 27 ± 4 mm. This was found to be statistically significant (p value < 0.001) (Table 2, Figure 2). Though the PAS and PNS-P did show deviation from normal values they were not statistically significant. The findings correlated with the severity of AHI.

3.1.2. Correlation at the Retroglossal Area. Here, group 1 had 43 patients and group 2 had 27 patients. Mean value of PNS-P increased from 30.7 (group 1) to 31.7 in group 2 (normal 17 mm). There was significant statistical association of retroglossal region with MP-H (p value < 0.001). This correlated well with severity of AHI (Table 4). In our study we could not find any statistical correlation between retroglossal

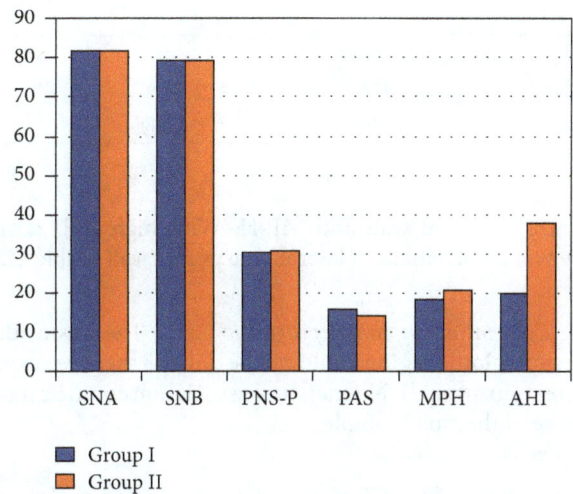

FIGURE 2: Bar diagram lateral cephalometric variables with retropalatal region.

region on flexible nasopharyngolaryngoscopy and the posterior airway space on lateral cephalogram (p value 0.934) (Table 3; Figure 3).

3.1.3. Correlation with Lateral Pharyngeal Wall Collapse. In our study, group I had 62 patients and group II had 8 patients and there was statistically significant association noted with

TABLE 4: Association of lateral pharyngeal wall on flexible nasopharyngolaryngoscopy with lateral cephalometric variables.

| Lateral cephalometric indices | Lateral pharyngeal wall | | | |
| | Group I <50% obstruction ($n = 62$) | | Group II >50% obstruction ($n = 8$) | |
	Mean	SD	Mean	SD
SNA	82.03	0.7	81.6	0.7
SNB	79.4	1.2	79.4	0.9
PNSP	30.6	3	31.5	1.9
PAS	14.6	5.2	16.9	8.4
MPH	19.3	3.3	24.1	2.5

TABLE 5: AHI with retropalatal collapse.

| AHI | Retropalatal region | | |
	Group I <50% obstruction ($n = 28$)	Group II >50% obstruction ($n = 42$)	p value
Mild	11 (39.28%)	1 (2.38%)	<0.016
Moderate	10 (35.71%)	18 (42.85%)	
Severe	7 (25.0%)	23 (54.76%)	

TABLE 6: AHI with retroglossal collapse.

| AHI | Retroglossal region | | |
	Group I <50% obstruction ($n = 43$)	Group II >50% obstruction ($n = 27$)	p value
Mild	12 (27.9%)		<0.001
Moderate	21 (48.83%)	7 (25.92%)	
Severe	10 (23.25%)	20 (74.07%)	

TABLE 7: AHI with Lateral pharyngeal wall collapse.

| AHI | Lateral pharyngeal wall | | |
	Group I <50% obstruction ($n = 62$) .	Group II >50% obstruction ($n = 8$)	p value
Mild	12 (19.35%)	0	0.002
Moderate	28 (45.16%)	0	
Severe	22 (35.48%)	8 (100%)	

TABLE 8: Correlations of MPH and PNS-P with AHI.

Variables	r	p value
MPH × AHI	0.938	<0.001
PNS-P × AHI	0.334	0.005

lateral pharyngeal wall and MP-H. With high AHI scores there was involvement of lateral pharyngeal wall (Table 4).

3.1.4. Correlation in the Supraglottic Area. The association with supraglottic region could not be done as there were only 2 patients in group II. No statistical association could be made because of the small sample size.

3.2. Association of AHI and Findings on Awake Endoscopy. There was significant involvement of retropalatal region with AHI. In mild OSA, 39.28% had retropalatal involvement in group I (Table 5) and only one in group II. In severe OSA the involvement was 25% and 54.76%, respectively.

There was a statistically significant correlation ($p <$ 0.001) of AHI with retroglossal collapse (74.07% in group II) (Table 6).

As per Table 7, the lateral pharyngeal wall showed correlation with increasing severity of OSA, though not statistically significant (p 0.002). In group I only 12 patients out of 62 had lateral pharyngeal wall collapse. The involvement was significant in moderate and severe OSA with 100% involvement in group II patients.

3.3. Association of AHI with Cephalometry (MP-H and PNS-P). A significant linear correlation between AHI and MP-H (Figure 4) and PNS-P (Figure 5) was noted (Table 8). Since MP-H was statistically significant in all areas, it was then analyzed by ROC curve to determine a cutoff value and was found to be 21.3 mm (Figure 6). Similarly, the cutoff value of PNS-P was found to be 31.5 mm (Figure 7).

4. Discussion

In the retropalatal area, in contrast to our observation, Koo et al.'s study [8] found no significant association between retropalatal region and MP-H. In the latter drug induced sleep endoscopy was performed. Besides, MP-H calculated in our study was manually done with a 0.1 mm calibration which may make it less specific than Jonathan's study where cephalometric software specifically designed for orthodontics was used. We do not have other studies with our background to compare with.

We found a statistically significant association of retroglossal region with PNS-P, MPH, and AHI (Tables 5 and 6). This is in accordance with many studies. This does show that hyoid is at a lower level in OSA patients and the length of soft palate is more. Our PAS was measured at C2 vertebral level. Hence, had we taken a lower level,

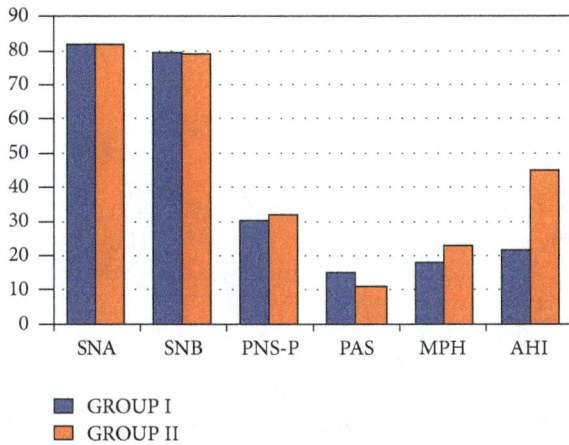

FIGURE 3: Bar diagram showing association of lateral cephalometric variables with retroglossal region.

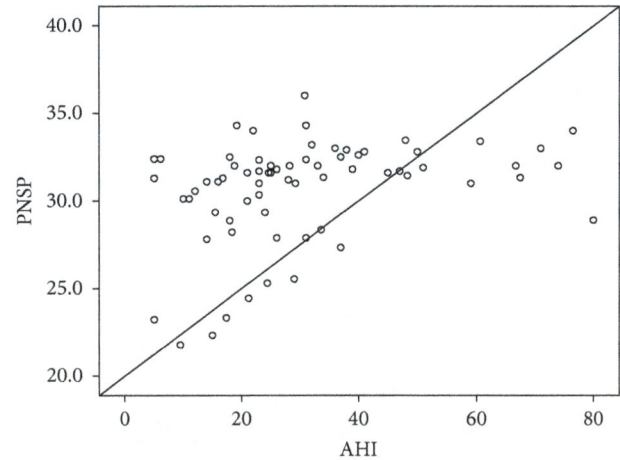

FIGURE 5: Positive correlation of AHI with PNS-P.

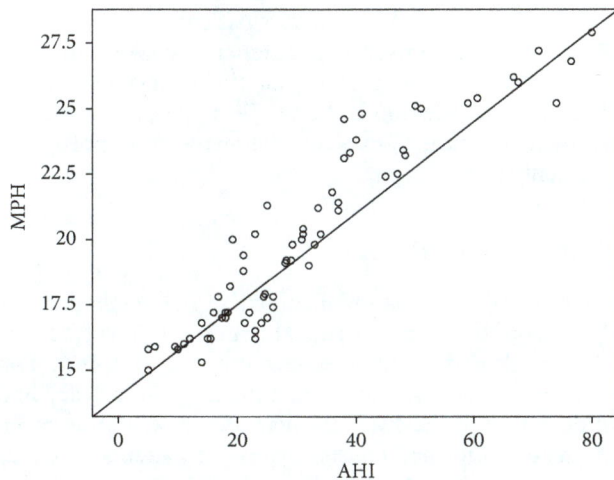

FIGURE 4: Positive correlation of AHI with MP-H.

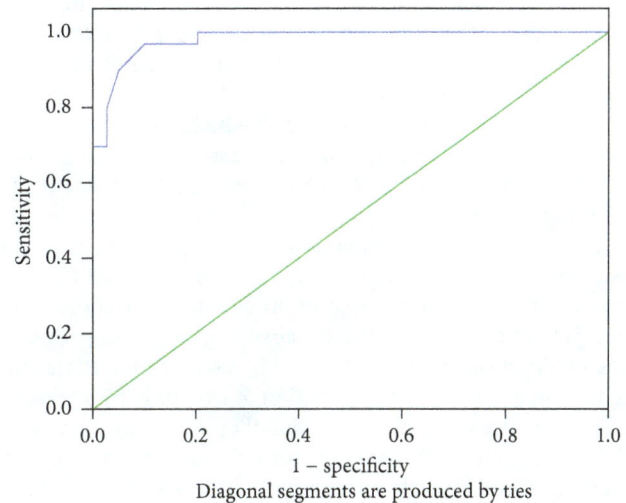

FIGURE 6: ROC curve for MP-H; area: 0.982.

the posterior airway space and retroglossal area may have shown significant correlation as in Jonathan's study. He measured PAS at multiple vertebral levels. In our study we could not find any statistical correlation between retroglossal region on flexible nasopharyngolaryngoscopy and the posterior airway space on lateral cephalogram (p value 0.935).

The relationship of lateral pharyngeal wall collapse in awake endoscopy with cephalometric variables is not possible theoretically since the latter provided only anteroposterior dimensions. But the analysis did show significant correlation with MP-H. This emphasizes interplay of various regions in bony framework and associated changes brought about in the soft tissue structures as a part of a compensatory mechanism. No comparison between these parameters has been done so far.

A significant statistical correlation of lateral pharyngeal wall, retropalatal region, and retroglossal region with AHI (p value < 0.001) was found in our study (Tables 5, 6, and 7). The observations matched with Koo et al. [8] study

though they used DISE. Pang et al. [9] reported that all 3 levels (palatal, lateral pharyngeal wall, and base of tongue) correlated very well with the severity of OSA. Hori et al. [10] reported that there was a significant correlation between the degree of narrowing of retropalatal area and apnea index. As regards to tongue base obstruction, Abdullah et al. [11] noted that there was a significant difference in the frequency and degree of base of tongue collapse in patients with severe OSA. They reported that only 6.9% of patients with mild OSA had more than 50% collapse of the base of the tongue region, as compared to 65.9% of patients with severe grade. In our study, we could find that there were no patients with more than 50% obstruction at the tongue base in the mild group but there were 74.07% of patients in the severe group. However, Ozdas et al. [12] reported that the obstruction and degree of the tongue base had no statistically significant correlation with AHI when examined by Muller's maneuver.

Angles SNA and SNB did not show any correlation in our studies. The results of correlation of AHI and MP-H

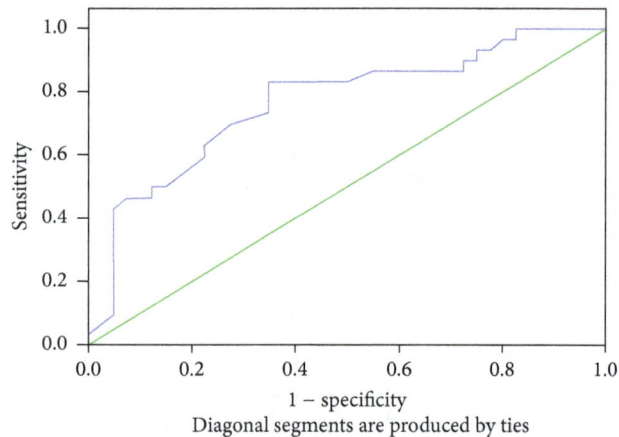

FIGURE 7: ROC curve area for PNS-P: 0.76.

and PNS-P are similar to Banhiran et al. [13]. There was no statistical significance with length of the palate and AHI which is similar to other studies even though elongated soft palate or excessive tissue in the soft palate is one of the most common causes of snoring and OSA [14–18].

There are anatomical changes which are interrelated explaining that a change in one variable also produces changes in another area in cephalometry or in nasopharyngolaryngoscopy.

Awake endoscopy diagnostically is quite sensitive in assessing the site of collapse in the abovementioned regions except in the supraglottic region. In our study we could only get 2 patients of supraglottic collapse in group II (more than 50% obstruction) which could not be assessed for statistical significance. This is in contradiction to the study by Soares et al. [6] which stated that assessment of awake endoscopy with Muller's maneuver alone is not a good method to detect the pharyngeal collapse site and predict UPPP success. They felt that such patients with retropalatal narrowing had surgical results short of what was expected [13]. Campanini et al. [19] showed, in a retrospective analysis of 250 patients, identical sites of obstruction during awake and sleep endoscopy in only 25% of patients as measured by the Nose Oropharynx Hypopharynx Larynx (NOHL) staging system, introduced by the same author. Soares et al. [20] retrospectively analyzed 53 patients with OSA and compared outpatient department assessment OPDA (endoscopy with and without Muller's maneuver) with DISE to assess the severity of collapse. These did not differ significantly regarding the presence of severe retropalatal collapse but did significantly differ in the incidence of severe retrolingual collapse (DISE 84.9%, OPDA 35.8%).

4.1. Limitations of the Study. Since the values in lateral cephalogram were manually traced and calculated to a maximum calibration of 0.1 mm, the accuracy may have been affected. This may explain certain disagreements with a few studies. Smaller sample size might oversubstantiate the findings. Since lateral cephalometry is a two-dimensional investigation, its correlation with a three-dimensional investigation

has certain disadvantages on practical aspects. Besides, findings of awake endoscopy involve the patient cooperation and so extrapolation of the findings may be limited.

5. Conclusions

There is significant correlation of lateral cephalogram and flexible nasopharyngolaryngoscopy with AHI in OSA.

At the retropalatal region, there was correlation with AHI and MPH of lateral cephalometry.

Retroglossal region showed significant correlation with MP-H, PNS-P, and AHI.

Lateral pharyngeal wall had correlation with MPH and AHI only in partial collapse. It is considered that the involvement of this region is usually secondary to other regions.

The lateral cephalometry parameters and flexiblescopy can predict possibilities of a snorer transforming into an OSA patient. Suitable lifestyle adjustments may prevent such event. Despite the fact that awake endoscopy may miss collapse at the supraglottic region in some cases, it may be used for primary screening of OSA patients. Further, lateral cephalometry can be used as an adjunct to awake endoscopy which captures whole anatomy of the pharyngeal airway with minimum radiation and cost. These should be assessed along with physical parameters for early and appropriate assessment of OSA.

Ethical Approval

Though the proposed study included an invasive procedure and radiography, no major ethical issues were involved. The study was cleared by Ethics committee on 10/05/2013 and was intended for publication maintaining the privacy and confidentiality of the study participants. It was undertaken after written informed consent from the patients that they were part of study and the study would not interfere with the optimum final treatment.

Conflict of Interests

There was no conflict of interests in this study.

Acknowledgments

This study was supported by the Department of Pulmonology at Amrita Institute of Medical Sciences, Kochi Amrita Dental College, Kochi.

References

[1] L. J. Epstein, D. Kristo, P. J. Strollo Jr. et al., "Clinical guideline for the evaluation, management and long-term care of obstructive sleep apnea in adults," *Journal of Clinical Sleep Medicine*, vol. 5, no. 3, pp. 263–276, 2009.

[2] American Academy of Sleep Medicine, *International Classification of Sleep Disorders: Diagnostic and Coding Manual*, American Academy of Sleep Medicine, Westchester, Ill, USA, 2nd edition, 2005.

[3] M. E. Bohlman, E. F. Haponik, P. L. Smith, R. P. Allen, E. R. Bleecker, and S. M. Goldman, "CT demonstration of pharyngeal narrowing in adult obstructive sleep apnea," *American Journal of Roentgenology*, vol. 140, no. 3, pp. 543–548, 1983.

[4] J. Rivlin, V. Hoffstein, J. Kalbfleisch, W. McNicholas, N. Zamel, and A. C. Bryan, "Upper airway morphology in patients with idiopathic obstructive sleep apnea," *American Review of Respiratory Disease*, vol. 129, no. 3, pp. 355–360, 1984.

[5] R. J. Schwab, W. B. Gefter, E. A. Hoffman, K. B. Gupta, and A. I. Pack, "Dynamic upper airway imaging during awake respiration in normal subjects and patients with sleep disordered breathing," *American Review of Respiratory Disease*, vol. 148, no. 5, pp. 1385–1400, 1993.

[6] M. C. M. Soares, A. C. R. Sallum, M. T. M. Gonçalves, F. L. M. Haddad, and L. C. Gregório, "Use of Muller's maneuver in the evaluation of patients with sleep apnea—literature review," *Brazilian Journal of Otorhinolaryngology*, vol. 75, no. 3, pp. 463–466, 2009.

[7] M. Cavaliere, F. Russo, and M. Iemma, "Awake versus drug-induced sleep endoscopy: evaluation of airway obstruction in obstructive sleep apnea/hypopnoea syndrome," *The Laryngoscope*, vol. 123, no. 9, pp. 2315–2318, 2013.

[8] S. K. Koo, J. W. Choi, N. S. Myung, H. J. Lee, Y. J. Kim, and Y. J. Kim, "Analysis of obstruction site in obstructive sleep apnea syndrome patients by drug induced sleep endoscopy," *American Journal of Otolaryngology*, vol. 34, no. 6, pp. 626–630, 2013.

[9] K. P. Pang, D. J. Terris, and R. Podolsky, "Severity of obstructive sleep apnea: correlation with clinical examination and patient perception," *Otolaryngology—Head and Neck Surgery*, vol. 135, no. 4, pp. 555–560, 2006.

[10] Y. Hori, H. Shizuku, A. Kondo, H. Nakagawa, B. Kalubi, and N. Takeda, "Endoscopic evaluation of dynamic narrowing of the pharynx by the Bernouilli effect producing maneuver in patients with obstructive sleep apnea syndrome," *Auris Nasus Larynx*, vol. 33, no. 4, pp. 429–432, 2006.

[11] V. J. Abdullah, Y. K. Wing, and C. A. Van Hasselt, "Video sleep nasendoscopy: the Hong Kong experience," *Otolaryngologic Clinics of North America*, vol. 36, no. 3, pp. 461–471, 2003.

[12] T. Ozdas, K. M. Ozcan, F. Ozdogan et al., "Investigation of lateral pharyngeal walls in OSAS," *European Archives of Oto-Rhino-Laryngology*, vol. 270, no. 2, pp. 767–771, 2013.

[13] W. Banhiran, P. Wanichakorntrakul, C. Metheetrairut, P. Chiewvit, and W. Planuphap, "Lateral cephalometric analysis and the risks of moderate to severe obstructive sleep-disordered breathing in Thai patients," *Sleep and Breathing*, vol. 17, no. 4, pp. 1249–1255, 2013.

[14] V. Tangugsorn, O. Skatvedt, O. Krogstad, and T. Lyberg, "Obstructive sleep apnoea: a cephalometric study. Part I. Cervico-craniofacial skeletal morphology," *European Journal of Orthodontics*, vol. 17, no. 1, pp. 45–56, 1995.

[15] M. Zucconi, L. Ferini-Strambi, S. Palazzi, C. Orena, S. Zonta, and S. Smirne, "Habitual snoring with and without obstructive sleep apnoea: the importance of cephalometric variables," *Thorax*, vol. 47, no. 3, pp. 157–161, 1992.

[16] F. Maltais, G. Carrier, Y. Cormier, and F. Series, "Cephalometric measurements in snorers, non-snorers, and patients with sleep apnoea," *Thorax*, vol. 46, no. 6, pp. 419–423, 1991.

[17] N. Pracharktam, S. Nelson, M. G. Hans et al., "Cephalometric assessment in obstructive sleep apnea," *American Journal of Orthodontics and Dentofacial Orthopedics*, vol. 109, no. 4, pp. 410–419, 1996.

[18] H. Gastaut, C. A. Tassinari, and B. Duron, "Polygraphic study of the episodic diurnal and nocturnal (hypnic and respiratory) manifestations of the pickwick syndrome," *Brain Research*, vol. 1, no. 2, pp. 167–186, 1966.

[19] A. Campanini, P. Canzi, A. De Vito, I. Dallan, F. Montevecchi, and C. Vicini, "Awake versus sleep endoscopy: personal experience in 250 OSAHS patients," *Acta Otorhinolaryngologica Italica*, vol. 30, no. 2, pp. 73–77, 2010.

[20] D. Soares, A. J. Folbe, G. Yoo, M. Safwan, J. A. Rowley, and H.-S. Lin, "Drug-induced sleep endoscopy vs awake Müller's maneuver in the diagnosis of severe upper airway obstruction," *Otolaryngology—Head and Neck Surgery*, vol. 148, no. 1, pp. 151–156, 2013.

Subclinical Hearing Loss, Longer Sleep Duration, and Cardiometabolic Risk Factors in Japanese General Population

Kei Nakajima,[1] Eiichiro Kanda,[2] Ami Hosobuchi,[1] and Kaname Suwa[3]

[1] Division of Clinical Nutrition, Department of Medical Dietetics, Faculty of Pharmaceutical Sciences, Josai University, 1-1 Keyakidai, Sakado, Saitama 350-0295, Japan
[2] Department of Nephrology, Tokyo Kyosai Hospital, Nakameguro 2-3-8, Meguroku, Tokyo 153-8934, Japan
[3] Saitama Health Promotion Corporation, 519 Kamiookubo, Saitama, Saitama 338-0824, Japan

Correspondence should be addressed to Kei Nakajima; keinaka@josai.ac.jp

Academic Editor: Myer III Myer

Hearing loss leads to impaired social functioning and quality of life. Hearing loss is also associated with sleeping disorders and cardiometabolic risk factors. Here, we determined whether subclinical hearing loss is associated with sleep duration and cardiometabolic risk factors in a cross-sectional and longitudinal study of healthy Japanese general population. 48,091 men and women aged 20–79 years who underwent medical checkups were included in a cross-sectional study, and 6,674 were included in an 8-year longitudinal study. The prevalence of audiometrically determined hearing loss (>25 dB) at 4000 and 1000 Hz increased significantly with increasing sleep duration in any age strata. Logistic regression analysis showed that compared with reference sleep duration (6 h) longer sleep duration (≥8 h) was significantly associated with hearing loss, even after adjusting for potential confounding factors. Simultaneously, hearing loss was significantly associated with male sex, diabetes, and no habitual exercise. In the longitudinal study, the risk of longer sleep duration (≥8 h) after 8 years was significantly greater in subjects with hearing loss at 4000 Hz at baseline. In conclusion, current results suggest a potential association of subclinical hearing loss with longer sleep duration and cardiometabolic risk factors in a Japanese general population.

1. Introduction

The progressive aging of society is leading to an increase in the prevalence of hearing loss worldwide. Although hearing loss is not directly life threatening, it may impair social functioning and quality of life, causing isolation, frustration, and impaired communication [1–6]. Meanwhile, several studies have revealed that sleeping disorders such as insomnia and daytime sleepiness are associated with hearing impairments, including hearing loss and tinnitus [7–10]. Therefore, some factors associated with sleep may be associated with hearing loss. To date, however, no study has examined the putative association between hearing loss and sleep duration.

In this context, we focused on subclinical objective hearing loss, which is often undetected and left untreated [4, 6], and investigated the lifestyles of individuals with subclinical hearing loss and the etiology of subclinical hearing loss. Because frequency of 500 to 4000 Hz is important range for speech processing [6], we determined whether hearing function at representative high (4000 Hz) and low (1000 Hz) frequencies, which are usually examined in a hearing screening test in Japan [11–13], was associated with lifestyle factors, including sleep duration per night and cardiometabolic risk factors, in a cross-sectional study of Japanese general population.

Because hearing loss has been shown to be associated with cardiometabolic risk factors, such as diabetes and smoking [11–16], we considered these factors as relevant confounding factors and also examined the associations between hearing loss and these cardiometabolic risk factors. To examine the effects of subclinical hearing loss on the incidence of longer sleep duration (8 h and ≥9 h), we performed a retrospective 8-year longitudinal study in an independent group of subjects whose sleep duration was classified as normal or short (≤7 h) at baseline.

2. Methods

2.1. Study Design.
This study was based on a composite research program that is being conducted to identify the factors associated with cardiometabolic and atherosclerotic diseases. The design of this study is described in more detail elsewhere [17]. This retrospective study consists of data recorded during annual medical checkups of asymptomatic individuals living or working in Saitama Prefecture, a suburb of Tokyo, Japan. The study started in 2011 and involves the collaboration of three institutions in Saitama: Jichi Medical University, Josai University, and Saitama Health Promotion Corporation. The protocol, which conforms to the Declaration of Helsinki, was approved by the Ethics Committee of Jichi Medical University and Josai University and by the Committee of the Saitama Health Promotion Corporation. Written informed consent was obtained from all participants. Since 1997, Saitama Health Promotion Corporation, a public interest corporation, has supported the health of individuals, including children and adolescents, living or working in Saitama Prefecture, primarily by carrying out various types of medical checkups [18].

2.2. Subjects

2.2.1. Cross-Sectional Study.
We digitally stored data from 83 286 apparently healthy subjects aged 20–79 years old who underwent medical checkups at Saitama Health Promotion Corporation between April 1, 2007, and March 31, 2008. Subjects with diagnosed or undiagnosed self-reported hearing loss ($n = 488$) were excluded from the analysis because the cause and treatment received (e.g., hearing aids and pharmacotherapy) were not available in this study. Subjects with self-reported depression and sleep apnea syndrome were also excluded because these conditions may affect sleep duration [19–22]. The exclusion criteria applied in this study and the disposition of subjects are shown in Figure 1. Subjects with self-reported tinnitus ($n = 1,396$) were included because tinnitus was usually mild and was not always diagnosed by a physician in this study. Consequently, 48 091 subjects were included in the cross-sectional study.

2.2.2. Longitudinal Study.
When we selected subjects for the longitudinal study from those included in the cross-sectional study, the number of subjects whose baseline sleep duration was normal or short (≤ 7 h) and who underwent the same checkup four times between April 1, 1999, and March 31, 2008 (8 years duration), was <1,000. Therefore, subjects included in the longitudinal study were identified from the original study population, which means the subjects included in the longitudinal study differed from those included in the cross-sectional study. However, the assessment of hearing loss and other laboratory tests were identical between the cross-sectional and longitudinal studies. After excluding subjects with incomplete data and those with known ear diseases, 6,774 subjects with normal or short sleep duration at baseline were included in the longitudinal study (Figure 1). During 8 years, many subjects abandoned the medical checkup held by Saitama Health Promotion Corporation (average

proportions of not undergoing the same checkup next year was approximately one-fourth to one-third during 1999~2008) and changed to other checkups because of house moving, resignation, or change of jobs, child care, or family reasons, resulting in the decreased number of subjects in the longitudinal study.

2.2.3. Anthropometric, Laboratory, and Audiometric Tests.
Anthropometric, laboratory, and audiometric tests were carried out in the morning. Serum parameters were measured using standard methods on Hitachi autoanalyzers (Tokyo, Japan) at Saitama Health Promotion Corporation. Hemoglobin (Hb) A1c was converted to national glycohemoglobin standardization program levels using a validated formula [23]. Unfortunately, fasting plasma glucose levels were not available in both studies. The hearing test was conducted in a quiet room by trained staff using an ordinary audiometer. Subclinical (objective) hearing loss was defined as a pure-tone average hearing loss of >25 dB at high (4000 Hz) and low (1000 Hz) frequencies.

2.2.4. Sleep Duration and Confounding Factors.
Self-reported sleep duration per night, which was obtained as a response to the simple question about sleep, was divided into five categories (≤ 5, 6, 7, 8, and ≥ 9 h) according to previous studies [24, 25]. The duration of daytime nap was not taken into consideration in this study. Subjects completed a form to record history of cardiovascular disease (including stroke), complications (hypertension, diabetes, or dyslipidemia), alcohol consumption (no, occasional, 1–3 times/week, 4–6 times/week, or daily), smoking status (no, past, or current), regular exercise (≥ 30 min per time; no, occasional, once/week, or at least twice/week), and work duration (≤ 6, 7, 8, 9, 10, or ≥ 11 h). The influence of body weight was evaluated in terms of body mass index (BMI), which was divided into six categories (≤ 18.9, 19.0–20.9, 21.0–22.9, 23.0–24.9, 25.0–26.9, and ≥ 27.0 kg/m^2). We took into consideration that WHO has proposed that BMI cutoff points for overweight and obesity for Asian populations should be lower (≥ 23.0 kg/m^2 and ≥ 27.5 kg/m^2, resp.) compared to Western populations [26]. Since the proportions of subjects classified as underweight (i.e., <18.5 kg/m^2) or obese (i.e., ≥ 30.0 kg/m^2) are very low (4.8% and 5.0%, resp.) in this study, we round up the low and high BMI cutoffs to 19 and 27 kg/m^2 (7.4% and 15.1%, resp.). The influence of systemic inflammation was roughly evaluated in terms of the circulating white blood cell count, a putative risk factor for cardiovascular disease [27–29], which was divided into quartiles. Because organic solvents can affect sleep duration [30, 31], the use of organic solvent in the workplace was taken into account, although the type was not recorded and the number of subjects was limited ($n = 39,691$).

2.2.5. Statistical Analysis.
Data are expressed as means (SD) or medians (interquartile range). Differences in clinical parameters and categorical variables between the five categories of sleep duration were examined by one-way analysis of variance (ANOVA) and χ^2 tests, respectively. The prevalence

Exclusion criteria of subjects and flow chart

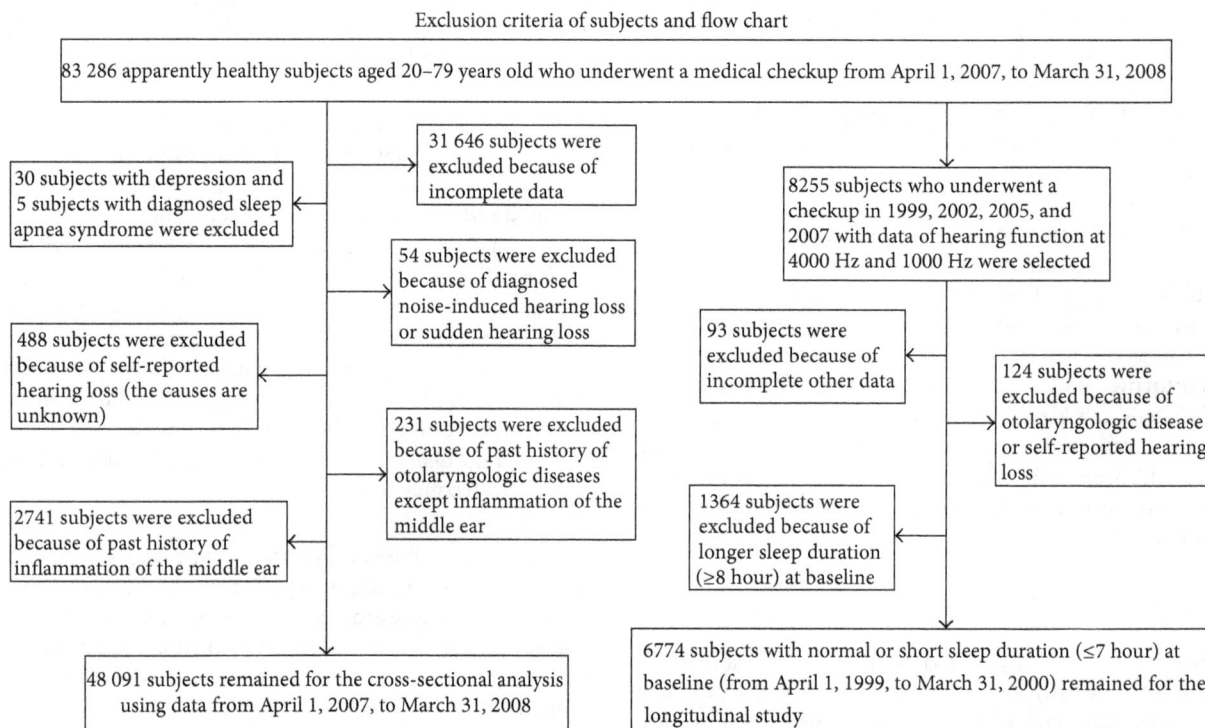

FIGURE 1: Exclusion criteria and subject disposition.

of hearing loss was first evaluated in four age groups (20–39, 40–49, 50–51, and 60–79 years) because advancing age is one of the main risk factors for hearing loss. In the cross-sectional study, multivariate logistic regression models were used to examine whether subclinical hearing loss was associated with lifestyle and cardiometabolic risk factors to calculate odds ratios (OR) and 95% confidence intervals (CI) with adjustment for relevant confounders. After sleep durations in five categories of sleep duration were coded as 5, 6, 7, 8, and 9 for ≤5 h, 6 h, 7 h, 8 h, and ≥9 h, respectively, associations between sleep duration as a continuous variable and hearing loss were examined. The associations between relevant confounders and hearing loss were also evaluated.

For the longitudinal analysis, multivariate logistic regression models were also used to examine the association between baseline hearing loss and risk of longer sleep duration (8 h and ≥9 h) after 9 years to calculate relative risk (RR) and 95% confidence interval (CI) because the incidence of longer sleep duration after 9 years was <10% and the ORs are expressed as relative risks in the longitudinal study [32]. In this analysis, the provisional reference BMI categories were defined as a BMI of 21.0–22.9 kg/m^2 based on the proposal by the World Health Organization regarding overweight and obese classifications for Asian populations [26]. Statistical analyses were performed using IBM-SPSS version 18.0 (PASW statistics 18; Chicago, IL, USA) and Statview version 5.0 (SAS Institute; Cary, NC, USA). Values of $P < 0.05$ were considered statistically significant.

3. Results

3.1. Cross-Sectional Study.
The clinical characteristics of the subjects are presented in Table 1. Subjects with longer sleep duration were more frequently men, were older, and had a shorter work duration, with increased numbers of cardiometabolic risk factors (especially decreased high-density lipoprotein cholesterol). BMI, white blood cell count, and the frequency of current smokers, no regular exercise, or use of organic solvents at work showed U- or J-shaped relationships with sleep duration. The prevalence of cardiovascular disease, hypertension, and diabetes increased with increasing sleep duration. Similarly, the prevalence of hearing loss increased with increasing sleep duration, irrespective of the left or right ear, or frequency. The proportions of manufacturing and construction workers were higher in the longer sleep duration groups (8 h and ≥9 h), whereas the opposite was true for the proportions of clerical, technical, and medical workers.

Figure 2 shows the prevalence of hearing loss according to age groups. The prevalence of hearing loss at 4000 Hz increased significantly with increasing sleep duration in any age strata except for younger age (20–39 years old). Likewise, the prevalence of hearing loss at 1000 Hz increased significantly with increasing sleep duration, particularly in the older age groups. However, there seemed to be a slight J-shaped relationship in subjects aged 60–79 years.

Multivariate logistic regression analyses showed that, compared with sleep duration of ≤5 h, the other categories of

TABLE 1: Clinical characteristics of subjects according to the five sleep duration categories.

Five categories by sleep duration	Total	≤5 h	6 h	7 h	8 h	≥9 h
N, (% of total)	48,091	5,049 (10.5)	22,386 (46.5)	15,106 (31.4)	5,176 (10.8)	374 (0.8)
Age, years	42.3 (12.1)	39.7 (11.2)	41.0 (11.7)	43.4 (12.3)	46.3 (12.8)	49.1 (15.5)
Men, n (%)	33,026 (68.7)	3,208 (63.5)	14,793 (66.1)	10,767 (71.3)	3,965 (76.6)	293 (78.3)
BMI, kg/m^2	23.5 (3.6)	23.7 (3.9)	23.5 (3.7)	23.4 (3.4)	23.5 (3.5)	23.6 (3.5)
Systolic blood pressure, mmHg	123 (17.3)	121 (16.7)	122 (16.9)	124 (17.5)	127 (18.4)	128 (18.5)
Diastolic blood pressure, mmHg	75 (13.3)	74 (13.5)	74 (13.1)	75 (13.5)	77 (13.3)	77 (13.7)
Total cholesterol, mg/dL	199 (35.5)	198 (35.7)	199 (35.5)	199 (35.2)	201 (35.7)	198 (38.8)
Triglyceride, mg/dL	96 (64–153)	88 (59–146)	93 (62–148)	100 (67–157)	107 (70–170)	103 (73–169)
HDL cholesterol, mg/dL	61.4 (15.5)	61.9 (15.6)	61.5 (15.6)	61.2 (15.4)	61.1 (15.9)	59.0 (15.1)
HbA1c, %, NGSP	5.5 (0.7)	5.5 (0.8)	5.5 (0.7)	5.5 (0.7)	5.6 (0.8)	5.7 (1.1)
White blood cell, ×10^2/μL	65.2 (17.6)	66.5 (18.5)	64.8 (17.4)	65.0 (17.6)	66.3 (18.1)	67.3 (19.4)
Past history of CVD, n (%)	711 (1.5)	72 (1.4)	301 (1.3)	229 (1.5)	100 (1.9)	9 (2.4)
Complication						
Hypertension, n (%)	3,697 (7.7)	264 (5.2)	1,436 (6.4)	1,325 (8.8)	623 (12.0)	49 (13.1)
Dyslipidemia, n (%)	2,187 (4.5)	164 (3.2)	969 (4.3)	756 (5.0)	280 (5.4)	18 (4.8)
Diabetes, n (%)	1,402 (2.9)	106 (2.1)	580 (2.6)	477 (3.2)	217 (4.2)	22 (5.9)
Subjects with high HbA1c (≥6.5%), n (%)	2,521 (5.2)	217 (4.3)	1,019 (4.6)	851 (5.6)	397 (7.7)	37 (9.9)
Alcohol consumption						
1~3/w/4~6/w/daily (%)	16.7/11.6/16.9	17.9/8.1/12.6	17.7/10.9/13.7	15.9/13.1/19.7	14.3/13.9/26.4	11.0/8.8/30.2
Smoker						
Past/current (%)	11.2/38.1	6.8/40.5	10.4/36.9	12.9/37.6	13.8/41.7	10.7/44.7
Having regular exercise						
No/occasional~1/w/≥2/w (%)*	51.0/31.8/17.2	57.4/28.4/14.3	51.4/32.2/16.4	48.4/33.2/18.4	49.9/30.2/20.0	57.0/24.9/18.2
Self-reported tinnitus, n (%)	1,396 (2.9)	121 (2.4)	635 (2.8)	457 (3.0)	170 (3.3)	13 (3.5)
Hearing loss at 4,000 Hz in the left ear, n (%)	3,068 (6.4)	188 (3.7)	1,013 (4.5)	1,100 (7.3)	675 (13.0)	92 (24.6)
Hearing loss at 4,000 Hz in the right ear, n (%)	2,883 (6.0)	158 (3.1)	952 (4.3)	1,012 (6.7)	656 (12.7)	105 (28.1)
Hearing loss at 1,000 Hz in the left ear, n (%)	1,097 (2.3)	90 (1.8)	404 (1.8)	367 (2.4)	192 (3.7)	44 (11.8)
Hearing loss at 1,000 Hz in the right ear, n (%)	1,070 (2.2)	81 (1.6)	390 (1.7)	338 (2.2)	225 (4.3)	36 (9.6)
Work duration, hour	8.6 (1.4)	9.2 (1.6)	8.7 (1.4)	8.4 (1.3)	8.3 (1.3)	8.1 (1.5)
Occupation, (%)*						
Clerical workers	21.2	17.5	22.4	22.5	17.0	7.2
Production workers	8.3	6.7	7.4	9.4	9.9	12.8
Service workers	10.6	11.7	10.8	9.8	10.2	15.8
Managerial workers	6.8	5.9	6.5	7.7	6.9	2.9
Technical workers	5.2	6.6	5.4	4.8	4.2	2.7
Construction workers	6.6	5.7	5.4	6.6	12.2	20.3
Medical workers	4.4	4.9	4.6	4.2	3.9	2.9
Transport workers	3.1	6.8	2.7	2.2	3.4	6.2
Workers not classifiable or nonemployed	33.8	34.1	34.8	32.9	32.4	29.1
Organic solvent workers, n (%) (total available $n = 39,691$)	1,053 (2.7)	109 (2.6)	427 (2.3)	371 (3.0)	134 (3.2)	12 (4.0)

The data are expressed as means (SD). Triglyceride is expressed as medians (interquartiles).
*Total sum is not 100% in some cases because of round-off to two decimal places.
Differences in parameters and categorical values between five sleep duration categories were significant (analysis of variance/χ^2 test; past history of CVD, and medical workers, both $P = 0.01$ and all others, $P < 0.001$), except self-reported tinnitus ($P = 0.06$).
BMI: body mass index, HDL: high-density lipoprotein, NGSP: national glycohemoglobin standardization program, CVD: cardiovascular disease (including stroke).

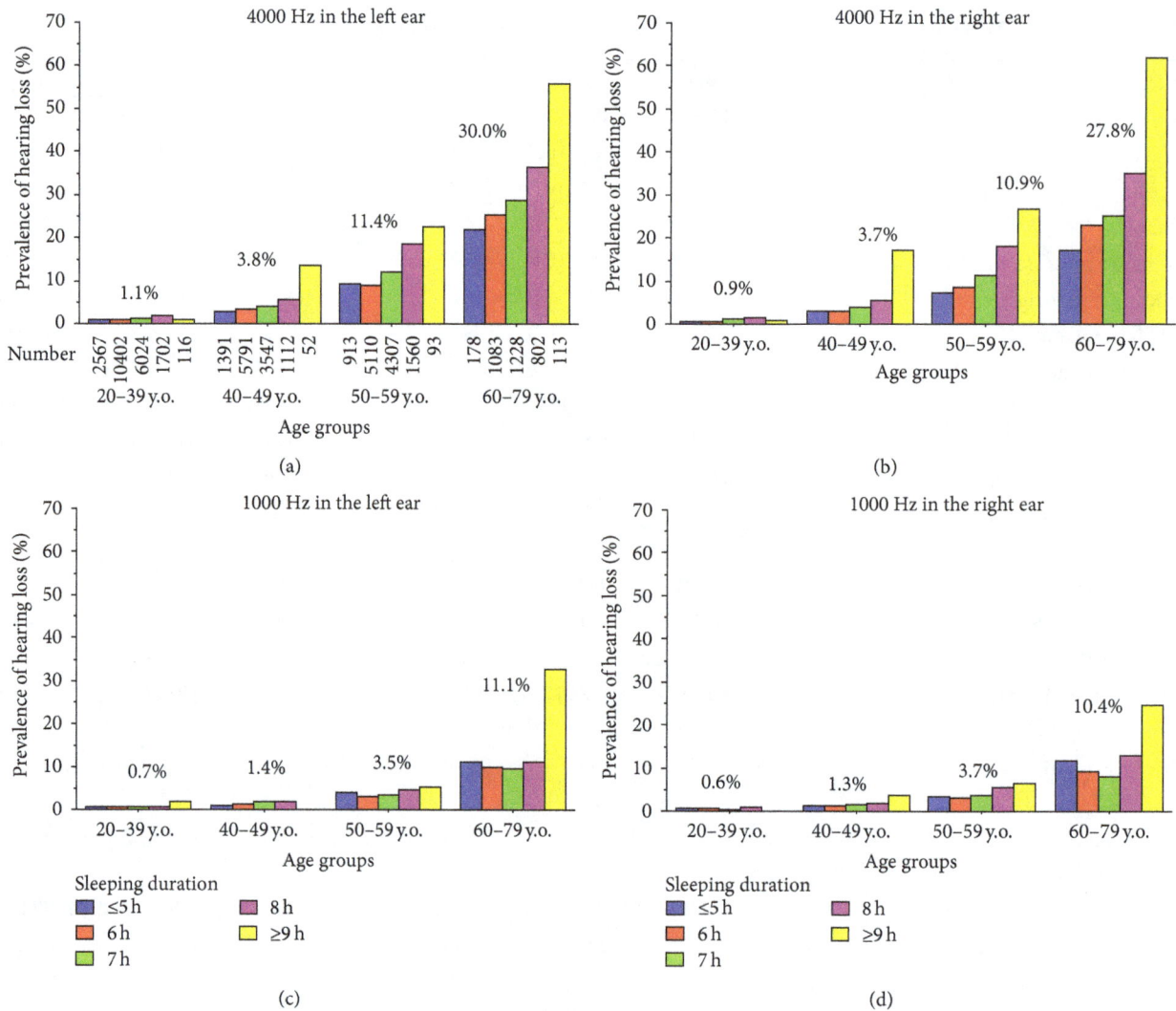

FIGURE 2: Prevalence of hearing loss according to age group. The number of subjects is shown under the column for hearing loss at 4000 Hz in the left ear (top-left panel). The numbers of subjects included in the other panels were identical. The percentage (%) above the column expresses the average of prevalence of hearing loss according to the age group. The prevalence of hearing loss at 4000 Hz, but not at 1000 Hz, increased significantly with increasing sleep duration in most age groups (χ^2 test). Left ear at 4000 Hz: 20–39 years, $P = 0.002$; all other age groups, $P < 0.001$. Right ear at 4000 Hz: all age groups, $P < 0.001$. Left ear at 1000 Hz: 20–39 years, $P = 0.51$; 40–49 years, $P = 0.20$; 50–59 years, $P = 0.08$; 60–79 years, $P < 0.001$. Right ear at 1000 Hz: 20–39 years, $P = 0.34$; 40–49 years, $P = 0.13$; 50–59 years, $P < 0.001$; 60–79 years, $P < 0.001$. y.o.: years old.

sleep duration were significantly associated with hearing loss at 4000 and 1000 Hz at least in one ear (Table 2). Adjustment for confounding factors, including age and sex, markedly attenuated the associations, but changing the reference sleep duration category from ≤5 h to 6 h (Model 2b) or additional adjustment for the use of organic solvents at work (Model 3) did not. Likewise, sleep duration as a continuous variable was also significantly associated with hearing loss at 4000 and 1000 Hz.

Table 3 shows the ORs for the confounding factors, except age, for hearing loss. Male sex, diabetes, no regular exercise, and tinnitus were significantly associated with hearing loss at both frequencies, whereas regular alcohol consumption, but not daily alcohol consumption, was inversely associated with hearing loss. Low body weight, the highest quartile of

white blood cell count ($\geq 88.9 \times 10^2/\mu L$), current smoking, and daily alcohol consumption were significantly associated with hearing loss at 4000 Hz. Work duration was significantly and inversely associated with hearing loss at 1000 Hz but not at 4000 Hz. Compared with clerical work, other work types, except managerial and medical work, were significantly associated with hearing loss at 4000 Hz (ORs 1.24–4.49) and 1000 Hz (ORs 1.34–1.90), even after controlling for confounding factors, including work duration (data not shown).

3.2. Longitudinal Study. The baseline clinical characteristics of subjects included in the longitudinal study (Table 4) are similar to those of the subjects included in the cross-sectional study (Table 1). Table 5 shows RRs of hearing loss at baseline for the longer sleep duration (≥8 hr) after 9 years. The risk of

TABLE 2: Odds ratios of each sleep duration for hearing loss.

Frequency	Sleep durations	≤5 h	6 h	7 h	8 h	≥9 h
4,000 Hz						
Model 1		1	1.27 (1.10–1.46)‡	2.06 (1.79–2.36)‡	3.92 (3.39–4.54)‡	8.38 (6.50–10.8)‡
Model 2	a	1	1.04 (0.90–1.21)	1.17 (1.01–1.37)*	1.38 (1.17–1.64)‡	1.82 (1.32–2.50)‡
	b	0.98 (0.84–1.14)	1	1.11 (1.01–1.21)*	1.30 (1.16–1.45)‡	1.72 (1.28–2.31)‡
Model 3		1	1.07 (0.90–1.27)	1.20 (1.01–1.43)*	1.36 (1.13–1.64)†	1.75 (1.22–2.50)†
1,000 Hz						
Model 1		1	1.08 (0.89–1.31)	1.42 (1.17–1.73)‡	2.41 (1.96–2.97)‡	6.80 (4.88–9.48)‡
Model 2	a	1	0.93 (0.77–1.14)	0.95 (0.77–1.16)	1.13 (0.90–1.41)	2.06 (1.43–2.97)‡
	b	1.07 (0.88–1.31)	1	1.02 (0.90–1.15)	1.21 (1.04–1.41)*	2.21 (1.60–3.07)‡
Model 3		1	1.00 (0.80–1.24)	1.00 (0.79–1.25)	1.16 (0.90–1.49)	2.20 (1.47–3.29)‡

*$P < 0.05$, †$P < 0.01$, and ‡$P < 0.001$.
The number of subjects in each group is the same as that in Table 1.
Hearing loss was defined as >25 dB hearing level in the right and/or left sides of ear.
Model 1: unadjusted.
Model 2: adjusted for age, sex, smoking, alcohol consumption, and having regular exercise, quartile of white blood cell counts, six tiles of body mass index, and past history of cardiovascular disease, complications (hypertension, dyslipidemia, and diabetes), self-reported tinnitus, working duration, and occupation. The reference sleep duration was ≤5 h in Model 2a and 6 h in Model 2b.
Model 3: Model 2a plus adjustments for organic solvent work (available $n = 39,691$).

long sleep duration was significantly greater in subjects with hearing loss at 4000 Hz at baseline compared with subjects without such hearing loss. This increased risk remained significant after adjusting for potential confounding factors at baseline. Although subjects with hearing loss at 1000 Hz at baseline had a significantly higher risk for longer sleep duration, this disappeared after adjusting for fundamental confounding factors (Model 2).

4. Discussion

Our cross-sectional and longitudinal studies provide robust evidence that subclinical hearing loss, especially at high frequencies, is associated with longer sleep duration, which was particularly depicted in older age, independently of relevant lifestyle factors, cardiometabolic risk factors, and the use of organic solvents at work. These associations were not weakened when the reference sleep duration was changed to 6 h, the major sleep duration category in this study. Although several epidemiological studies have shown U- or J-shaped relationships between sleep duration and clinical disorders, such as obesity and diabetes [24, 33, 34], the relationship between hearing loss at 4000 Hz and sleep duration in our study was nearly linear in all of the age categories. Because many studies have shown that noise-induced hearing loss, a major form of acquired hearing loss [35], gradually begins around the frequency of 4000 Hz [36, 37], currently observed hearing loss might be attributable to a great extent to the long-term noise exposure, which was not measured in this study.

Regarding the cause-effect relationship, considering the results of our longitudinal study, it is likely that longer sleep duration may occur because of or in conjunction with hearing loss. In other words, subclinical hearing loss may be a predictor of long sleep duration, which may be related to the development of cardiometabolic disease [24, 33–38]. Hearing loss is also associated with dementia and cognitive

impairment [39–42], whereas cognitive impairments, including Alzheimer disease, are associated with sleep and circadian problems [43–45]. Therefore, it is possible that long sleep duration might reflect other clinical conditions that were not examined in this study and that the currently observed associations may be spurious and unknown factors might mediate two conditions. Frustration and uneasiness associated with hearing loss or noisy daytime environments may reduce sleep quality and provoke insomnia [9, 10, 46] and may result in longer sleep durations. By contrast, once individuals with hearing loss do fall asleep, they could maintain good sleep without waking during the night. Hearing loss might also protect sleep by reducing the subjects' awareness of environmental noise during sleep [8] and might prolong sleep duration [46–48].

Meanwhile, many previous studies have provided evidence that diabetes, cardiometabolic disease, and smoking are associated with hearing loss [11–16], plausibly through diabetic micro- and macroangiopathy [14, 49, 50]. Thus, like typical diabetic complications, hearing loss may be one of complications following diabetic or atherosclerotic etiologies. Nevertheless, there is also a possibility that long-time sleep in turn may deteriorate the pathophysiology of diabetes and atherosclerosis because of putative associations between long-time sleep and diabetes [24, 33–38]. Intriguingly, low BMI (i.e., low body weight rather than obesity) was associated with hearing loss at 4000 Hz. Underweight might be associated with increased risk for hearing loss through inadequate intake of dietary nutrients, especially vitamin B_{12} and antioxidants [51–55], or other factors that were previously reported to be associated with increased mortality in underweight people [56–58]. In our study, hearing loss at 4000 Hz was also associated with current smoking, daily alcohol consumption, and high white blood cell count, which are all generally classified as cardiovascular risk factors [27–29, 59–62]. Recently, Ronksley et al. [60] have shown that

TABLE 3: Odds ratio of cardiovascular risk factors for hearing loss.

Models	4,000 Hz		1,000 Hz	
	Unadjusted	Multivariate adjusted	Unadjusted	Multivariate adjusted
Gender				
Men (versus women)	5.69 (5.07–6.37)[‡]	4.47 (3.87–5.15)[‡]	1.22 (1.09–1.36)[‡]	1.18 (1.01–1.37)[*]
Body mass index six categories				
$\leq$19.0 kg/m^2	0.73 (0.63–0.86)[‡]	1.22 (1.02–1.47)[*]	0.98 (0.79–1.20)	1.23 (0.99–1.53)
19.1–21.0 kg/m^2	0.80 (0.71–0.89)[‡]	1.06 (0.93–1.20)	0.81 (0.69–0.96)[*]	0.94 (0.80–1.11)
21.1–22.9 kg/m^2	1	1	1	1
23.0–24.9 kg/m^2	1.37 (1.25–1.50)[‡]	1.05 (0.94–1.17)	1.05 (0.91–1.21)	0.89 (0.77–1.03)
25.0–26.9 kg/m^2	1.46 (1.32–1.62)[‡]	1.06 (0.95–1.19)	1.10 (0.94–1.28)	0.89 (0.76–1.05)
$\geq$27.0 kg/m^2	1.00 (0.90–1.11)	0.95 (0.84–1.08)	0.88 (0.74–1.03)	0.88 (0.74–1.05)
White blood cell				
<25% tile	1	1	1	1
25–49.9% tile	1.29 (1.17–1.42)[‡]	1.08 (0.96–1.21)	1.15 (1.00–1.33)	1.10 (0.95–1.28)
50–75% tile	1.38 (1.25–1.52)[‡]	1.07 (0.95–1.19)	1.13 (0.98–1.31)	1.07 (0.92–1.24)
>75% tile ($\geq$88.9 $\times 10^2/\mu$L)	1.67 (1.52–1.83)[‡]	1.15 (1.03–1.29)[*]	1.18 (1.02–1.36)[*]	1.08 (0.92–1.26)
Past history of cardiovascular disease[a,b]	2.08 (1.70–2.55)[‡]	1.08 (0.85–1.36)	1.91 (1.40–2.58)[‡]	1.15 (0.83–1.58)
Complication of				
Hypertension[b]	3.14 (2.85–3.45)[‡]	1.00 (0.90–1.11)	2.46 (2.15–2.81)[‡]	1.07 (0.92–1.23)
Dyslipidemia[b]	1.27 (1.10–1.46)[†]	0.81 (0.70–0.95)[†]	1.51 (1.24–1.84)[‡]	1.00 (0.82–1.23)
Diabetes[b]	3.71 (3.27–4.21)[‡]	1.53 (1.32–1.76)[‡]	3.06 (2.54–3.68)[‡]	1.56 (1.28–1.90)[‡]
Tinnitus				
Present[b]	4.51 (3.99–5.09)[‡]	3.13 (2.71–3.62)[‡]	3.13 (2.60–3.77)[‡]	2.03 (1.67–2.47)[‡]
Smoking				
No smoker	1	1	1	1
Past smoker	1.89 (1.71–2.09)[‡]	0.98 (0.87–1.11)	1.19 (1.02–1.39)	0.96 (0.81–1.13)
Current smoker	2.04 (1.90–2.18)[‡]	1.29 (1.18–1.41)[‡]	1.15 (1.04–1.28)[†]	1.08 (0.95–1.22)
Alcohol consumption				
No drinker	1	1	1	1
Occasional drinker	0.54 (0.48–0.60)[‡]	0.95 (0.84–1.07)	0.49 (0.42–0.56)[‡]	0.87 (0.74–1.01)
1~3/week drinker	0.77 (0.69–0.86)[‡]	0.85 (0.75–0.96)[†]	0.62 (0.52–0.73)[‡]	0.85 (0.72–1.01)
4~6/week drinker	1.31 (1.18–1.46)[‡]	0.93 (0.83–1.06)	0.82 (0.70–0.97)[*]	0.82 (0.69–0.98)[*]
Daily drinker	2.40 (2.21–2.62)[‡]	1.17 (1.05–1.30)[†]	1.37 (1.20–1.55)[‡]	1.04 (0.90–1.20)
Exercise				
$\geq$2/week exerciser	1	1	1	1
1/week exerciser	0.94 (0.84–1.05)	0.99 (0.87–1.13)	0.83 (0.71–0.99)[*]	0.93 (0.78–1.10)
Occasional exerciser	0.88 (0.78–0.99)[*]	1.12 (0.97–1.29)	0.72 (0.59–0.87)[‡]	0.99 (0.81–1.21)
No exerciser	1.13 (1.03–1.23)[*]	1.18 (1.06–1.31)[†]	1.10 (0.96–1.25)	1.18 (1.02–1.36)[*]
Work duration				
$\leq$6 h	1	1	1	1
7 h	1.58 (1.34–1.85)[‡]	1.05 (0.86–1.29)	0.89 (0.73–1.10)	0.90 (0.72–1.11)
8 h	1.27 (1.12–1.45)[‡]	1.00 (0.85–1.18)	0.61 (0.52–0.70)[‡]	0.85 (0.71–1.01)
9 h	0.96 (0.83–1.11)	0.87 (0.72–1.06)	0.45 (0.37–0.55)[‡]	0.76 (0.61–0.95)[*]
10 h	0.93 (0.79–1.08)	0.92 (0.76–1.11)	0.40 (0.32–0.49)[‡]	0.71 (0.56–0.90)[†]
$\geq$11 h	0.70 (0.60–0.82)[‡]	0.87 (0.72–1.06)	0.29 (0.24–0.36)[‡]	0.62 (0.48–0.79)[‡]

[*]$P < 0.05$, [†]$P < 0.01$, and [‡]$P < 0.001$.
[a]Cardiovascular disease including heart disease and stroke.
[b]Present versus absent.
Confounding factors in multivariate adjustments include those listed in Model 2a of Table 2.
Numbers in exercise express the times of exercise (>30 min per session).

TABLE 4: Baseline clinical characteristics of subjects and prevalence of longer sleep duration eight years later in the longitudinal study.

Categories by sleep duration	Total	≤5 h	6 h	7 h	P values
N, (% of total)	6,774	450 (10.5)	3,063 (46.6)	3,261 (31.4)	—
Age (years)	41.6 ± 9.0	40.2 ± 9.5	41.2 ± 9.1	42.1 ± 8.8	<0.0001
Men, n (%)	4,639 (68.5)	268 (59.6)	1,959 (64.0)	2,412 (74.0)	<0.0001
BMI (kg/m^2)	23.2 ± 3.3	23.3 ± 3.6	23.3 ± 3.4	23.2 ± 3.1	0.67
Systolic blood pressure (mmHg)	123 ± 16.0	122 ± 15.7	123 ± 16.0	124 ± 16.0	<0.0001
Diastolic blood pressure (mmHg)	74 ± 12.2	72 ± 12.2	74 ± 12.2	75 ± 12.1	<0.0001
HbA1c (%, NGSP)	5.4 ± 0.6	5.4 ± 0.8	5.4 ± 0.6	5.4 ± 0.6	0.39
White blood cell (×10^2/μL)	65.0 ± 17.4	64.0 ± 16.4	64.9 ± 17.7	65.3 ± 17.1	0.32
Past history of CVD, n (%)	84 (1.2)	10 (2.2)	36 (1.2)	38 (1.2)	0.15
Medication for					
Hypertension, n (%)	259 (3.8)	13 (2.9)	113 (3.7)	133 (4.1)	0.41
Dyslipidemia, n (%)	71 (1.0)	0 (0.0)	33 (1.1)	38 (1.2)	—*
Diabetes, n (%)	66 (1.0)	5 (1.1)	32 (1.0)	29 (0.9)	—*
Alcohol consumption					
No~occasional/1~3/w/4~6/w/daily (%)*	45/23/11/22	48/26/8/17	48/23/11/18	41/22/12/26	<0.0001
Current smoker, n (%)	2,606 (38.5)	171 (38.0)	1,120 (36.6)	1,315 (40.3)	0.009
Having regular exercise					
No/occasional/1/w/≥2/w (%)*	50/13/18/20	54/14/14/18	50/13/18/20	47/14/19/20	0.09
Hearing loss at least in one ear at 4,000 Hz, n (%)	457 (6.7)	19 (4.2)	175 (5.7)	263 (8.1)	<0.0001
Hearing loss at least in one ear at 1,000 Hz, n (%)	168 (2.5)	8 (1.8)	77 (2.5)	83 (2.5)	0.61
Work duration (hour) (available n = 6,703)	8.5 ± 1.2	8.9 ± 1.4	8.6 ± 1.2	8.4 ± 1.1	<0.0001
Prevalence of longer sleep duration eight years later, n (%)	452 (6.7)	11 (2.4)	109 (3.6)	332 (10.2)	<0.0001

The data are expressed as means ± SD. Triglyceride is expressed as medians (interquartiles).
Individuals with longer sleep duration (≥8 hour) at baseline were not enrolled in the longitudinal study.
*Total sum is not 100% in some cases because of decimal points.
BMI: body mass index, HDL: high-density lipoprotein, NGSP: national glycohemoglobin standardization program, and CVD: cardiovascular disease (including stroke).

TABLE 5: Relative risks for longer sleep duration according to baseline hearing loss.

| | Baseline hearing loss at 4000 Hz | | Baseline hearing loss at 1000 Hz | |
	Absent	Present	Absent	Present
Baseline	6317	457	6606	168
Long-time sleep in 2008	394	58	433	19
	Relative risk (95% CI)		Relative risk (95% CI)	
Model 1	1	2.19 (1.63–2.93)[†]	1	1.82 (1.12–2.96)*
Model 2	1	1.56 (1.14–2.13)*	1	1.50 (0.92–2.47)
Model 3	1	1.53 (1.11–2.10)*	1	1.52 (0.92–2.50)

*P < 0.01 and [†]P < 0.001.
Longer sleep duration at the time point of 9 years was defined as ≥8 h. Hearing loss was defined as loss of hearing of >25 dB in at least one ear.
The number of subjects in each group is the same as that in Table 3.
Model 1: unadjusted.
Model 2: adjusted for age, sex, smoking, alcohol consumption, and regular exercise.
Model 3: Model 2 plus baseline medications for hypertension, dyslipidemia, and diabetes; baseline past history of cardiovascular disease; and baseline body mass index and white blood cell count (total available n = 6250).

neutrophil-lymphocyte ratio, white blood cell count, and C-reactive protein may be associated with hearing loss of diabetic patients. Taken together, although noise-induced hearing loss commonly begins at frequency of 4000 Hz [35–37], our results demonstrates that some cardiovascular risk factors might aggravate the pathophysiology of such noise-induced hearing loss. Then, long-term noise exposure and cardiovascular risk factors might provoke and aggravate a pivotal health damage of hearing loss and sequentially sleep disorder, which needs to be confirmed in further study.

5. Limitations

Several limitations should be mentioned. First, we assessed self-reported sleep duration but not the quality of sleep or other related factors. Nocturnal awakening, insomnia, nocturia, daytime napping, and difficulties with falling sleep may interfere with the observed associations [8, 63, 64]. Future studies should also include objective assessments of sleep duration, preferably made using actigraphy, because such factors may be important confounding factors. Second, we did not assess socioeconomic status in terms of education or annual income. It is possible that the site of residence, work duration, or shift work could shift the endogenous sleeping duration to an exogenously restricted sleeping duration [41, 65–67]. However, adjustment for the type or duration of work did not markedly alter the associations. Third, subclinical hearing loss was only determined using an audiometric test. Other screening methods, such as whispered voice, finger rubbing, and watch tick tests, can detect subclinical hearing loss that may not be identified with audiometric tests [6, 68]. Finally, our results may not be applicable to other populations who have different sleep durations, socioeconomic status, morbidities, and longevities, because these are likely to affect both sleep duration and subclinical hearing loss.

6. Conclusion

Our results suggest that subclinical hearing loss, especially at a high frequency, was independently associated with longer sleep duration and cardiometabolic risk factors in Japanese general population. Current findings remain to be warranted in further study.

Conflict of Interests

The authors declare that they have no competing interests.

Authors' Contribution

K. Nakajima designed the overall study and confirmed the ethicality of the study; K. Suwa identified eligible subjects from the database; K. Nakajima, A. Hosobuchi, and K. Suwa analyzed the data; K. Nakajima, E. Kanda, and A. Hosobuchi reviewed the literature and discussed the results; and K. Nakajima wrote the paper. All authors reviewed and edited the paper and approved the final version of the paper.

Acknowledgment

The authors wish to thank all of the staff of Saitama Health Promotion Corporation for their kind cooperation with this study.

References

[1] A. Howarth and G. R. Shone, "Ageing and the auditory system," *Postgraduate Medical Journal*, vol. 82, no. 965, pp. 166–171, 2006.

[2] X. Z. Liu and D. Yan, "Ageing and hearing loss," *Journal of Pathology*, vol. 211, no. 2, pp. 188–197, 2007.

[3] Q. Huang and J. Tang, "Age-related hearing loss or presbycusis," *European Archives of Oto-Rhino-Laryngology*, vol. 267, no. 8, pp. 1179–1191, 2010.

[4] H. S. Li-Korotky, "Age-related hearing loss: quality of care for quality of life," *Gerontologist*, vol. 52, no. 2, pp. 265–271, 2012.

[5] A. Ciorba, C. Bianchini, S. Pelucchi, and A. Pastore, "The impact of hearing loss on the quality of life of elderly adults," *Clinical Interventions in Aging*, vol. 7, pp. 159–163, 2012.

[6] V. A. Moyer and U.S. Preventive Services Task Force, "Screening for hearing loss in older adults: U.S. preventive services task force recommendation statement," *Annals of Internal Medicine*, vol. 157, no. 9, pp. 655–661, 2012.

[7] R. S. Hallam, "Correlates of sleep disturbance in chronic distressing tinnitus," *Scandinavian Audiology*, vol. 25, no. 4, pp. 263–266, 1996.

[8] R. Asplund, "Sleepiness and sleep in elderly subjects with hearing complaints," *Archives of Gerontology and Geriatrics*, vol. 36, no. 1, pp. 93–99, 2003.

[9] K. I. Hume, "Noise pollution: a ubiquitous unrecognized disruptor of sleep?" *Sleep*, vol. 34, no. 1, pp. 7–8, 2011.

[10] T. Test, A. Canfi, A. Eyal, I. Shoam-Vardi, and E. K. Sheiner, "The influence of hearing impairment on sleep quality among workers exposed to harmful noise," *Sleep*, vol. 34, no. 1, pp. 25–30, 2011.

[11] K. Ito, R. Naito, T. Murofushi, and R. Iguchi, "Questionnaire and interview in screening for hearing impairment in adults," *Acta Oto-laryngologica*, vol. 559, pp. 24–28, 2007.

[12] N. Nakanishi, M. Okamoto, K. Nakamura, K. Suzuki, and K. Tatara, "Cigarette smoking and risk for hearing impairment: a longitudinal study in Japanese male office workers," *Journal of Occupational and Environmental Medicine*, vol. 42, no. 11, pp. 1045–1049, 2000.

[13] Y. Takata, "Hearing loss associated with smoking in male workers," *Journal of UOEH*, vol. 33, no. 1, pp. 35–40, 2011.

[14] V. Kakarlapudi, R. Sawyer, and H. Staecker, "The effect of diabetes on sensorineural hearing loss," *Otology and Neurotology*, vol. 24, no. 3, pp. 382–386, 2003.

[15] D. F. Austin, D. Konrad-Martin, S. Griest, G. P. McMillan, D. McDermott, and S. Fausti, "Diabetes-related changes in hearing," *Laryngoscope*, vol. 119, no. 9, pp. 1788–1796, 2009.

[16] K. E. Bainbridge, Y. J. Cheng, and C. C. Cowie, "Potential mediators of diabetes-related hearing impairment in the U.S. population: National Health and Nutrition Examination Survey 1999–2004," *Diabetes Care*, vol. 33, no. 4, pp. 811–816, 2010.

[17] T. Muneyuki, H. Sugawara, K. Suwa et al., "Design of the Saitama Cardiometabolic Disease and Organ Impairment Study (SCDOIS): a multidisciplinary observational epidemiological study," *Open Journal of Endocrine and Metabolic Diseases*, vol. 3, no. 2, pp. 144–156, 2013.

[18] Saitama Health Promotion Corporation, (Japanese), http://www.saitama-kenkou.or.jp/.

[19] N. Tsuno, A. Besset, and K. Ritchie, "Sleep and depression," *Journal of Clinical Psychiatry*, vol. 66, no. 10, pp. 1254–1269, 2005.

[20] Y. Kaneita, T. Ohida, M. Uchiyama et al., "The relationship between depression and sleep disturbances: a Japanese nationwide general population survey," *Journal of Clinical Psychiatry*, vol. 67, no. 2, pp. 196–203, 2006.

[21] E. J. Mezick, M. Hall, and K. A. Matthews, "Are sleep and depression independent or overlapping risk factors for cardiometabolic disease?" *Sleep Medicine Reviews*, vol. 15, no. 1, pp. 51–63, 2011.

[22] J. S. Loredo, X. Soler, W. Bardwell, S. Ancoli-Israel, J. E. Dimsdale, and L. A. Palinkas, "Sleep health in U.S. Hispanic population," *Sleep*, vol. 33, no. 7, pp. 962–967, 2010.

[23] A. Kashiwagi, M. Kasuga, E. Araki et al., "International clinical harmonization of glycated hemoglobin in Japan: from Japan Diabetes Society to National Glycohemoglobin Standardization Program values," *Journal of Diabetes Investigation*, vol. 3, no. 1, pp. 39–40, 2012.

[24] C. Sabanayagam and A. Shankar, "Sleep duration and cardiovascular disease: results from the National Health Interview Survey," *Sleep*, vol. 33, no. 8, pp. 1037–1042, 2010.

[25] A. Shankar, S. Charumathi, and S. Kalidindi, "Sleep duration and self-rated health: the National Health Interview Survey 2008," *Sleep*, vol. 34, no. 9, pp. 1173–1177, 2011.

[26] WHO Expert Consultation, "Appropriate body-mass index for Asian populations and its implications for policy and intervention strategies," *The Lancet*, vol. 363, pp. 157–163, 2004.

[27] M. P. Weijenberg, E. J. M. Feskens, and D. Kromhout, "White blood cell count and the risk of coronary heart disease and all-cause mortality in elderly men," *Arteriosclerosis, Thrombosis, and Vascular Biology*, vol. 16, no. 4, pp. 499–503, 1996.

[28] H. J. Sun, Y. P. Jung, H. Kim, Y. L. Tae, and J. M. Samet, "White blood cell count and risk for all-cause, cardiovascular, and cancer mortality in a cohort of Koreans," *The American Journal of Epidemiology*, vol. 162, no. 11, pp. 1062–1069, 2005.

[29] E. Jia, Z. Yang, B. Yuan et al., "Relationship between leukocyte count and angiographical characteristics of coronary atherosclerosis," *Acta Pharmacologica Sinica*, vol. 26, no. 9, pp. 1057–1062, 2005.

[30] E. Kiesswetter, A. Seeber, R. Nat, K. Golka, and B. Sietmann, "Solvent exposure, shiftwork, and sleep," *International Journal of Occupational and Environmental Health*, vol. 3, supplement 2, pp. S61–S66, 1997.

[31] M. Viaene, G. Vermeir, and L. Godderis, "Sleep disturbances and occupational exposure to solvents," *Sleep Medicine Reviews*, vol. 13, no. 3, pp. 235–243, 2009.

[32] C. Zocchetti, D. Consonni, and P. A. Bertazzi, "Relationship between prevalence rate ratios and odds ratios in cross-sectional studies," *International Journal of Epidemiology*, vol. 26, no. 1, pp. 220–223, 1997.

[33] K. L. Knutson, "Sleep duration and cardiometabolic risk: a review of the epidemiologic evidence," *Best Practice and Research: Clinical Endocrinology and Metabolism*, vol. 24, no. 5, pp. 731–743, 2010.

[34] C. Chao, J. Wu, Y. Yang et al., "Sleep duration is a potential risk factor for newly diagnosed type 2 diabetes mellitus," *Metabolism: Clinical and Experimental*, vol. 60, no. 6, pp. 799–804, 2011.

[35] O. Hong, "Hearing loss among operating engineers in American construction industry," *International Archives of Occupational and Environmental Health*, vol. 78, no. 7, pp. 565–574, 2005.

[36] B. Bergström and B. Nyström, "Development of hearing loss during long-term exposure to occupational noise. A 20-year follow-up study," *Scandinavian Audiology*, vol. 15, pp. 227–234, 1986.

[37] M. Mostaghaci, S. J. Mirmohammadi, A. H. Mehrparvar, M. Bahaloo, A. Mollasadeghi, and M. H. Davari, "Effect of workplace noise on hearing ability in tile and ceramic industry workers in Iran: a 2-year follow-up study," *The Scientific World Journal*, vol. 2013, Article ID 923731, 7 pages, 2013.

[38] C. J. Williams, F. B. Hu, S. R. Patel, and C. S. Mantzoros, "Sleep duration and snoring in relation to biomarkers of cardiovascular disease risk among women with type 2 diabetes," *Diabetes Care*, vol. 30, no. 5, pp. 1233–1240, 2007.

[39] M. I. Wallhagen, W. J. Strawbridge, and S. J. Shema, "The relationship between hearing impairment and cognitive function: a 5-year longitudinal study," *Research in Gerontological Nursing*, vol. 1, no. 2, pp. 80–86, 2008.

[40] F. R. Lin, L. Ferrucci, E. J. Metter, Y. An, A. B. Zonderman, and S. M. Resnick, "Hearing loss and cognition in the Baltimore Longitudinal Study of Aging," *Neuropsychology*, vol. 25, no. 6, pp. 763–770, 2011.

[41] L. Xu, C. Q. Jiang, T. H. Lam et al., "Short or long sleep duration is associated with memory impairment in older chinese: the Guangzhou Biobank Cohort Study," *Sleep*, vol. 34, no. 5, pp. 575–580, 2011.

[42] F. R. Lin, K. Yaffe, J. Xia et al., "Hearing loss and cognitive decline in older adults," *JAMA Internal Medicine*, vol. 173, no. 4, pp. 293–299, 2013.

[43] E. I. Most, S. Aboudan, P. Scheltens, and E. J. van Someren, "Discrepancy between subjective and objective sleep disturbances in early- and moderate-stage Alzheimer disease," *The American Journal of Geriatric Psychiatry*, vol. 20, no. 6, pp. 460–467, 2012.

[44] D. R. Mazzotti, C. Guindalini, A. L. Sosa, C. P. Ferri, and S. Tufik, "Prevalence and correlates for sleep complaints in older adults in low and middle income countries: a 10/66 Dementia Research Group study," *Sleep Medicine*, vol. 13, no. 6, pp. 697–702, 2012.

[45] Y. S. Ju, J. S. McLeland, C. D. Toedebusch et al., "Sleep quality and preclinical Alzheimer disease," *JAMA Neurology*, vol. 70, no. 5, pp. 587–593, 2013.

[46] B. Fruhstorfer, M. G. Pritsch, and H. Fruhstorfer, "Effects of daytime noise load on the sleep-wake cycle and endocrine patterns in man: I. 24 hours neurophysiological data," *International Journal of Neuroscience*, vol. 39, no. 3-4, pp. 197–209, 1988.

[47] F. Abad-Alegría and M. Gutiérrez, "Characteristics of sleep in deafness," *Revue Neurologique*, vol. 26, no. 154, pp. 959–961, 1998.

[48] A. L. Rios and G. Alves da Silva, "Sleep quality in noise exposed Brazilian workers," *Noise and Health*, vol. 7, no. 29, pp. 1–6, 2005.

[49] P. A. Wackym and F. H. Linthicum Jr., "Diabetes mellitus and hearing loss: clinical and histopathologic relationships," *The American Journal of Otology*, vol. 7, no. 3, pp. 176–182, 1986.

[50] T. L. Smith, E. Raynor, J. Prazma, J. E. Buenting, and H. C. Pillsbury, "Insulin-dependent diabetic microangiopathy in the inner ear," *Laryngoscope*, vol. 105, no. 3 I, pp. 236–240, 1995.

[51] Z. Shemesh, J. Attias, M. Ornan, N. Shapira, and A. Shahar, "Vitamin B12 deficiency in patients with chronic-tinnitus and noise-induced hearing loss," *American Journal of Otolaryngology—Head and Neck Medicine and Surgery*, vol. 14, no. 2, pp. 94–99, 1993.

[52] D. K. Houston, M. A. Johnson, R. J. Nozza et al., "Age-related hearing loss, vitamin B-12, and folate in elderly women," *American Journal of Clinical Nutrition*, vol. 69, no. 3, pp. 564–571, 1999.

[53] J. Shargorodsky, S. G. Curhan, R. Eavey, and G. C. Curhan, "A prospective study of vitamin intake and the risk of hearing loss in men," *Otolaryngology—Head and Neck Surgery*, vol. 142, no. 2, pp. 231–236, 2010.

[54] A. O. Lasisi, F. A. Fehintola, and O. B. Yusuf, "Age-related hearing loss, vitamin B12, and folate in the elderly," *Otolaryngology-Head and Neck Surgery*, vol. 143, no. 6, pp. 826–830, 2010.

[55] B. Gopinath, V. M. Flood, C. M. McMahon et al., "Dietary antioxidant intake is associated with the prevalence but not incidence of age-related hearing loss," *Journal of Nutrition, Health and Aging*, vol. 15, no. 10, pp. 896–900, 2011.

[56] S. H. Jee, J. W. Sull, J. Park, S. Y. Lee, H. Ohrr, and E. Guallar, "Body-mass index and mortality in Korean men and women," *The New England Journal of Medicine*, vol. 355, no. 8, pp. 779–787, 2006.

[57] A. B. de Gonzalez, P. Hartge, J. R. Cerhan et al., "Body-mass index and mortality among 1.46 million white adults," *The New England Journal of Medicine*, vol. 363, no. 23, pp. 2211–2219, 2010.

[58] W. Zheng, D. F. McLerran, B. Rolland et al., "Association between body-mass index and risk of death in more than 1 million Asians," *The New England Journal of Medicine*, vol. 364, no. 8, pp. 719–729, 2011.

[59] J. Rehm, C. Mathers, S. Popova, M. Thavorncharoensap, Y. Teerawattananon, and J. Patra, "Global burden of disease and injury and economic cost attributable to alcohol use and alcohol-use disorders," *The Lancet*, vol. 373, no. 9682, pp. 2223–2233, 2009.

[60] P. E. Ronksley, S. E. Brien, B. J. Turner, K. J. Mukamal, and W. A. Ghali, "Association of alcohol consumption with selected cardiovascular disease outcomes: a systematic review and meta-analysis," *BMJ*, vol. 342, article d671, 2011.

[61] H. Iso, "Lifestyle and cardiovascular disease in Japan," *Journal of Atherosclerosis and Thrombosis*, vol. 18, no. 2, pp. 83–88, 2011.

[62] R. Gupta and P. Deedwania, "Interventions for cardiovascular disease prevention," *Cardiology Clinics*, vol. 29, no. 1, pp. 15–34, 2011.

[63] Y. Udo, M. Nakao, H. Honjo, O. Ukimura, H. Kitakoji, and T. Miki, "Sleep duration is an independent factor in nocturia: analysis of bladder diaries," *BJU International*, vol. 104, no. 1, pp. 75–79, 2009.

[64] J. Cohen-Mansfield and R. Perach, "Sleep duration, nap habits, and mortality in older persons," *Sleep*, vol. 35, no. 7, pp. 1003–1009, 2012.

[65] S. Y. Ryu, K. S. Kim, and M. A. Han, "Factors associated with sleep duration in Korean adults: Results of a 2008 community health survey in Gwangju Metropolitan City, Korea," *Journal of Korean Medical Science*, vol. 26, no. 9, pp. 1124–1131, 2011.

[66] K. A. Ertel, L. F. Berkman, and O. M. Buxton, "Socioeconomic status, occupational characteristics, and sleep duration in African/Caribbean immigrants and US white health care workers," *Sleep*, vol. 34, no. 4, pp. 509–518, 2011.

[67] T. Lallukka, L. Sares-Jäske, E. Kronholm et al., "Sociodemographic and socioeconomic differences in sleep duration and insomnia-related symptoms in Finnish adults," *BMC Public Health*, vol. 12, no. 1, article 565, 2012.

[68] R. Chou, T. Dana, C. Bougatsos, C. Fleming, and T. Beil, "Screening adults aged 50 years or older for hearing loss: a review of the evidence for the U.S. preventive services task force," *Annals of Internal Medicine*, vol. 154, no. 5, pp. 347–355, 2011.

3

From Inpatient Notes to Outpatient Followup: Enhancing the Rhinology Service in a Tertiary Centre through Student Led Projects

M. Sayma, R. Hyne, M. Sharma, L. Kyle, M. Abo Khatwa, I. MacKay-Davies, A. Poulios, and H. S. Khalil

Plymouth Hospitals NHS Trust and Peninsula College of Medicine and Dentistry, Plymouth, UK

Correspondence should be addressed to M. Sayma; meelad.sayma@students.pcmd.ac.uk

Academic Editor: David W. Eisele

Introduction. Medical students can use systems to help improve the quality of care in a unit. Following the review of care within the ENT department at a tertiary centre a number of quality improvement projects were put in place. *Methods*. The following interventions were established: (1) creation of an outpatient telephone enquiry clinic, (2) development of a rhinology database, (3) introduction of operative note templates, and (4) construction of electronic discharge summary templates (eDSTs). *Discussion and Outcomes*. (1) Consultant telephone inquiry clinics were successfully organised and showed high levels of patient satisfaction. (2) A database to collect patient reported outcome measures was piloted within rhinology outpatients; the results suggest that such a database would be simple to introduce and yield benefits for patients and the department. (3) Operative note templates for FESS procedures were implemented with a view to improving the continuity of care onto the ward; these have become well established and further steps to integrate these into routine care are being taken. (4) eDSTs specific to FESS and septorhinoplasty procedures were introduced with a view to increasing completion speed of templates and adherence to Royal College of Physician Guidance.

1. Introduction

Medical students have been shown to have the ability to improve patient care outcomes when given the opportunity to be involved in quality improvement in healthcare settings [1]. Senior medical students were offered the opportunity as part of a student selected component in rhinology to undertake a series of quality improvement project assessing the efficacy of a number of processes in a British rhinology unit. This series was selected to sequentially assess and improve points of patient care from recording operative data to reviewing these patients as outpatients.

1.1. Creation of an Outpatient Telephone Enquiry Clinic. With pressured clinical resources failing to accommodate the increasing backlog of follow-up appointments, telephone clinics have been proposed as a novel alternative of reducing the vast number of patients waiting for routine followup [2]. Traditionally, surgeons have reviewed postoperative patients

face to face (FTF) as this postoperative outpatient review is important not only for patient reassurance but also for auditing the efficacy and complications of surgical procedures [3, 4]. However, reports performed in 2008/2009 and 2010/2011 stated that many follow-up appointments are unnecessary for patients undergoing routine surgery [2]. With "best practice" defined as having a "no wait culture," the South West Strategic Health Authority (SW SHA) aims to improve the time in which care is delivered through safely and effectively substituting specific FTF follow-up appointments with telephone consultations [2].

1.2. Development of a Rhinology Database. Standardisation and comparison of surgical outcomes are important to ensure best patient care and are a requirement for revalidation. At present many departments report surgical outcomes via data collected from coding. Although this may not necessarily reflect patient reported outcomes, departments may have little other options. Patient-reported outcome measures (PROMs) are increasingly gaining acceptance as important and valid measures of symptoms, experiences, and quality of life. Patient communication, care, and outcomes have been shown to improve as a result of integrating their collection into routine clinical practice [5].

Since 2009, the BRS has provided an online tool for recording outcomes and evaluating performance against national averages. However, problems with access and a large number of obligatory fields have inhibited its use [6]. Therefore, this project aimed to pilot and evaluate an in-house, computerised database for collection of PROMs, introduced as a means of assessing the effect of interventions and aiding reporting of outcomes.

1.3. Operative Note Templates for FESS Procedures. Operative notes are the only comprehensive documented evidence of what happens in surgery [7]. They serve as a method of communication between theatre staff and ward staff. Accurate and detailed notes are important to provide satisfactory postoperative care and serve as proficient evidence in medicolegal situations [7–12]. The GMC states that good note keeping is an essential part of good medical care [7, 13], and the Royal College of Surgeons (RCS) says that medical records are "fundamental for clinical care and audit of surgical services" [14]. The RCS published guidelines on the basic components that all operative notes should include in order to communicate the necessary information and produce a medicolegally safe document [10, 14].

Problems arise with hand-written operative notes, such as legibility of the surgeons' handwriting [7]. Up to 11.4% of drug errors made on wards are due to illegible handwriting in operative notes [12]. Handwritten operative notes may not be complete; a template devised for use in kidney cancer showed an increase in completion rates from 68% in dictated notes to 92% in the online template [15].

Through introducing an operative note template for functional endoscopic sinus surgery (FESS) and nasal polypectomy procedures, we aim to improve the completeness of operative notes, create a safer communication pathway between surgical staff and ward based staff, and save time taken to fill out operative notes.

1.4. eDSTs Specific Production. Discharge summaries communicate essential clinical information from inpatient settings to primary care. Information transmission was previously conducted through dictated letters completed by administrative staff. This often resulted in poor quality information being given to primary care providers, in an untimely manner [16]. As a result GP's called for the introduction of "electronic discharge summaries" (eDSs) to increase quality and speed of information transfer [17].

The hospital involved in this project introduced an eDS system in 2008 and in 2010 the "Clinical Data Standards Assurance programme" began a project to deliver national, clinically assured eDSs [18]. Despite implementation of eDSs, problems have still arisen regarding their timeliness and content and these have been well discussed in the literature [19–21]. Further literature analysis highlighted that these issues

may lead to deficits regarding patient safety and continuity of care [22]. The Royal College of Physicians recommends that a DS should be produced for every patient and should contain a set of key subheadings [23].

Recent evidence has suggested that the addition of "prompting systems" to electronic discharge summaries may improve their content quality, resulting in improved patient safety [24, 25].

For these reasons, the quality of electronic discharge summaries in Rhinology at Derriford Hospital was analysed, with a view to the introduction of a "prompting system" or custom eDS templates to improve their quality.

2. Methods

2.1. Creation of Outpatient Telephone Enquiry Clinic. In order to maximise the possibility of successfully contacting patients, whilst utilising clinician time efficiently five patients were selected using the inclusion and exclusion criteria. The inclusion criteria comprised of surgical procedures with low-risk complications such as functional endoscopic sinus surgery (FESS), diathermy of inferior turbinates (DITs), polypectomy, and septoplasty. Sinonasal tumours, endoscopic dacryocystorhinostomy (DCR), nasal biopsies, and septorhinoplasty were excluded due to the expected need for regular followup. During each consultation, patients were asked questions relevant to their procedure using either a Sino-Nasal Outcome Test (SNOT22) or Nasal Obstruction and Septoplasty Effectiveness (NOSE) scale and this was completed using the ENT electronic database. The time taken per consult was recorded and a mixed methodology approach, including telephone and FTF interviews, was used to obtain patient views on suitability of the TIC and monitor patient satisfaction.

2.2. Development of a Rhinology Database. A Microsoft access database was developed for use in rhinology outpatients. This database allows recording of patient ID, demographics, diagnosis, surgery performed, and date of surgery in addition to the appropriate PROM. Two validated PROMs were included: Sino-Nasal Outcome Test 22 for use in rhinosinusitis and Nasal Obstruction Symptom Evaluation for use in nasal obstruction.

This database was piloted in two settings: outpatients and a telephone follow-up clinic. In each clinic the database was completed for four patients and the time taken was recorded. In addition, an opinion on the database was sought from an ENT surgeon with expertise in database design.

2.3. Introduction of Operative Note Templates. A pilot study trialling the use of an operative note template for FESS and nasal polypectomy was conducted. The template was developed using the RCS operative note guidelines to ensure the 14 points in RCS guidelines were included. The template was piloted in theatre by four surgeons and then evaluated straight after using Likert scales. The operative notes entered the patient notes, where four recovery nurses evaluated them. Following evaluation from both groups, the template was adapted to appease their suggestions and include important information. The template was repiloted by the same four surgeons and recovery ward nurses to see if opinions and the usability of the template had improved, with the eventual aim of computerising the template. The inclusion criterion was any FESS, nasal polypectomy, and functional endoscopic nasal surgery (FENS) taking place. Exclusion criteria included any operations not stated above.

2.4. Construction of Electronic Discharge Summary Template. A prospective case note review was conducted of sequential patients who had undergone rhinology procedures. The entries on the generic eDSs to the GP were compared to the information in clinical records. Discrepancies were noted. The content of each eDSs was assessed against RCP generic record guidance to screen for omissions. Five clinicians were timed when completing eDSs to assess completion time. Following the audit, a custom eDS template was designed using lists of common symptoms, risks, and warnings (among other subheadings) prompting clinicians to complete all required data.

3. Discussion and Outcomes

3.1. Creation of Outpatient Telephone Enquiry Clinic. The TEC for postoperative rhinology patients appears to be a safe and cost-effective alternative to FTF followup, both acceptable to and appreciated by patients. The initial pilot study has shown that TECs can avoid unnecessary outpatient appointments and increase the availability of clinic slots by providing a quicker method of reviewing patients. Our experience suggests that future TECs should be led by a senior clinician to adequately address the complexity of questions asked and maintain patient safety. Patient views regarding the TEC proved promising, with patients stating the preference for telephone consultations as it reduced waiting and travel times and minimised the need to take time of work and the cost of hospital parking.

Overall, the proposed intervention is a safe and effective substitution of FTF consultations that provides efficient health care which is equitable and patient-centred, validating its future sustainability of the inclusion of TEC in routine follow-up care.

3.2. Development of a Rhinology Database. The pilot provided information about the utility of the database. The mean time taken to complete the database was 3.25 minutes in the outpatient clinic and 4 minutes in the telephone clinic. In addition the pilot, together with the opinion of our database expert, allowed a range of positive and negative aspects of the database to be identified.

Positive aspects included

(i) ease of use,

(ii) time efficiency,

(iii) PROM simple for patients to understand.

Negative aspects included

(i) not available on the network,

(ii) no ability to delete entries from database if incorrectly entered,

(iii) no easy access to database tables.

The results from this pilot suggest that a fit for purpose database would not greatly increase the time taken for outpatient appointments and has the potential to improve patient care and allow the department to accurately report outcomes.

Further development and liaison with the IT department is now recommended to overcome the identified limitations and integrate the use of such a database into routine clinical practice.

3.3. Introduction of Operative Note Templates. The staff involved in the pilot study found the use of a template to be safer, especially the recovery nurses who found the consistent order of the notes easier to follow than hand-written notes. They found that the tick box sections and reduction in writing made the template more legible and therefore they felt safer administering the postoperative care required. The surgical team did not rate the original template as highly as the nursing staff but found the second template quicker to fill out, safer, and more comprehensive.

The surgical team found the original FESS template unclear, and some disliked the illustrations. The surgeons found the modified form incorporating their feedback to be quicker, safer, and preferable to writing out their operative notes. They preferred the use of colour to stratify sections. They preferred to use their own drawings to illustrate intraoperative findings. The surgeons found the modified template to be quicker than hand-written notes. The sample of four templates showed complete, comprehensive notes which follow the RCS guidelines.

Following the introduction of the operative note template, we intend to compare hand-written operative notes with the operative note template for completeness when a sufficient number of templates have been used.

3.4. Construction of Electronic Discharge Summary Template. All discharges had adequate information but there was noncompliance with the RCP guidance; highlights included the following:

(i) 12 of the 15 eDSs were available for analysis;

(ii) 7 out of 12 contained inconsistencies when compared to patient notes;

(iii) half of all eDSs assessed contained "incomplete information" when compared to RCP guidance (see Table 1 for summary of detail);

(iv) clinicians took a mean time of 5 minutes 25 seconds completing each electronic discharge summary.

This audit highlighted that there was room for improvement in the content quality of eDSs in rhinology. As a result custom "prompting" templates were constructed for FESS and septoplasty/turbinate surgery with a view to improving these parameters, improving patient safety, and saving time

TABLE 1

Information subheading	% of records containing complete information
GP details	100%
Patient details	65.47%
Admission details	100%
Discharge details	75%
Clinical information	46.70%
Advice, recommendations, and future plan	55.55%
Person completing summary	100%

and money. These templates where constructed with two ideas in mind as follows.

(1) Addition of prewritten "delete as appropriate suggestions" for each subheading to aid clinicians to speed up completion of forms (see the following list).

Please delete as appropriate suggestions:

   (i) chronic sinusitis refractory to medical treatment,
   (ii) recurrent sinusitis,
   (iii) nasal polyposis,
   (iv) antrochoanal polyps,
   (v) sinus mucoceles,
   (vi) excision of tumour,
   (vii) cerebrospinal fluid (CSF) leak closure,
   (viii) orbital decompression,
   (ix) optic nerve decompression,
   (x) dacryocystorhinostomy (DCR),
   (xi) choanal atresia repair,
   (xii) foreign body removal,
   (xiii) epistaxis control.

(2) "Prompting words" to remind clinicians regarding certain content that had previously been omitted. See the following list for sample of new template:

   please include a brief clinical narrative and summary of advice for patients' GP, including medication recommendations,

   please include any RISKS and WARNINGS,

   what information has been given to patient regarding procedure?

   did the patient have the mental capacity to consent to this procedure? Y/N.

Following the introduction of these templates, a pilot study was conducted on patients undergoing septoplasty and turbinate surgery. An eDS was observed for completion time. The summary was then compared against RCP guidance using the same methodology as the initial audit.

Despite having a small sample, the audit of this pilot showed a 1-minute improvement in speed of completion of eDS (mean time taken was 4 minutes and 30 seconds). Prompting words improved adherence to RCP recommendations. A proposal has been put forward with a view to creating specific EDST's for common procedures across ENT.

4. Conclusion

Student-led interventions in specialist units can improve the quality of care given to patients. These four projects have shown the potential to ensure the delivery of safe, patient-centred healthcare that is both efficient and equitable and offer examples for other national units to consider in their practice.

Disclosure

Hisham Khalil takes overall responsibility for the integrity of the paper.

Conflict of Interests

The authors declare that there is no conflict of interests regarding the publication of this paper.

References

[1] B. E. Gould, M. R. Grey, C. G. Huntington et al., "Improving patient care outcomes by teaching quality improvement to medical students in community-based practices," *Academic Medicine*, vol. 77, no. 10, pp. 1011–1018, 2002.

[2] The National Institute for Health Research (NIHR) Collaboration for Leadership in Applied Health Research and Care (CLAHRC) South West Peninsula, "Telecon-Thyroid: are telephone consultations safe and effective in the management of thyroid disease?" 2010, http://clahrc-peninsula.nihr.ac.uk/research/telecon-thyroid.

[3] M. R. McVay, K. R. Kelley, D. L. Mathews, R. J. Jackson, E. R. Kokoska, and S. D. Smith, "Postoperative follow-up: is a phone call enough?" *Journal of Pediatric Surgery*, vol. 43, no. 1, pp. 83–86, 2008.

[4] R. T. Gray, M. K. Sut, S. A. Badger, and C. F. Harvey, "Postoperative telephone review is cost-effective and acceptable to patients," *Ulster Medical Journal*, vol. 79, no. 2, pp. 76–79, 2010.

[5] S. Marshall, K. Haywood, and R. Fitzpatrick, "Impact of patient-reported outcome measures on routine practice: a structured review," *Journal of Evaluation in Clinical Practice*, vol. 12, no. 5, pp. 559–568, 2006.

[6] K. Kapoor and C. Hopkins, "Underutilisation of the British Rhinological Society minimum electronic dataset in an age of mandatory reporting; an investigation," *Clinical Otolaryngology*, vol. 40, no. 2, pp. 140–142, 2015.

[7] Y. Ghani, R. Thakrar, D. Kosuge, and P. Bates, "'Smart' electronic operation notes in surgery: an innovative way to improve patient care," *International Journal of Surgery*, vol. 12, no. 1, pp. 30–32, 2014.

[8] L. Moore, R. Churley-Strom, B. Singal, and S. O'Leary, "Laparotomy operative note template constructed through a modified Delphi method," *American Journal of Obstetrics & Gynecology*, vol. 200, no. 5, pp. e16–e17, 2009.

[9] D. A. Cowan, M. B. Sands, S. M. Rabizadeh et al., "Electronic templates versus dictation for the completion of Mohs micrographic surgery operative notes," *Dermatologic Surgery*, vol. 33, no. 5, pp. 588–595, 2007.

[10] D. Moegan, N. Fisher, A. Ahmad, and F. Alam, "Improving operation notes to meet British orthopaedic association guidelines," *Annals of the Royal College of Surgeons of England*, vol. 91, no. 3, pp. 217–219, 2009.

[11] A. W. Barritt, L. Clark, A. M. Cohen, N. Hosangadi-Jayedev, and P. A. Gibb, "Improving the quality of procedure-specific operation reports in orthopaedic surgery," *Annals of the Royal College of Surgeons of England*, vol. 92, no. 2, pp. 159–162, 2010.

[12] N. D. Bateman, A. S. Carney, and K. P. Gibbin, "An audit of the quality of operation notes in an otolaryngology unit," *Journal of the Royal College of Surgeons of Edinburgh*, vol. 44, no. 2, pp. 94–95, 1999.

[13] GMC, *Good Medical Practice*, GMC, London, UK, 2011.

[14] The Royal College of Surgeons of England, *Good Surgical Practice*, The Royal College of Surgeons of England, London, UK, 2010.

[15] D. N. Hoffer, A. Finelli, R. Chow et al., "Structured electronic operative reporting: comparison with dictation in kidney cancer surgery," *International Journal of Medical Informatics*, vol. 81, no. 3, pp. 182–191, 2012.

[16] K. J. O'Leary, D. M. Liebovitz, J. Feinglass et al., "Creating a better discharge summary: improvement in quality and timeliness using an electronic discharge summary," *Journal of Hospital Medicine*, vol. 4, no. 4, pp. 219–225, 2009.

[17] K. J. O'Leary, D. M. Liebovitz, J. Feinglass, D. T. Liss, and D. W. Baker, "Outpatient physicians' satisfaction with discharge summaries and perceived need for an electronic discharge summary," *Journal of Hospital Medicine*, vol. 1, no. 5, pp. 317–320, 2006.

[18] HSCIC, *Electronic 24-Hour Discharge Summary Implementation*, HSCIC, 2010, http://systems.hscic.gov.uk/clinrecords/24hour.

[19] L. I. Horwitz, G. Y. Jenq, U. C. Brewster et al., "Comprehensive quality of discharge summaries at an academic medical center," *Journal of Hospital Medicine*, vol. 8, no. 8, pp. 436–443, 2013.

[20] J. P. Mamo, "Electronic discharge summaries—are they being done and do they have the required information?" *Irish Medical Journal*, vol. 107, no. 3, pp. 88–90, 2014.

[21] E. A. Hammad, D. J. Wright, C. Walton, I. Nunney, and D. Bhattacharya, "Adherence to UK national guidance for discharge information: an audit in primary care," *British Journal of Clinical Pharmacology*, vol. 78, no. 6, pp. 1453–1464, 2014.

[22] S. Kripalani, F. LeFevre, C. O. Phillips, M. V. Williams, P. Basaviah, and D. W. Baker, "Deficits in communication and information transfer between hospital-based and primary care physicians: implications for patient safety and continuity of care," *Journal of the American Medical Association*, vol. 297, no. 8, pp. 831–841, 2007.

[23] Academy of Medical Royal Colleges, *Standards for the Clinical Structure and Content of Patient Records*, Academy of Medical Royal Colleges, Health and Social Care Information Centre, London, UK, 2013, https://www.rcplondon.ac.uk/sites/default/files/standards-for-the-clinical-structure-and-content-of-patient-records.pdf.

[24] A. P. Maurice, S. Chan, C. W. Pollard et al., "Improving the quality of hospital discharge summaries utilising an electronic prompting system," *BMJ Quality Improvement Reports*, vol. 3, no. 1, 2014.

[25] E. Ladds, F. Betteridge, S. Yamamoto, and T. Gupta-Jessop, "Improving the quality of discharge summaries for elective surgical procedures at North Bristol NHS Trust," *BMJ Quality Improvement Reports*, vol. 4, no. 1, 2015.

Effect of Preoperative Mastoid Ventilation on Tympanoplasty Success

Mehmet Metin,[1] Zeynep Kizilkaya Kaptan,[2] Sedat Dogan,[3] Hasmet Yazici,[4] Cem Bayraktar,[3] Hakan Gocmen,[2] and Etem Erdal Samim[2]

[1] *Hendek State Hospital, 54300 Sakarya, Turkey*
[2] *Ankara Research and Training Hospital, Ministry of Health, 06340 Ankara, Turkey*
[3] *Faculty of Medicine, Adiyaman University, Ear Nose Throat Clinic, 02200 Adiyaman, Turkey*
[4] *Faculty of Medicine, Balikesir University, Ear Nose Throat Clinic, 10145 Balikesir, Turkey*

Correspondence should be addressed to Sedat Dogan; sdtdgn1981@hotmail.com

Academic Editor: Jeffrey P. Pearson

Purpose. This study was conducted with the aim of investigating the relationship between mastoid air cell volumes and graft success after tympanoplasty. *Material and Methods*. This study was performed retrospectively with patients undergoing type I tympanoplasty and antrostomy. A total of 57 patients (20–35.09% female and 37–64.91% male) with a mean age of $29.69 \pm SD$ (range 12–56 years) were included in the study. The patients were invited for a control at the 1st, 3rd, and 12th months, and otoscopic examinations and audiometric tests were performed. The temporal bone computed tomography images were screened with the 4800 Dpi optic resolution scanner and transferred to the computer environment in JPG format in order to calculate the mastoid air cell volume, and the volumes were calculated using the Autocad 2007 program. *Results*. Although, the graft success was determined to be better in the well-ventilated group, no significant difference could be found between the groups in terms of graft success at the 1st, 3rd, and 12th months ($P > 0.05$). No statistically significant difference could be found between the three groups in terms of the preoperative and postoperative hearing gains ($P > 0.05$).

1. Introduction

Chronic otitis media (COM) is a common problem. Genetic and environmental factors affect the progression of otitis media to chronicity. A decrease in the mastoid air cells has been shown to be related with atelectatic ear diseases, cholesteatoma, and chronic otitis media with effusion [1, 2]. Whether poorly developed mastoid cells are the reason or a result of otitis media has not been proven yet. Whether mastoid cell ventilation affects the outcomes of tympanoplasty is an issue which has not been discussed sufficiently and on which only a limited number of studies have been performed. The effect of preoperative mastoid ventilation on tympanoplasty results is controversial.

In this study, the relationship between the mastoid air cell volumes and the graft success after tympanoplasty was investigated. The relationships between the preoperative mastoid air cell ventilation and the obtained hearing gains, air-bone gaps, and ventilation degrees according to gender and the patient ages were also investigated.

2. Material and Methods

Patients who had been diagnosed with chronic otitis media for whom surgery had been planned, and on whom temporal bone computed tomographies had been performed, were included in the study. Patients who had undergone otoscopy, microscopy, audiometry, and computed tomography tests and who had undergone type I tympanoplasty and antrostomy were included in the study. Patients who were determined to have cholesteatoma intraoperatively, revision cases, and patients whose follow-up findings were missing were excluded from the study. Patients underwent type 1 tympanoplasty and surgeries are done by the same surgeon

TABLE 1

	Mastoid volume (cm^3)	Patient number	%	Mean volume
Group I	10 cm^3 and above	7	12.28%	11.7322 cm^3
Group II	Between 5 and 10 cm^3	14	24.56%	7.1755 cm^3
Group III	Between 0 and 5 cm^3	36	69.91%	2.1237 cm^3

and the same operative technique is used. Only antrostomy was performed following a postauricular incision (as pathology was not detected in the other cells). Patients whose ossicles were intact and mobile were included in the study. Patients who were found to have encountered complications such as bleeding and infection were excluded from the study. Temporal muscle fascia was used as graft in all the patients. On the control visits, otoscopy examinations and audiometry tests were performed and the results were recorded. Of the 57 patients who met the criteria of the study, 20 (35.09%) were male and 37 (64.91%) were female, with a mean age of 29.69 (range 12–56).

Temporal bone computed tomographies were performed using a Hitachi-Pronto AR HP spiral scanner. The tomography sections were 2 mm in thickness and parallel to the orbitomeatal line. The temporal bone computed tomography images were scanned using the 4800 Dpi optic resolution scanner and transferred to the computer environment in JPG format in order to calculate the mastoid bone volume using the Cavalieri technique. The mastoid volumes of CT images which had been transferred to the computer environment were calculated using the Autocad 2007 program. On CT, the air cell area in the mastoid bone on the operated side was calculated and the bony part of the mastoid was not included in this calculation. Air cells containing soft tissue areas in which inflammatory activity was present were not included in the volume calculation of the air cells. The patients were divided into three groups as the poorly ventilated group, the moderately ventilated group, and the well ventilated group according to the mastoid air cell ventilations detected on the preoperatively performed temporal bone CT.

3. Statistical Analysis and Results

The data were analyzed using the SPSS for Windows 11.5 package program. Whether the distribution of constant variables was near normal or not was analyzed using the Shapiro Wilk test. The descriptive statistics were shown as mean ± standard deviation for constant variables, and the nominal variables were shown as numbers and percentages (%). The presence or absence of a significant change between the air-bone gap levels in the preoperative period and at the postoperative 12th month was evaluated using the Dependent t-test. The nominal variables were analyzed using the Pearson's Chi-square test. A P level of <0.05 was accepted as statistically significant.

Mastoid Volume. The total mastoid cell ventilations were divided to three groups as the result of the measurements was made according to the Cavalieri principle, benefiting from

TABLE 2: Graft success rates of the mastoid ventilation groups at the 12th month.

Mastoid ventilation	Graft success
Group I ($n = 7$)	6 (85.7%)
Group II ($n = 14$)	11 (78.6%)
Group III ($n = 36$)	23 (63.9%)
$P^\dagger$	0.352

†Pearson Chi-square test.

the preoperative temporal CT (Table 1): Group I: ventilated, Group II: moderately ventilated, and Group III: poorly ventilated (Table 1). The average mastoid volume of all the patients was measured as 3.8486 cm^3 (range 0.7765 cm^3–14.891 cm^3). The mean volume was 11.7322 cm^3 for Group I, 7.1755 cm^3 for Group II, and 2.1237 cm^3 for Group III. Statistical analyses were performed between the mastoid ventilation groups and the graft success (Table 2).

Graft success was analyzed at the 1st, the 3rd, and the 12th months in the mastoid cell groups. In Group I, the graft success in 7 patients was 85.71% at the 1st, the 3rd, and the 12th month. In Group II, the graft success in 14 patients was 85.71% (12/14 patients) at the 1st month, 78.57% (11/14 patients) at the 3rd Month, and 78.57% (11/14 patients) at the 12th month. In Group III, the graft success of 36 patients was 75% (27/36 patients) at the 1st month, 69.44% (25/36 patients) at the 3rd month, and 63.88% (23/36 patients) at the 12th month.

No statistically significant difference was determined between the mastoid ventilation groups in terms of graft success rates at the 1st, the 3rd, and the 12th months ($P = 0.352$).

Audiometry Results. In the preoperative audiometries of the patients, the mean threshold values of the side which would be operated and the mean threshold values of the air conduction and bone conduction thresholds at the 1st, 3rd, and 12th months were measured (Table 3).

Statistical analyses including air-bone gaps and air conduction gains were performed between the mastoid ventilation groups (Table 3).

A statistically significant decrease was found between the mean air-bone gaps and the air conduction thresholds at the postoperative 12th month compared to the preoperative values ($P < 0.001$). However there was no significant difference between ventilation groups in terms of audiometry results at the end of the 12th month ($P > 0.05$).

Age and Gender Groups. 20 (35%) of the patients were male and 37 (65%) were female, with a mean age of 19.69 (range 12–56). The mean age of the patients was 24.14 years in Group I,

TABLE 3: Preoperative and postoperative hearing threshold averages and air-bone gaps measured in all the patients and the mastoid ventilation groups.

	Preoperative			1st month			3rd month			12th month		
	ac (dB)	bc (dB)	abg (dB)	ac (db)	bc (dB)	abg (dB)	ac (dB)	bc (dB)	abg (dB)	ac (dB)	bc (dB)	abg (dB)
Patients	48	22	26	36.3	15.6	20.6	32.3	15.9	16.4	30.8	15.3	15.5
Group I	39.71	16.85	22.86	34.4	13	21.4	26.1	13	13.1	22.9	11.9	11
Group II	45.14	24.35	20.79	35.3	18.3	17	31.1	17.1	13.9	31.1	17.6	13.4
Group III	46.69	21.86	24.83	37.2	17.6	19.5	34.2	18.1	16.1	32.8	17.6	17.6

ac: air way conduction; bc: bone conduction; abg: air bone gap.

25.57 years in Group II, and 29.27 years in Group III. No statistically significant difference was found between the gender groups in terms of graft success rates at the end of the 12th month ($P = 0.217$).

Operated Side. The right ears of 27 patients and the left ears of 30 patients were operated.

No statistically significant difference was determined between the right and the left sides in terms of graft success rates at the end of the 12th month ($P = 0.234$).

4. Discussion

The mastoid air cell system has a great importance in middle ear physiology. Tumarkin and Holmquist claimed that mastoid cells provided an air reservoir for the middle ear and demonstrated that they played a role in the pressure regulation of the middle ear [3, 4]. This hypothesis was also supported by Sade and Fuchs [2]. Frisberg et al. was the first who analyzed the relationship between the mastoid air cell size and the prognosis of middle ear disease [5]. Holmquist and Bergstrom also studied that issue later. Holmquist and Bergstroem showed that the success of middle ear surgery depended on mastoid cell ventilation. In his study, Holmquist and Bergstroem measured the mastoid volumes using Schüller X-Rays performed preoperatively. They showed that middle ear retraction was greater in patients who had undergone tympanomastoidectomy compared to those who had undergone tympanoplasty without mastoidectomy [6]. Therefore, they advocated that well ventilated mastoid cells should not be intervened during surgery [6]. Bonding suggested that the reason for unsuccessful tympanomastoidectomy in children depended on the mastoid cell system [7]. However, Siedentop, Palva, and Gimenez did not find such a relationship in the studies they carried out with 63, 61, and 52 chronic otitis media patients, respectively [8–10]. In the study of Onur et al. carried out with 255 patients, they observed that the graft success obtained in ears with diploic mastoiditis was more favorable compared to the pneumatic ones and they concluded that there was no relationship between the mastoid ventilation amount and the myringoplasty success [11]. The authors used Schüller X-Ray as the imaging method for measurement of the mastoid volume. In our study, mastoid volumes were evaluated as three-dimensional through calculating the mastoid volumes using high resolution computed tomography and Autocad.

As the Schüller X-Ray provides a two-dimensional imaging, the technique used in our study may provide more precise results. Moreover previous studies authors [2, 6, 11]. investigated effect of mastoid ventilation on tympanoplasty success but they performed mastoidectomy in their studies but it is known that mastoidectomy decreases mastoid volume and affects middle ear pressure. Based on this opinion some authors studied regeneration of mastoid air cells. Kanemaru et al. reported that regeneration of mastoid air cells (MACs) can effectively eliminate intractable COM [12–14]. In another study, Kanemaru et al. investigated the ability of regenerated MACs to restore gas exchange function and contribute to the improvement of eustachian tube function and indicated that tissue-engineered regeneration of MACs improves eustachian tube function and gas exchange in the middle ear [15]. In our study all the patients had undergone only antrostomy without mastoidectomy and relationship between preoperative mastoid volume and tympanoplasty success is evaluated.

The results of studies about mastoid ventilation are controversial. Holmquist and Bonding carried out studies indicating that mastoid ventilation affected the surgical results [7, 16]; however, there are also researchers who did not detect this relationship [8–11]. Similar results were obtained also in our study. Although we assessed better results in well-ventilated group there was no statistically significant difference between the well-ventilated group and the poorly ventilated group in terms of graft success. Furthermore, no statistically significant differences were determined between the mastoid cell ventilation and the postoperative airway gains.

5. Conclusion

In conclusion, no statistically significant relationship could be found between the preoperative mastoid cell ventilation and the postoperative graft success in patients who had undergone only antrostomy together with tympanoplasty as chronic otitis surgery. In addition, no statistically significant difference could be determined between the mastoid ventilation and the postoperative hearing gains.

Disclosure

The work was done in Ankara Research and Training Hospital, Ministry of Health tertiary reference hospital.

Conflict of Interests

The authors declare that there is no conflict of interests regarding the publication of this paper.

References

[1] I. Bayramoglu, F. N. Ardic, and C. O. Kara, "Importance of mastoid pneumatization on secretory otitis media," *International Journal of Pediatric Otorhinolaryngology*, vol. 40, pp. 60–65, 1997.

[2] J. Sade and C. Fuchs, "A comparison of mastoid pneumatization in adults and children with cholesteatoma," *European Archives of Oto-Rhino-Laryngology*, vol. 251, no. 4, pp. 191–195, 1994.

[3] A. Tumarkin, "On the nature and vicissitudes of the accessory air spaces of the middle ear," *The Journal of Laryngology and Otology*, vol. 71, no. 2, pp. 65–99, 1957.

[4] J. Holmquist, "Aeration in chronic otitis media," *Clinical Otolaryngology and Allied Sciences*, vol. 3, no. 3, pp. 279–284, 1978.

[5] K. Frisberg, S. Ingelstedt, and U. Ortegren, "On middle ear pressure," *Acta Oto-Laryngologica: Supplementum*, vol. 182, pp. 43–56, 1963.

[6] J. Holmquist and B. Bergstroem, "Eustachian tube function and size of the mastoid air-cell system in middle ear surgery," *Scandinavian Audiology*, vol. 6, no. 2, pp. 87–89, 1977.

[7] P. Bonding, "Tympanoplasty in children," *Acta Oto-Laryngologica*, vol. 106, no. 449, pp. 199–201, 1988.

[8] F. Gimenez, J. Marco-Algarra, R. Carbonell, A. Morant, and S. Cano, "Prognostic factors in tympanoplasty: a statistical evaluation," *Revue de Laryngologie Otologie Rhinologie*, vol. 114, no. 5, pp. 335–337, 1993.

[9] T. Palva and H. Virtanen, "Ear surgery and mastoid air cell system," *Archives of Otolaryngology*, vol. 107, no. 2, pp. 71–73, 1981.

[10] K. H. Siedentop, L. R. Hamilton, and S. B. Osenar, "Predictability of tympanoplasty results. Preoperative eustachian tube function and size of mastoid air cell system," *Archives of Otolaryngology*, vol. 95, no. 2, pp. 146–150, 1972.

[11] Ç. Onur, Y. Şinasi, G. Üzeyir, K. Turgut, S. Nihat, and Ç. Tufan, "Miringoplastiler: 255 Olgunun Sonuçlari," *Kulak Burun Boğaz ve Baş Boyun Cerrahisi Dergisi*, vol. 5, no. 3, pp. 171–175, 1997.

[12] S.-I. Kanemaru, T. Nakamura, K. Omori, A. Magrufov, M. Yamashita, and J. Ito, "Regeneration of mastoid air cells in clinical applications by in situ tissue engineering," *Laryngoscope*, vol. 115, no. 2, pp. 253–258, 2005.

[13] S.-I. Kanemaru, T. Nakamura, K. Omori et al., "Regeneration of mastoid air cells: clinical applications," *Acta Oto-Laryngologica, Supplement*, no. 551, pp. 80–84, 2004.

[14] A. Magrufov, S.-I. Kanemaru, T. Nakamura et al., "Tissue engineering for the regeneration of the mastoid air cells: a preliminary in vitro study," *Acta Oto-Laryngologica*, vol. 124, no. 551, pp. 75–79, 2004.

[15] S.-I. Kanemaru, H. Umeda, M. Yamashita et al., "Improvement of eustachian tube function by tissue-engineered regeneration of mastoid air cells," *The Laryngoscope*, vol. 123, no. 2, pp. 472–476, 2013.

[16] J. Holmquist, "Size of the mastoid air cell system in relation to healing after myringoplasty and to eustachian tube function," *Acta Oto-Laryngologica*, vol. 69, no. 1, pp. 89–93, 1970.

5

Evaluation of the Nasal Surgical Questionnaire for Monitoring Results of Septoplasty

Rolf Haye,[1] **Magnus Tarangen,**[2] **Olga Shiryaeva,**[2] **and Liv Kari Døsen**[1]

[1]*The Department of Oto-Rhino-Laryngology, Lovisenberg Diakonale Hospital, Norway*
[2]*The Department of Quality, Lovisenberg Diakonale Hospital, Norway*

Correspondence should be addressed to Rolf Haye; rolf.haye@medisin.uio.no

Academic Editor: David W. Eisele

Monitoring the results of surgery is important. The otorhinolaryngology department of our hospital currently uses preoperative and postoperative versions of the Nasal Surgical Questionnaire (NSQ) for continuous evaluation of nasal septoplasty. In this study, 55 patients undergoing septoplasty answered the preoperative version twice to assess the NSQ's test-retest precision, and 75 patients answered the preoperative questionnaire before and the postoperative one 6 months after surgery to evaluate the NSQ's ability to detect change in symptoms following surgery. Both the pre- and postoperative versions of the NSQ use separate visual analogue scales (VAS) to assess nasal obstruction during the day, at night, and during exercise. Other nasal symptoms are graded as secondary outcomes using 4-point Likert scales. The mean VAS scores for the two preoperative obstruction ratings were not significantly different. The scores were significantly higher than in a normal population. There were also significant differences between preoperative and postoperative ratings. The mean pre- and postoperative scores at night for those who reported complete improvement were 66.1 and 8.4, substantial improvement 74.5 and 24.2, and no improvement 83.3 and 76.4. The NSQ reliably assesses nasal symptoms in patients and may be useful for both short and long term prospective studies of septoplasty.

1. Introduction

The results of septoplasty are reported in many different studies, with improvement in obstruction varying from 47% to 98% [1–4]. It is, however, difficult to compare studies as so many different instruments are used to detect changes in obstruction after surgery. Few investigations are concerned with continuous monitoring of the results of nasal septoplasty. Otolaryngology departments in every hospital in Sweden report their nasal septal surgeries to a central register, which performs a six-month follow-up of the patients. The results are open to public survey [5]. As the success of surgery diminishes over time [1], the central register has increased the follow-up time to 1 year. The ear-nose-throat department of our hospital has initiated a 6-month quality control assessment using mailed questionnaires and plans to follow this up with another assessment at 4 years after surgery. Given this long follow-up period, it will be necessary to use a scoring system that does not rely on one's memory of the preoperative symptoms.

Ideally, all patients undergoing septoplasty would be recalled for a postoperative consultation, but this is neither feasible financially nor feasible in terms of human resources. The best alternative may be to implement a quality assurance program that continuously and prospectively monitors septoplasty outcomes. This can be easily done by using preoperative questionnaires and mailed postoperative questionnaires. Our intention is to recall only patients whose responses indicate no improvement or worsening of symptoms. The results will be presented on the hospital's website and individual patient results will be provided to the operating surgeon so he/she can correlate them with the surgery performed.

There are many questionnaires available; some of them only contain items related to nasal symptoms whereas others also include general quality of life items. We want to focus on the surgical results per se and would therefore prefer a questionnaire that specifically assesses nasal symptoms. The Nasal Obstruction Symptom Evaluation (NOSE) questionnaire [3] has been validated and used in many countries, but one item is difficult to translate into the Norwegian language. Questionnaires using a single visual analogue scale (VAS) for obstruction have been used in several studies [6]. We believe that use of separate and continuous scales for obstruction in different situations (day, night, and during exercise) will yield clinically relevant information about the patients' symptoms and how they change in response to surgery. Other nasal symptoms and the use of nasal medication should also be taken into account in surveying the results. We constructed the preoperative version of the Nasal Surgical Questionnaire (NSQ), which has separate VAS for obstruction during the day, at night, and during exercise, and used Likert scales for other nasal symptoms and for the use of nasal medication [7]. The preoperative questionnaire was favourably assessed in normal volunteers but has not yet been evaluated in a patient population. For the purpose of this study, a postoperative version of the NSQ (NSQ after operation) (see the questionnaire) has also been developed. It is the purpose of this study to assess both versions of the NSQ in septoplasty patients in order to evaluate the precision of the instrument and its ability to detect change in pre- and postoperative symptoms.

2. Materials and Methods

The study was conducted at Lovisenberg Diakonale Hospital in Oslo, Norway, and was approved by the ethical committee of the hospital. Included in the study are patients 16 years of age or older undergoing septoplasty with or without surgery to the inferior concha. The exclusion criteria were inadequate command of the Norwegian language, any other concomitant nasal or sinus surgery, and any other nasal disease except nasal allergy.

The pre- and postoperative versions of the NSQ have separate VAS for obstruction during day, night, and exercise. The scales are 10 cm long with markings of *0 = completely open* and *10 = completely obstructed* at either end. The patients are asked to mark their sense of obstruction on this scale. Scores are the distance between the mark and the left end of the line (measured in mm) and can range from 0 to 100. The VAS scores are measured and recorded manually, whereas answers to the rest of the questions, which are marked in boxes, are recorded automatically by scanning. There are 4-point (1 = no, 2 = mild, 3 = moderate, and 4 = severe) Likert scales for five other nasal symptoms (crusting, bleeding, sneezing, secretion, and nasal pain) and for nasal medication (vasoactive drugs, topical steroids, and antihistamines). In addition, the instrument includes items about smoking habits and allergy. The postoperative NSQ is supplemented with the following 5-point retrospective rating of perceived improvement: Is your nasal breathing completely, substantially, mildly, or not improved, or has it deteriorated? Patients are asked to answer the questionnaire based on a normal day without nasal infection. It was intended to be self-explanatory and to a large extent it was. However, in some cases, we had to instruct the patients in how to complete the questionnaire and in a few others we had to call up the patients to clarify

ambiguous responses. As a result of this, we began checking each questionnaire preoperatively.

To ensure the quality of the manual VAS scoring, the markings of the scales of 50 patients were rescored by a second person. The mean difference in scores between the first and the second measurements was 0.9 (0–5) on a scale from 0 to 100. In only two cases was the difference in scores more than 2 mm. Ten percent of the patients recorded the scores on the scale with numbers with or without a mark. For these, we recorded the number and not the marking.

2.1. Test-Retest Precision. During 2014, the preoperative version of the NSQ was administered twice to patients who were scheduled for septoplasty with or without surgery to the inferior concha. They were administered at least four weeks apart to ensure that patients would not recollect the precise location of their responses to the first questionnaire. At the time of the second preoperative questionnaire, the patients were also asked if they regarded the intensity of their nasal symptoms as stronger, weaker, or equal to the first questionnaire. Only those who perceived their symptoms to be equal on both occasions were included in the test-retest analysis. Patients who had received treatment for nasal symptoms in the interim period were also excluded. Both positive and negative differences between the two questionnaires were given a positive numerical value. To reduce the influence of nasal allergy on the results, we collected most of the questionnaires for this study from October 2013 to April 2014 and from October to December 2014.

2.2. Results of Surgery. All patients who had adequately answered the questionnaire preoperatively were presented with the postoperative questionnaire by mail six to eight months after surgery. Only patients who had their septoplasty performed endonasally were included in the analysis. Included patients were operated on from February to mid-August 2014, and the postoperative questionnaires were collected in the pollen-free time, October 2014 to February 2015, 6–8 months after surgery. Patients in our department are never operated on during their pollen allergy season.

2.3. Statistical Analysis. Continuous data are presented as means and standard deviation (SD) and categorical data as frequencies and percentages. Group comparisons of VAS scores were performed using the Mann-Whitney U test. The Wilcoxon Signed Ranks Test was applied to evaluate the difference in responses between the first and second presentation of the preoperative version of the questionnaire and between the pre- and postoperative versions on the VAS items for nasal obstruction during the day, at night, and during exercise. For the other nasal symptoms measured on a four-point scale, marginal homogeneity tests were performed to estimate the difference in responses between the first and second questionnaire. Cronbach's alpha was used to assess the internal consistency of the three VAS items (at day, at night, and during exercise). Data were analyzed with SPSS software (version 22.0 for Windows, IBM Corp., Armonk, NY). All tests were two-sided, and p values < 0.05 were considered statistically significant.

TABLE 1: Preoperative test-retest VAS scores.

		Questionnaire 1			Questionnaire 2	
	N	VAS (mean)	[SD]	N	VAS (mean)	[SD]
Day	55	(61.8)	[20.4]	55	(63.4)	[18.8]
Night	55	(73.7)	[18.3]	54	(74.3)	[16.8]
Exercise	52	(66.2)	[24.4]	53	(65.7)	[24.2]

3. Results

3.1. Test-Retest Precision. Fifty-five patients, 37 male and 18 female with a mean age of 40.4 (SD 12.9) years, completed the preoperative version of the NSQ twice prior to surgery. There were 8 smokers and 18 with self-reported nasal allergy. The results from both preoperative questionnaires are presented in Table 1. The sample sizes vary because a few patients left one or more questions unanswered. The three different VAS items were highly correlated, both in the first (Cronbach's alpha = 0.824) and in the second (Cronbach's alpha = 0.800) questionnaire. For both questionnaires, the mean score for obstruction at night was significantly higher than during the day ($p < 0.001$) and during exercise ($p < 0.05$). The mean difference in scores between the first and second questionnaire was 7.7 (SD 5.7) for day, 6.9 (SD 5.8) for night, and 8.5 (SD 7.7) for exercise. The Wilcoxon Signed Ranks Tests showed that there was no significant difference between these scores. The Mann-Whitney U test showed that the scores for males versus females, smokers versus nonsmokers, and allergic patients versus nonallergic patients were not significantly different. The Likert scale scores for the other nasal symptoms and nasal medication were not significantly different between the first and second questionnaire.

3.2. Results of Surgery. Of the 102 patients who had responded to the preoperative questionnaire and were operated for nasal septal deviation with or without surgery to the inferior concha, 75 (73.5%) answered the postoperative questionnaire and were included in the comparison of pre- and postoperative scores. These 75 patients included 48 males and 27 females and had a mean age of 41.6 (SD 13.8) years. There were 14 (19%) smokers and 23 (33.8%) with self-reported allergy.

The mean preoperative and postoperative VAS obstruction scores indicated significant improvement following surgery: 62.8 versus 33.8 for day, 75.6 versus 37.9 for night, and 65.0 versus 37.9 for exercise, respectively, all $p < 0.05$. The three VAS scales were correlated with each other both preoperatively (Cronbach alpha = 0.79) and postoperatively (0.96). We compared the VAS scores with the 5-point retrospective rating of improvement (complete, substantial, mild, or no improvement or worsening of symptoms). The results for preoperative, postoperative, and improvement scores are presented in Table 2. The mean differences in VAS scores before and after the operation compare favourably to the retrospective rating of improvement. There was no statistically significant difference in VAS scores for day, night, or exercise between males and females, smokers and nonsmokers, and

allergic and nonallergic patients, in either the preoperative or postoperative questionnaire.

The pre- and postoperative differences in the 4-point Likert scale scores for the other nasal symptoms are shown in Table 3. There was a statistically significant change in scores for bleeding, crusting, sneezing, and nasal pain ($p < 0.05$). Most of the differences indicate symptom improvement but a few patients had worse symptoms postoperatively.

4. Discussion

The results of these two analyses provide evidence of the NSQ's precision in assessing nasal symptoms and its ability to detect change in symptoms following nasal surgery. These findings suggest that it may be a useful tool for efficiently monitoring surgery results and identifying patients who need further follow-up.

The VAS obstruction scores obtained in this study using the NSQ are comparable to those reported in other studies. Rhee and colleagues [6] have established normative VAS obstruction scores in normal people and patients before and after nasal surgery by critically reviewing prior studies using VAS to assess nasal obstruction. One of the studies [8] used four-point scales for nasal obstruction, which were converted to VAS scores of 0 to 10. To facilitate comparison with our results, we have taken the liberty of further converting the normative VAS scores to a scale from 0 to 100. All of the reviewed studies used only a single VAS item to assess nasal obstruction and did not distinguish between symptoms experienced during the day, at night, or during exercise. The mean preoperative VAS score in these articles [4, 8–15] was 67, which is comparable to the VAS scores we obtained using the NSQ. In our studies using three items to assess obstruction in different situations, the preoperative VAS score for obstruction at night was significantly higher than the scores for day and exercise. In the present test-retest study, these scores from the first questionnaire were 73.7 for night, 61.8 for day, and 66.2 for exercise. Given the relatively high scores, symptoms during the night may be the most important for patients and should be included in future studies. Our study has shown that the differences in nasal obstruction scores between first and second administration of the NSQ were very small, only 7.7 for day scores, 6.9 for night, and 8.5 for exercise. We have not found comparable data in the other articles [4, 8–15].

Our evaluation of the results of surgery showed that the patient's short term (6 months) retrospective perception of their improvement in breathing was comparable to the prospective VAS scores. Not surprisingly, patients who reported their breathing as completely improved had mean VAS score close to 0 postoperatively. The same is apparent in those who rated their breathing as substantially improved; their mean VAS scores were 20.9 (day) and 24.2 (night), regardless of the relative improvement in scores. Patients reporting mild improvement scored 65.5 (day) and 76.7 (night) preoperatively and improved by 21.2 and 27.2, respectively. These results lend credence to the values for both the 6-month retrospective improvement rating and the prospective change in VAS scoring. For short term results being presented

TABLE 2: Results of surgery. Pre- to postoperative change in day and night VAS scores for each level of perceived improvement in nasal breathing.

Perceived improvement	N	Day VAS scores			N	Night VAS scores		
		Preop Mean (SD)	Postop Mean (SD)	Difference Mean (SD)		Preop Mean (SD)	Postop Mean (SD)	Difference Mean (SD)
Complete	8	57.8 (19.3)	5.9 (5.1)	51.9 (21.0)	8	66.1 (21.6)	8.4 (6.2)	57.8 (22.1)
Substantial	34	60.9 (19.7)	20.9 (16.5)	39.9 (24.4)	34	74.5 (19.4)	24.2 (15.9)	50.3 (23.3)
Mild	21	65.5 (17.4)	44.3 (15.8)	21.2 (16.2)	19	76.7 (15.0)	49.9 (18.6)	27.2 (17.1)
No	11	69.5 (22.3)	72.3 (19.8)	2.7 (15.2)	10	83.3 (16.7)	76.4 (25.9)	7.3 (13.6)
Worse	1	33.0 (—)	47.0 (—)	14.0 (—)	1	88.0 (—)	87.0 (—)	1.0 (—)
Total	75	62.8 (19.6)	33.8 (25.7)	29.0 (27.0)	72	75.6 (18.2)	37.9 (27.9)	38.4 (26.4)

TABLE 3: Differences between pre- and postoperative scores on the 4-point Likert scales for other nasal symptoms.

Symptoms	N	Deterioration		No change	Improvement		
		2 points N (%)	1 point N (%)	0 points N (%)	1 point N (%)	2 points N (%)	3 points N (%)
Crusting	72	1 (1.4)	10 (13.9)	36 (50.0)	16 (22.2)	6 (8.3)	3 (4.2)
Bleeding	74	2 (2.7)	7 (9.5)	38 (51.4)	19 (25.7)	6 (8.1)	2 (2.7)
Sneezing	69	1 (1.4)	7 (10.1)	32 (46.4)	20 (29.0)	9 (13.0)	0 (0.0)
Secretion	73	2 (2.7)	15 (20.5)	31 (42.5)	16 (21.9)	8 (11.0)	1 (1.4)
Nasal pain	72	1 (1.4)	6 (8.3)	41 (54.7)	20 (27.8)	3 (4.2)	1 (1.4)

Statistically significant changes for all symptoms ($p < 0.05$, marginal homogeneity tests) except for secretion.

to the public, it may be sufficient to use a 5-point retrospective scale. For our prospective long term studies, however, we believe that recollection of the state of their preoperative obstruction will be spurious. We found that the prospective VAS scoring reliably reflects the patients' assessment of their obstruction. At 3 to 5 years this prospective recording will be unaffected by patients' recollection.

Although there were differences between the VAS scores for obstruction during the day, at night, and during exercise, the scores were highly correlated. One or two of the scales may therefore be superfluous. As the highest scores are seen at night, one might choose this as the scale best representing the patients' situation. There are, however, patients who are more bothered with symptoms during the day or during exercise than at night. The patient reporting worse symptoms after surgery, for instance, had a negative change in the VAS score during the day and no change at night. Individual differences may not influence the overall group score but may be relevant to the surgeons. We will therefore continue with separate scales.

Rhee et al. [6] did not identify the minimal clinically significant difference in VAS score that would signify an improvement after therapy. However, we have found that the change in VAS scores after surgery in the patients reporting mild improvement was 21.2 during the day and 27.2 at night. Patients reporting no improvement had a mean difference in score of 2.7 during the day and 7.3 at night. In a prior study [7] using the NSQ in a normal population, we found that the mean change in scores between two administrations was 5.09 during the day and 6.22 at night. The present study showed that the score between the two preoperative administrations were 7.7 for day and 6.9 at night. Together, these data indicate

that the minimal significant change in VAS score is likely somewhere between 10 and 20 during the day and at night. We are not aware of other attempts to identify this, and further studies are needed to supplement these results.

Questionnaires, such as the NSQ, are often used for group comparisons, but differences across studies can make comparisons between them difficult. In prior studies [4, 8–15], patients typically served as their own control, but personal factors, such as gender, age, weight, smoking, and allergy, may still influence the results [16], particularly if study populations vary considerably in composition. The individual result of surgery may also depend on the influence of these other factors. Studies have also included different surgical procedures, such as rhinoplasty, septoplasty, turbinoplasty, polypectomy, and sinus surgery, used either alone or in combination, which may have influenced the results reported. Two studies [8, 14] only included patients with allergy, another [12] had patients rate their preoperative symptoms retrospectively, and a fourth [13] showed patients their preoperative ratings before asking them to rate their postoperative symptoms. In our study, we asked the patients to answer the questionnaire based on a normal day when they were free of nasal infection to eliminate spontaneous variations and the influence of nasal infection. However, it is not clear whether other studies used a similar approach. These differences need to be considered when comparing findings with the current study.

Smoking may reduce surgery results, as clinical studies have shown that smoking negatively influences nasal breathing [17–19]. This, however, was not apparent in our study, probably because the structural deformities were so prominent preoperatively and still present to various degrees postoperatively. To overcome the influence of smoking, one study excluded smokers [14]. Other studies have not examined the influence of smoking.

A large part of the population has allergy, which may influence the results of surgery [20]. Two studies addressed this problem by only including patients with allergy [8, 14], while other studies took no measures to circumvent the confounding influence of allergy [4, 9–13, 15]. For this study, we have taken care to reduce the influence of allergy by collecting the questionnaire outside of the pollen seasons. However, as we plan to run permanent quality control throughout the year, this problem may occur and we have therefore included questions about allergy status and the use of medication in the NSQ. This will be helpful in assessing the results, which may vary by time of year. To reduce the influence of allergy, it might be preferable to postpone the postoperative assessment from 6 to 12 months after the surgery so that influence of allergy season will be the same for both the pre- and postoperative assessments.

A study using only allergic patients compared the result of septoplasty with or without turbinoplasty [8]. There was no change in scores, regardless of whether the inferior concha had been operated upon, but the use of nasal steroid medication did substantially decrease after surgery. They did not evaluate the quantitative influence that the medication might have had on nasal obstruction. A patient who is able to stop taking medication may be satisfied, even though the obstruction is not completely relieved. The use of nasal medication was also reduced in our study.

Our surgeons would like to review not only the overall results of surgery but also the individual pre- and postoperative questionnaires for assessing their surgical praxis. The NSQ allows them to take into account not only the VAS scores but also the change in the intensity of the other nasal symptoms and the use of medication.

In a prior study [7], we evaluated the preoperative NSQ in a normal population. Many persons had no breathing problem and scored 0 on the VAS, whereas others had some nasal obstruction for which they did not seek medical attention. The mean VAS scores for obstruction in the normal population were 9.99 during day, 12.95 at night, and 11.67 during exercise. When we compare these to the preoperative scores in surgical patients, we find that the preoperative NSQ significantly differentiates between patients and normal persons. This is reconfirmed by the substantial change in scores after surgery.

5. Conclusion

We developed the pre- and postoperative NSQ to prospectively and continuously monitor the results of septoplasty. The difference in VAS scores for nasal obstruction between two preoperative administrations of the NSQ was minimal, indicating reliability and precision in scoring. The changes in VAS scores after surgery were comparable to the retrospective improvement ratings, indicating that the VAS scoring is representative of the results. There is also a substantial difference between preoperative scores in patients and those seen in a normal population, indicating that the NSQ has useful

discriminatory power. These findings indicate that the NSQ may be useful for short and long term quality control of nasal septal surgery.

Nasal Surgical Questionnaire after Operation (Answer When Free of a Cold/Nasal Infection)

Is Your Nasal Breathing

    ☐ Completely improved

    ☐ Substantially improved

    ☐ Mildly improved

    ☐ Unchanged

    ☐ Worse

Rate your sense of obstruction	Open	Put a mark on this scale (*0 = completely open. 10 = completely blocked.*)	Blocked
On a normal day	0	———————————	10
At night	0	———————————	10
During exercise	0	———————————	10

Rate These Nasal Symptoms

Crusting

    ☐ None

    ☐ Slight

    ☐ Moderate

    ☐ Severe

Bleeding

    ☐ None

    ☐ Slight

    ☐ Moderate

    ☐ Severe

Sneezing

    ☐ None

    ☐ Slight

    ☐ Moderate

    ☐ Severe

Secretion

    ☐ None

    ☐ Slight

    ☐ Moderate

    ☐ Severe

Nasal Pain

    ☐ None

□ Slight

□ Moderate

□ Severe

Rate Your Use of Nasal Medication

Nonprescriptional Nasal Spray/Drops (Naso/Nazaren/Otrivin/ Rhinox/Zymelin/Zycomb)

□ None

□ Slight

□ Moderate

□ Daily

Corticosteroid Nasal Spray/Drops (Avamys/Budesonid/Flutide nasal/Nasacort/Nasonex/Rhinocort)

□ None

□ Slight

□ Moderate

□ Daily

Antihistamines (Aerius/Alzyr/Cetrizin/Clarityn/Kestine/ Loratadin/Telfast/Zyrtec/Xyzal)

□ None

□ Slight

□ Moderate

□ Daily

Smoking

□ None

□ 1–10 daily

□ 11 or more daily

Do You Suffer from Nasal Allergy

□ Yes

□ No

□ Uncertain

If yes

do you have nasal allergy at present

□ Yes

□ No

do you use allergy medication at present

□ Yes

□ No

Conflict of Interests

The authors declare that there is no conflict of interests.

Authors' Contribution

Rolf Haye contributed to overall design and is the main author; Magnus Tarangen contributed to data collection; Olga Shiryaeva contributed to statistics and is part author; and Liv Kari Døsen contributed to design and is part author.

Acknowledgment

The authors thank Caryl Gay, Ph.D., for English language editing.

References

[1] C. Sundh and O. Sunnergren, "Long-term symptom relief after septoplasty," *European Archives of Oto-Rhino-Laryngology*, vol. 272, no. 10, pp. 2871–2875, 2015.

[2] P. Illum, "Septoplasty and compensatory inferior turbinate hypertrophy: long-term results after randomized turbino-plasty," *European Archives of Oto-Rhino-Laryngology*, vol. 254, supplement 1, pp. S89–S92, 1997.

[3] M. G. Stewart, T. L. Smith, E. M. Weaver et al., "Outcomes after nasal septoplasty: results from the Nasal Obstruction Septo-plasty Effectiveness (NOSE) Study," *Otolaryngology—Head and Neck Surgery*, vol. 130, no. 3, pp. 283–290, 2004.

[4] H.-Y. Li, Y. Lin, N.-H. Chen, L.-A. Lee, T.-J. Fang, and P.-C. Wang, "Improvement of quality of life after nasal surgery alone for patients with obstructive sleep apnea and nasal obstruction," *Archives of Otolaryngology: Head and Neck Surgery*, vol. 134, no. 4, pp. 429–433, 2008.

[5] M. Holmstrøm, "The use of objective measures in selecting patients for septal surgery," *Rhinology*, vol. 48, no. 4, pp. 387–393, 2010.

[6] J. S. Rhee, C. D. Sullivan, D. O. Frank, J. S. Kimbell, and G. J. M. Garcia, "A systematic review of patient-reported nasal obstruction scores: defining normative and symptomatic ranges in surgical patients," *JAMA Facial Plastic Surgery*, vol. 16, no. 3, pp. 219–225, 2014.

[7] R. Haye, E. Amlie, O. Shiryaeva, and L. K. Døsen, "Evaluation of a nasal surgical questionnaire designed for monitoring surgical outcomes and comparing different techniques," *The Journal of Laryngology & Otology*, vol. 129, no. 07, pp. 656–661, 2015.

[8] M. Lavinsky-Wolff, H. L. Camargo Jr., C. R. Barone et al., "Effect of turbinate surgery in rhinoseptoplasty on quality-of-life and acoustic rhinometry outcomes: a randomized clinical trial," *Laryngoscope*, vol. 123, no. 1, pp. 82–89, 2013.

[9] S. Yoo and S. P. Most, "Nasal airway preservation using the autospreader technique: analysis of outcomes using a disease-specific quality-of-life instrument," *Archives of Facial Plastic Surgery*, vol. 13, no. 4, pp. 231–233, 2011.

[10] K. Zhao, K. Blacker, Y. Luo, B. Bryant, and J. Jiang, "Perceiving nasal patency through mucosal cooling rather than air temperature or nasal resistance," *PLoS ONE*, vol. 6, no. 10, Article ID e24618, 2011.

[11] M. Reber, F. Rahm, and P. Monnier, "The role of acoustic rhinometry in the pre- and postoperative evaluation of surgery

for nasal obstruction," *Rhinology*, vol. 36, no. 4, pp. 184–187, 1998.

[12] R. Mahlon, M. R. Van Delden, P. R. Cook, and W. E. Davis, "Endoscopic partial inferior turbinoplasty," *Otolaryngology: Head and Neck Surgery*, vol. 121, no. 4, pp. 406–409, 1999.

[13] D. S. Utley, R. L. Goode, and I. Hakim, "Radiofrequency energy tissue ablation for the treatment of nasal obstruction secondary to turbinate hypertrophy," *Laryngoscope*, vol. 109, no. 5, pp. 683–686, 1999.

[14] C. J. Nease and G. A. Krempl, "Radiofrequency treatment of turbinate hypertrophy: a randomized, blinded, placebo-controlled clinical trial," *Otolaryngology—Head and Neck Surgery*, vol. 130, no. 3, pp. 291–299, 2004.

[15] S. P. Most, "Analysis of outcomes after functional rhinoplasty using a disease-specific quality-of-life instrument," *Archives of Facial Plastic Surgery*, vol. 8, no. 5, pp. 306–309, 2006.

[16] T. Kjærgaard, M. Cvancarova, and S. K. Steinsvåg, "Does nasal obstruction mean that the nose is obstructed?" *Laryngoscope*, vol. 118, no. 8, pp. 1476–1481, 2008.

[17] P. Dessi, R. Sambuc, G. Moulin, V. Ledoray, and M. Cannoni, "Effect of heavy smoking on nasal resistance," *Acta Oto-Laryngologica*, vol. 114, no. 2, pp. 305–310, 1994.

[18] T. Kjaergaard, M. Cvancarova, and S. K. Steinsvaag, "Smoker's nose: structural and functional characteristics," *Laryngoscope*, vol. 120, no. 7, pp. 1475–1480, 2010.

[19] P. Virkkula, M. Hytönen, A. Bachour et al., "Smoking and improvement after nasal surgery in snoring men," *American Journal of Rhinology*, vol. 21, no. 2, pp. 169–173, 2007.

[20] A. D. Karatzanis, G. Fragiadakis, J. Moshandrea, J. Zenk, H. Iro, and G. A. Velegrakis, "Septoplasty outcome in patients with and without allergic rhinitis," *Rhinology*, vol. 47, no. 4, pp. 444–449, 2009.

6

Effects of Sacrificing Tensor Tympani Muscle Tendon When Manubrium of Malleus Is Foreshortened in Type I Tympanoplasty

Sohil Vadiya

Pramukhswami Medical College and Shree Krishna Hospital, Karamsad, Gujarat 388325, India

Correspondence should be addressed to Sohil Vadiya; sohilv81@gmail.com

Academic Editor: Vittorio Rinaldi

The current study aims at observing effects of sacrificing the tensor tympani tendon when manubrium of malleus is foreshortened or retracted on graft uptake, hearing improvement, and occurrence of complications if any during type I tympanoplasty surgery for central perforations. 42 patients were included in group A where the tensor tendon was sectioned and 42 patients were included in group B where the tensor tympani tendon was retained and kept intact. Graft uptake rates are very good in both groups but hearing improvement was found significantly better in group A than group B. No unusual or undesired complications were seen in any of the cases. Sectioning of tensor tympani tendon is safe and effective procedure in cases where manubrium is foreshortened.

1. Introduction

It is not unusual to find medially retracted or foreshortened handle of malleus (manubrium) during tympanoplasty. Apart from posing difficulties in placement of graft during underlay technique, it can affect orientation during surgery as the manubrium is one of the important landmarks in middle ear. Sectioning of the tensor tympani tendon near the neck of malleus would lateralize the manubrium to a significant extent and add to mobility of malleus as well. Arviso and Todd Jr. [1] have studied adult crania without clinical otitis and concluded that foreshortened malleus is an anatomic variant, not a sign of pathology. The current study aims at evaluating results of type I tympanoplasty for central perforations where manubrium was found foreshortened preoperatively or during surgery and the tensor tympani tendon (TT) was cut during surgery and comparing these results with those cases where manubrium was foreshortened and TT was kept intact.

2. Material and Methods

A total of 84 cases were included in the study with inclusion criteria being a dry central perforation where the manubrium of malleus was found to be medially rotated and touching the medial wall of the middle ear. Cases with perforation size more than 4 mm (measured by placing graph paper on the perforation) are included. Cases where all the three ossicles were intact and mobile and where a type I tympanoplasty was performed were included. Cases with ossicular erosion or with cholesteatoma or with a marginal perforation were excluded. All subjects with mucosal chronic otitis media were clinically evaluated thoroughly including tuning fork tests and otoendoscopy done when ear is dry for more than 2 weeks. A pure tone audiogram was done for all the subjects. In some of them, a medially rotated malleus could be found during otoendoscopy (Figure 1) whereas, in many others, it was found during surgery. Odd numbered patients were included in group A where TT was cut during surgery (Figure 2). Even numbered patients were included in group B where TT was not cut. All cases were operated on under general anesthesia. Postauricular skin incision was used in all the cases in both groups. Vascular strip incision was used for canal wall skin and after middle ear contents were observed and after necessary disease removal, malleus was carefully made free of all attachments from remnant of tympanic membrane (TM). Ossicular mobility and intactness were also checked. If the subject met the inclusion criteria, decision of

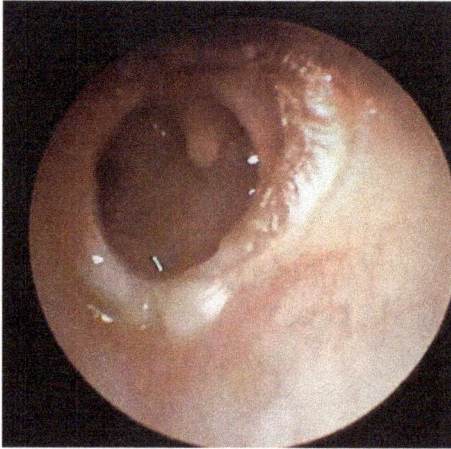

FIGURE 1: Foreshortened manubrium seen on otoendoscopy.

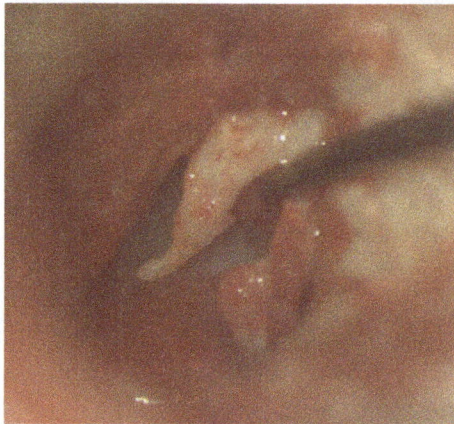

FIGURE 2: Tensor tympani tendon being cut during surgery.

TABLE 1: Hearing evaluation in both groups (ABG: air bone gap).

Average ABG	Group A	Group B	Significance
Preop ABG (db)	35.60	36.76	$P = 0.264$
Postop ABG (db)	14.92	19.88	$P < 0.00001$
Hearing gain (db)	20.68	16.88	$P < 0.00001$

3. Results

42 patients were included in group A where manubrium was found medialised and TT was cut near the neck of malleus and 42 patients belonged to group B where TT was not cut. All patients were between 20 and 40 years of age and there were 29 males and 13 females in group A and 27 males and 15 females in group B. There were 40 patients in group A where graft was successfully taken up and 2 cases where there was residual perforation at 8 weeks and they required revision surgery. In group B, graft uptake was complete in 39 patients and in one patient there was a tiny residual anterior perforation that healed with conservative management and two patients required revision surgery. So graft uptake rate is 95.24% for group A and 92.86% for group B. Medialisation was not seen in any patients in group A whereas 2 cases in group B developed graft medialisation where the neotympanic membrane was touching the promontory at 6 months postoperatively as evident on otoendoscopy. Blunting of anterior angle was not seen in any of the patients in both groups. The results of hearing thresholds are given in Table 1. Hearing thresholds at 500 Hz, 1000 Hz, and 2000 Hz were considered for hearing evaluation. The average preop ABG in group A was 35.60 db whereas in group B it was 36.76 db ($P = 0.264$). Average postop ABG in group A was 14.92 db and in group B was 19.88 db with statistically significant difference between the two groups ($P < 0.000001$) (Supplementary Material, available online at http://dx.doi.org/10.1155/2015/531296). Three cases in group A and 14 cases in group B had postoperative ABG more than 20 db. None of the patients in both groups had bone conduction threshold more than 15 db suggestive of sensorineural hearing loss. Average hearing gain in group A is 20.68 db whereas in group B it is 16.88 db. This shows clearly that hearing improvement in group A is significantly better than in group B.

Statistical analysis was performed with application of Student's t-test for the ABG values. No other complications were seen in any of the cases in both groups.

4. Discussion

Handle of malleus is longer than the long process of incus and this provides additional impedance matching function of middle ear and adds to improved conduction of sound through middle ear. When the handle is retracted severely, this should affect conduction of sound as well. Hol et al. [4] have used autologous interposition of incus to overcome severely retracted handle of malleus and stated that patients presenting with COM (chronic otitis media), a (central) perforation, a medially rotated malleus, and intact ossicular

sectioning of TT was taken if the patient is in group A and TT was kept intact in patients of group B. Temporalis fascia was used as the graft material and kept lateral to the handle of malleus and medial to the annulus [2, 3]. Anterior tucking was done in all the cases in both groups. It was made sure during surgery that the annulus at the anterior canal wall is reposited back in the original position in the sulcus. Plenty of gelfoam was kept in middle ear, around ossicles especially medial to manubrium and also in the external ear canal in all cases. Cases were followed up regularly for the next 6 months minimum and audiometry results were recorded at 6 months postoperatively. Otoendoscopy picture at 6 months was taken into consideration. The same Amplaid A177 dual channel audiometer with standard calibration was used in all the cases to avoid errors. Parameters compared include graft uptake, medialisation suggested by graft touching the medial wall of middle ear, lateralisation suggested by blunting of anterior angle, air bone gap (ABG) at 6 months, and occurrence of squamous pearls.

TABLE 2: Comparison of graft uptake rates of different authors.

Author	Graft material	Take-up (%)
Dabholkar et al. [7]	Temporalis fascia	84
Dornhoffer [8]	Perichondrium	85
Indorewala [9]	Fascia lata	95
Indorewala [9]	Temporalis fascia	66
Batni and Goyal [10]	Temporalis fascia	88
Present series	Temporalis fascia group A	95.24
Present series	Temporalis fascia group B	92.86

chain are a treatment challenge. Lateralizing the malleus handle may require disconnection of the ossicular chain and an autologous incus interposition to bring back the reconstructed tympanic membrane in its original position and improve the hearing. According to Todd [5], orientation of manubrium is inexplicably widely variable. Deng et al. [6] have concluded that the section of the tensor tympani muscle tendon in canal wall-down tympanoplasty with ossiculoplasty had no statistically significant influence on sound transmission and can be a safe maneuver in middle ear surgery.

It is well known, and we can see it in our cases; after cutting the tensor tympani tendon, the anterior tympanic membrane remnant becomes pleated, so we need to completely separate it from the manubrium. It will also make it easy to place the graft. The manubrium will support the graft from medial side, so the chances of medialisation should also be reduced. By cutting the tensor tympani tendon, the graft is more lateral thus increasing the middle ear volume. This will also help the ossicles to move more freely and it should improve hearing as adequate volume of middle ear is an important consideration for successful conduction of sound.

The current study aims to evaluate effect of sectioning the tensor tympani tendon in type I tympanoplasty surgery without mastoidectomy where the canal wall was preserved and the results are compared. Table 2 shows comparison of graft uptake rates of different authors.

5. Conclusion

Graft uptake rates are adequate if tensor tympani is cut or preserved, whereas hearing improvements are better in patients where tensor tendon was cut and the difference is statistically significant. No other complications were observed in the current study in both groups. Sectioning of tensor tympani tendon is safe and effective procedure during tympanoplasty if manubrium is severely retracted and it brings good improvement in hearing also.

Consent

Informed consent was obtained from all individual participants included in the study.

Disclosure

Animals were not involved in this study.

Conflict of Interests

The author of this paper declares that he has no conflict of interests.

References

[1] L. C. Arviso and N. W. Todd Jr., "The foreshortened malleus: anatomic variant, not pathologic sign," *Otolaryngology—Head and Neck Surgery*, vol. 143, no. 4, pp. 561–566, 2010.

[2] R. J. Yawn, M. L. Carlson, D. S. Haynes, and A. Rivas, "Lateral-to-malleus underlay tympanoplasty: surgical technique and outcomes," *Otology and Neurotology*, vol. 35, no. 10, pp. 1809–1812, 2014.

[3] O. Yigit, S. Alkan, E. Topuz, B. Uslu, O. Unsal, and B. Dadas, "Short-term evaluation of over-under myringoplasty technique," *European Archives of Oto-Rhino-Laryngology*, vol. 262, no. 5, pp. 400–403, 2005.

[4] M. K. S. Hol, D. Q. Nguyen, C. Schlegel-Wagner, G. Pabst, and T. E. Linder, "Tympanoplasty in chronic otitis media patients with an intact, but severely retracted malleus: a treatment challenge," *Otology and Neurotology*, vol. 31, no. 9, pp. 1412–1416, 2010.

[5] N. W. Todd, "Orientation of the manubrium mallei: inexplicably widely variable," *Laryngoscope*, vol. 115, no. 9, pp. 1548–1552, 2005.

[6] R. Deng, X. Ou, D. Tao, Y. Fang, W. Liuyang, and B. Chen, "Is it necessary to retain the tensor tympan tendon in tympanoplasty?" *Laryngoscope*, vol. 125, no. 10, pp. 2358–2361, 2015.

[7] J. P. Dabholkar, K. Vora, and A. Sikdar, "Comparative study of underlay tympanoplasty with temporalis fascia and tragal perichondrium," *Indian Journal of Otolaryngology and Head and Neck Surgery*, vol. 59, no. 2, pp. 116–119, 2007.

[8] J. L. Dornhoffer, "Hearing results with cartilage tympanoplasty," *Laryngoscope*, vol. 107, no. 8, pp. 1094–1099, 1997.

[9] S. Indorewala, "Dimensional stability of free fascia grafts: clinical application," *Laryngoscope*, vol. 115, no. 2, pp. 278–282, 2005.

[10] G. Batni and R. Goyal, "Hearing outcome after type I tympanoplasty: a retrospective study," *Indian Journal of Otolaryngology and Head & Neck Surgery*, vol. 67, no. 1, pp. 39–42, 2015.

7

Aerodigestive Foreign Bodies in Adult Ethiopian Patients: A Prospective Study at Tikur Anbessa Hospital, Ethiopia

Abebe Bekele

Department of Surgery, School of Medicine, Addis Ababa University, Ethiopia

Correspondence should be addressed to Abebe Bekele; abebesurg@yahoo.com

Academic Editor: Charles Monroe Myer

Introduction. Foreign bodies (FBs) in the aerodigestive tract are important causes of morbidity and mortality and pose diagnostic and therapeutic challenges. The best method of removal of an esophageal and tracheobronchial FB is endoscopic guided extraction. *Objective.* To present our experience of the removal of aerodigestive FBs in adult Ethiopian patients using rigid endoscopes. *Methods.* A hospital-based prospective study, at Tikur Anbessa Referral and Teaching Hospital, from January 2011 to December 2012 (over two years). *Results.* A total of 32 patients (18 males and 14 females) with a mean age of 28.0 ± 12.74 years were treated for FB ingestion and aspiration at Tikur Anbessa Hospital. The FBs were impacted at the esophagus in 18 (56.2%) patients, at the pharynx in 7 (21.8%), and at the air way in 7 (21.8%) patients. Pieces of bones were the commonest objects found in the esophagus (17/18 of the cases) and the pharynx (4/7), while fractured tracheostomy tubes and needles were frequently seen in the air way (3/7 cases each). The foreign bodies were visible in plain radiographs of 26 (81.2%) patients. Successful extraction of FBs was achieved by using Mc gill forceps in 11 cases, rigid esophagoscopes in 9 patients, and bronchoscopes in 4 cases. Four cases required open surgery to remove the foreign bodies. Two complications (one pneumothorax and one esophageal perforation) occurred. All patients were discharged cured. *Discussion and Recommendations.* Aerodigestive FBs are not so rare in the hospital and timely diagnosis and removal of accidentally ingested and aspirated foreign body should be performed so as to avoid the potentially lethal complications associated. Rigid esophagoscopy requires general anesthesia and is associated with its own complications, but our experience and outcome of its use are encouraging.

1. Introduction

Foreign bodies (FBs) in the aerodigestive tract are important causes of morbidity and mortality in the two extremes of life and pose diagnostic and therapeutic challenges [1]. The ingestion and aspiration of FBs occur most commonly in children's population, especially in their first six years of life [1–3]. However, they are not so uncommon in adults [4, 5]. Most FB ingestions in adults are related to eating, leading to either bone or meat bolus impaction, while poor dentition, inadequate chewing, and eating while being sedated can precipitate this problem [5, 6]. Food impaction may also indicate obstructive esophageal preexisting lesions such as esophageal (mucosal) ring, peptic or malignant esophageal stricture, or eosinophilic esophagitis [6, 7].

Adults account for only about 20% of the reported cases of aspirations [8]. The leading causes are associated with altered mental status, trauma with a decreased level of consciousness, and impaired airway reflexes, when airway protective mechanisms function inadequately or facial traumas. However, there is a distinct group of patients such as young Muslim ladies who frequently use Hijab pins who are being recognized and are at risk [8–11].

The best method of removal of an esophageal and tracheobronchial FB is endoscopic guided extraction [3–5]. However, the endoscopic method of choice has remained controversial. Over the past decade, the flexible fiberoptic esophagoscope has gained great popularity [2–4]. However, the rigid endoscope is equally effective in the hands of an experienced surgeon. Both rigid and flexible bronchoscopes can attain above 90–95% success rate [8], but there is no consensus as to which is better.

The most commonly used method in our hospital for removal of such FBs has been rigid endoscopy, mainly due to the lack of flexible scopes [12]. Hence, the purpose of this study is to present our experience of the removal of aerodigestive FBs in adult Ethiopians using rigid endoscopes under general anesthesia, with a review of the pertinent literature.

2. Methods

This is a prospective analysis of patients admitted for removal of FBs from the aerodigestive tract at Tikur Anbessa Hospital from January 2011 to December 2012. The hospital is the main teaching and referral hospital of Addis Ababa University, where patients with aspirated and swallowed FBs are mainly referred to and treated. Data collected in the study included age and sex of the patient, time elapsed before presenting to the hospital, type and location of the foreign bodies, diagnostic and treatments techniques utilized, and short-term follow-up of the patients. The FBs locations were recorded as pharyngeal, upper esophageal (between 15 and 28 cm from the incision teeth), middle esophageal (between 28 cm and 34 cm), distal esophageal (34 cm to the lower esophageal sphincter), tracheal, and main bronchial regions.

All procedures were performed after patients were admitted to the hospital and under general anesthesia. When FBs were visible in the pharynx or in the accessible segment of the upper esophagus, extraction was performed by Mc gill forceps. Rigid bronchoscopes and rigid esophagoscopes were utilized when the objects were deeper in the aerodigestive tract or when Mc gill forceps extraction was impossible. Esophagotomy and bronchotomy were also required in some cases (see Table 4). After each procedure, patients were observed in the hospital to see whether complications occurred or not. One follow-up visit one month after discharge was arranged for all patients. Data was collected using a structured questionnaire and analysis done by using EP-INFO-2002 statistical software.

3. Results

A total of 32 patients (18 males and 14 females) were treated in the hospital during the study period and included in the study. Their mean age was 28.0 ± 12.74 (range, 15–70) years. Twenty-one (65.4%) of patients were aged between 15 and 30. Nineteen (59.3%) patients presented to the hospital within 24 hours and 4 (12.5%) patients came after five days. One particular patient came after 2 months (see Table 1). The FBs were impacted at the esophagus in 18 (56.2%) patients (9 in the upper esophagus and 9 in the middle esophagus), at the pharynx in 7 (21.8%) patients, and at the air way in 7 (21.8%) patients (3 left main bronchi, 3 right main bronchi, and 1 trachea) (see Tables 2 and 3).

All patients with pharyngeal and esophageal foreign bodies presented with dysphagia and odynophagia, while one patient complained of additional severe left-sided neck pain. All patients with airway foreign bodies had cough and shortness of breath, one patient presented with severe upper airway obstruction, and one presented with recurrent respiratory tract infection.

Pieces of bones were the commonest objects found in the esophagus (17/18 of the cases) and the pharynx (4/7), while

TABLE 1: Sociodemographic features of patients who underwent foreign body extraction at Tikur Anbessa Hospital, 2011-2012.

Characteristics	Frequency ($N = 32$)	Percentage (100%)
Age in years		
15–20	11	34.3
21–30	10	31.1
31–40	8	25
41–50	1	3.1
51–60	1	3.1
61–70	1	3.1
Sex		
Male	18	56.3
Female	14	43.7
Time between incident and presentation		
<6 hours	12	37.5
6–24 hours	7	21.8
24–48 hours	5	15.6
>48 hours	8	25

fractured tracheostomy tubes and needles were frequently seen in the air way (3/7 cases each). The tracheostomy tubes were permanently inserted for complicated thyroidectomy (1 patient), previous cut throat injury (1 patient), and unidentified indication (1 patient). Since all were not performed on in the study hospital, details of the patient were not available. Other impacted foreign bodies included Hijab pins, leech, and metal pieces in 1 (3.1%) patient each. Plain CXR was performed in all patients and foreign bodies were visible in 26 (81.2%). The six (18.8%) nonvisualized objects included 2/21 of the bone fragments, 2/2 of the wooden pieces, 1/3 of the broken plastic tracheostomy tubes, and 1/1 of the leech.

In all the 7 patients with the foreign body stuck in the pharynx and 4/9 of the proximal esophageal foreign bodies, the objects were successfully removed with the help of Mc gill forceps and laryngoscopes. These include 8/21 of the bone pieces, 1/2 of the pieces of wood, and 1/1 of leech and piece of metal (see Tables 2 and 3). Rigid endoscopy was used in 14 patients with esophageal foreign bodies and successful foreign body removal was accomplished in 9 patients (4/9 upper esophagus and 5/9 midesophagus). Four were disimpacted and were found difficult to grasp and hence were pushed to the stomach (all midesophageal).

One patient with a proximal esophageal FB required esophagotomy and extraction of the object. This was a 33-year-old male who swallowed a bone fragment 8 days before presentation complaining of dysphagia, severe neck pain, and neck swelling. His neck X-ray revealed a big bony lesion in the cervical esophagus and endoscopy showed a sharp speculated big piece of bone stuck at the proximal esophagus, perforating it at 3 and 9 o'clock. Therefore, left lateral neck incision was done and there was collected pus which was drained, the foreign body extracted with difficulty and the esophageal lacerations were debrided and repaired over an NG tube.

TABLE 2: Patters and location of foreign bodies extracted from patients who underwent endoscopic foreign body extraction in Addis Ababa, 2011-2012.

Foreign bodies extracted	Trachea	Right main bronchus	Left main bronchus	Pharynx	Upper esophagus	Middle esophagus	Frequency ($N = 32$)	Percentage %
Bone	—	—	—	4	8	9	21	65.6
Hijab pins	—	1	—	—	—	—	1	3.1
Leech	—	—	—	1	—	—	1	3.1
Metal pieces	—	—	—	1	—	—	1	3.1
Needle	—	—	3	—	—	—	3	9.4
Tracheostomy tube	1	2	—	—	—	—	3	9.4
Piece of wood	—	—	—	1	1	—	2	6.2
Total	1	3	3	7	9	9	32	

TABLE 3: Types of foreign bodies and techniques of extraction in Addis Ababa, 2011-2012.

Foreign body	Esophagoscopy	Esophagotomy	Mc gill forceps	Dislodged and pushed	Tracheotomy	Bronchotomy	Bronchoscopy	Total
Bone	8	1	8	4				21
Hijab pins							1	1
Leech			1					1
Metal pieces			1					1
Needle						1	2	3
Tracheostomy tube					1	1	1	3
Piece of wood	1		1					2
Total	9	1	11	4	1	2	4	32

The neck incision was drained and a feeding gastrostomy was placed. The incision drained for about two weeks and the patient showed gradual but complete recovery within three weeks and was discharged cured. Follow-up after 3 and 6 months revealed a completely healthy patient with no complications (see Tables 2 and 3).

Two-thirds of main bronchial bodies in each side were successfully removed with a rigid bronchoscope, while thoracotomy and bronchotomy were required in two patients (one long needle on the left and one fractured tracheostomy tube on the right). There was one tracheal fractured piece of a tracheostomy tube in the trachea that required emergency tracheotomy.

There were two complications seen. One patient developed pneumothorax after the extraction of a sharp Hijab pin from the left main bronchus which required chest tube drainage for three days. One esophagoscopy to remove a midesophageal bone fragment that was stuck for two months was successful but was complicated by esophageal perforation. This was successfully treated with prolonged right-sided chest drainage and a gastrostomy tube feeding. None of the patients died. All patients were followed up for one month after discharge and there were no short-term complications seen.

4. Discussion

Endoscopy has been the mainstay of management of aerodigestive foreign bodies [3, 4, 10–17]. Both rigid and fiberoptic esophagoscopes reportedly have similar success and morbidity rates [14]. The literature recommends flexible endoscopy (esophagoscopy and bronchoscopy) as cost effective because it is performed on an outpatient basis without general anesthesia, but, when sharp, penetrating, or difficult foreign bodies are present, rigid esophagoscopy is required [3, 4]. However, endoscopy does pose its own risks of complications, including failure of the procedure, bleeding, bronchospasm, accidental extubation, postprocedure stridor, hypoxia, esophageal perforation, and mediastinitis [10, 11].

Rigid endoscopy has a larger lumen and allows removal of most objects under direct vision [13]. The endotracheal intubation also provides an adequate airway and minimizes the incidence of aspiration during the procedure. Weisberg and Refaely and Al-Qudah et al. have also recommended the use of the rigid endoscope as the instrument of choice for extracting foreign bodies from the esophagus [14, 15]. Our method of endoscopic extraction has been the rigid scope, primarily because this has been the traditional approach in the hospital and the availability of flexible scopes was not regular. However, as reported by other studies done in the country [4], timely diagnosis and removal of accidentally ingested foreign body by flexible endoscopes can be practiced in Ethiopia.

Plain radiography on two planes has been recommended as an initial screening method in patients suspected with foreign bodies [7, 8]; our diagnostic yield has been 81.2%. Other studies have reported a detection rate of 47–75% [5, 10]. The use of barium swallow is discouraged by some authors

TABLE 4: Site of impaction and the techniques of foreign body extraction utilized in Addis Ababa, 2011-2012.

Techniques of extraction	Trachea	Right main bronchus	Left main bronchus	Pharynx	Upper esophagus	Middle esophagus	Total
Bronchotomy	0	1	1	0	0	0	2
Bronchoscopy	0	2	2	0	0	0	4
Esophagoscopy	0	0	0	0	3	6	9
Esophagotomy	0	0	0	0	1	0	1
Mc gill forceps	0	0	0	7	4	0	11
Pushed down	0	0	0	0	1	3	4
Tracheotomy	1	0	0	0	0	0	1
Total	1	3	3	7	9	9	32

since it may impair subsequent endoscopic visualization and increase the patient's aspiration risk [6].

Upper airway FBs are not frequently occurring phenomena in adults. As reported by Ramos et al. of the 9781 bronchoscopies performed in one center, only 32 involved cases of bronchoaspiration of FBs [10]. One of the largest series published identified 65 adults with tracheobronchial FB aspiration over a period of 12 years [18]. In our series FBs in the respiratory tract only represented 21% of the cases. Risk factors in adults include older age, abuse of sedative medications, neurological disorders (vascular dementia, Parkinson's), mental retardation, trauma with loss of consciousness, dental manipulations and procedures, alcoholism, and medical procedures, such as those resulting from cleaning or manipulating tracheostomy cannulas [9–12]. However, in contrast to these reports, our patients were found to be significantly younger and the only identifiable risk factor was the presence of tracheostomy tubes. The other types of FBs aspirated were sharp pins (needles and Hijab pins). Aspiration of such objects may occur when the pins are held between the lips and the individual forcefully inhales or coughs.

Air way FBs are potentially life threatening conditions that need to be addressed as soon as they are diagnosed or suspected. In most published series, the FBs tended to localize in the right bronchial tree [10, 18]. This right-side predominance can be explained by the vertical nature of the right main bronchus, its larger diameter, the greater air flow through it, and the localization of the carina to the left of the midline of the trachea [10]. In our series, 42.8% of the FBs were situated on each main bronchus and 14.4% were in the trachea.

In our series, we could remove the FB by bronchoscopy in 3 (42.8%) of the cases and open surgical techniques (bronchotomy and tracheotomy) were required in 4 (57.2%). A high incidence of surgical treatment is also reported by other studies [10]. This fact could be explained by scarring and dense adhesion of the FB to the airway following recurrent infections, the special nature of some FBs that makes them difficult to grasp by forceps, and maybe our very low threshold for operative extraction when faced with difficult bronchoscopies. However, none of the patients were complicated with atelectasis or pneumonia.

A FB which failed to progress distally in the esophagus should be removed as soon as possible [1–5]. The rationale includes the following. Once an object is impacted in the esophagus the chance of spontaneous passage is small, edema from local trauma tends to grip the object more firmly making later manipulation increasingly difficult, and perforation of the esophagus is much more serious and dangerous than perforation of any other part of the gastrointestinal tract. Delay in presentation, diagnosis, or treatment will also result in complications [6–8]. This is supported by the fact that one of our patients who has swallowed a sharp piece of bone and presented after 5 days with esophageal perforation and cervical abscess collection. Some authors recommend that when cervical esophageal perforation is diagnosed after 48 hours, the treatment of preference is lateral neck incision, abscess drainage, foreign body extraction, limited attempt of esophageal repair, and prolonged drainage of the incision with nutritional support [16]. We have followed this protocol and our patient showed a complete recovery.

Fracture of tracheostomy tube with subsequent migration into the tracheobronchial tree is very uncommon and carries the potentially fatal risk of respiratory obstruction causes of FBs in the airway [17]. However, from our 7 patients with airway FBs, three had aspirated the fractured distal limb of a plastic tube. In one patient, the tube was lodged at the trachea and caused sudden potentially lethal airway obstruction. As these tubes can induce inflammation in the mucosal wall and cause fibrous adhesion, endoscopic extraction was not possible in 2 patients. Therefore, patients with tracheostomy must receive adequate information about this complication, in addition to their regular follow-up care.

In conclusion, aerodigestive FBs are not so rare in the hospital and timely diagnosis and removal of accidentally ingested and inhaled foreign body should be performed so as to avoid the potentially lethal complications associated. Rigid esophagoscopy requires general anesthesia and is associated with its own complications, but our experience and outcome of its use are encouraging.

Conflict of Interests

The author declares that there is no conflict of interests regarding the publication of this paper.

References

[1] P. Nandi and G. B. Ong, "Foreign body in the esophagus: review of 2394 cases," British Journal of Surgery, vol. 65, no. 1, pp. 5–9, 1978.

[2] J. M. Gilyoma and P. L. Chalya, "Endoscopic procedures for removal of foreign bodies of the aerodigestive tract: the Bugando Medical Centre experience," *BMC Ear, Nose and Throat Disorders*, vol. 11, no. 1, article 2, 2011.

[3] H. Ekim, "Management of esophageal foreign bodies: a report on 26 patients and literature review," *Eastern Journal of Medicine*, vol. 15, no. 1, pp. 21–25, 2010.

[4] A. Bane and A. Bekele, "Management of gastrointestinal foreign bodies using flexible endoscopy: an experience from Addis Ababa, Ethiopia," *East and Central African Journal of Surgery*, vol. 17, no. 3, 2012.

[5] J. Roura, A. Morello, J. Comas, F. Ferran, M. Colome, and J. Traserra, "Esophageal foreign bodies in adults," *Journal for Oto-Rhino-Laryngology and Its Related Specialties*, vol. 52, no. 1, pp. 51–56, 1990.

[6] T. George and R. Andrew, "Update on foreign bodies in the esophagus: diagnosis and management," *Current Gastroenterology Reports*, vol. 15, article 317, 2013.

[7] P. Ambe, S. A. Weber, M. Schauer, and W. T. Knoefel, "Swallowed foreign bodies in adults," *Deutsches Ärzteblatt International*, vol. 109, no. 50, pp. 869–875, 2012.

[8] N. Al-Sarraf, H. Jamal-Eddine, F. Khaja, and A. K. Ayed, "Headscarf pin tracheobronchial aspiration: a distinct clinical entity," *Interactive Cardiovascular and Thoracic Surgery*, vol. 9, no. 2, pp. 187–190, 2009.

[9] T.-H. Wu, Y.-L. Cheng, C. Tzao, H. Chang, C.-M. Hsieh, and S.-C. Lee, "Longstanding tracheobronchial foreign body in an adult," *Respiratory Care*, vol. 57, no. 5, pp. 808–810, 2012.

[10] M. B. Ramos, A. Fernández-Villar, J. E. Rivo et al., "Extraction of airway foreign bodies in adults: experience from 1987–2008," *Interactive Cardiovascular and Thoracic Surgery*, vol. 9, no. 3, pp. 402–405, 2009.

[11] M. Boyd, A. Chatterjee, C. Chiles, and R. Chin Jr., "Tracheobronchial foreign body aspiration in adults," *Southern Medical Journal*, vol. 102, no. 2, pp. 171–174, 2009.

[12] M. Derbew and E. Ahmed, "The pattern of pediatric surgical conditions in Tikur Anbessa Unversity Hospital, Addis Ababa, Ethiopia," *Ethiopian Medical Journal*, vol. 44, no. 4, pp. 331–338, 2006.

[13] K. Athanassiadi, M. Gerazounis, E. Metaxas, and N. Kalantzi, "Management of esophageal foreign bodies: a retrospective review of 400 cases," *European Journal of Cardio-Thoracic Surgery*, vol. 21, no. 4, pp. 653–656, 2002.

[14] D. Weissberg and Y. Refaely, "Foreign bodies in the esophagus," *Annals of Thoracic Surgery*, vol. 84, no. 6, pp. 1854–1857, 2007.

[15] A. Al-Qudah, S. Daradkeh, and M. Abu-Khalaf, "Esophageal foreign bodies," *European Journal of Cardio-Thoracic Surgery*, vol. 13, no. 5, pp. 494–499, 1998.

[16] J. Jiang, T. Yu, Y. F. Zhang, J. Y. Li, and L. Yang, "Treatment of cervical esophageal perforation caused by foreign bodies," *Diseases of the Esophagus*, vol. 25, no. 7, pp. 590–594, 2012.

[17] S. S. Qureshi, D. Chaukar, and A. Dcruz, "Fractured tracheostomy tube in the tracheo-bronchial tree," *Journal of the College of Physicians and Surgeons Pakistan*, vol. 16, no. 4, pp. 303–304, 2006.

[18] K. L. Swanson, U. B. Prakash, J. C. McDougall et al., "Airway foreign bodies in adults," *Journal of Bronchology*, vol. 10, no. 2, pp. 107–111, 2003.

8

Evaluation of Etiology and Treatment Methods for Epistaxis: A Review at a Tertiary Care Hospital in Central Nepal

Ramesh Parajuli

Department of Otorhinolaryngology, Chitwan Medical College Teaching Hospital, P.O. Box 42, Chitwan, Nepal

Correspondence should be addressed to Ramesh Parajuli; drrameshparajuli@gmail.com

Academic Editor: Michael D. Seidman

Introduction. Epistaxis is one of the most common emergencies in Otorhinolaryngology. It is usually managed with simple conservative measures but occasionally it is a life threatening condition. Identification of the cause is important, as it reflects the management plan being followed. *Aims and Objectives.* To analyze the etiology and treatment methods for patients with epistaxis. *Methods.* A retrospective study was done in a tertiary care hospital in central Nepal. The study period was from May 2014 to April 2015. *Results.* A total of 84 patients had epistaxis; 52 were males and 32 were females. The most common cause of epistaxis was idiopathic (38.09%) followed by hypertension (27.38%), trauma (15.47%), and coagulopathy (8.33%). Regarding treatment methods, most (52.38%) of our patients required anterior nasal packing. Chemical cautery was sufficient to stop bleeding in 14.28% of patients while electrocautery and posterior nasal packing were performed in 2.38% and 16.66% patients, respectively. Two (2.38%) patients required endoscopic sphenopalatine arterial ligation. *Conclusion.* Hypertension, trauma and coagulopathy were the most common etiological factors among the patients in whom etiology was found although in most of the patients etiology could not be found. Anterior nasal packing was the most common treatment method applied to these patients.

1. Introduction

Epistaxis is defined as the bleeding from inside the nose or nasal cavity. It is one of the most common emergencies in Otorhinolaryngology worldwide which often requires admission to the hospital [1]. Its incidence is difficult to assess but it is expected that approximately 60% of the population will be affected by epistaxis at some point in their lifetime, with 6% requiring medical attention [2]. Epistaxis can be classified as anterior and posterior epistaxis based on the site of origin [3]. Anterior epistaxis is more common than posterior epistaxis [4]. It usually arises either from kiesselbach's plexus, a rich vascular anastomotic area formed by end arteries, or from vein (retrocolumellar vein). As the bleeding site is accessible, anterior epistaxis which occurs more frequently in children and young adults is rarely serious. On the other hand posterior epistaxis arises from the area supplied by sphenopalatine artery (SPA) in the posterior part of nasal cavity, which is more frequent in elderly people. Usually there is profuse bleeding with difficulty in accessing the site of bleed so it poses challenge in the management.

Anterior epistaxis is usually controlled by local pressure or anterior nasal packing while posterior epistaxis often requires posterior nasal packing or arterial ligation.

Epistaxis can be due to both systemic and local factors. Local causes include inflammatory, infective, traumatic, anatomical (deviated nasal septum, septal spur), chemical, or climatic changes, neoplasm, and foreign body. Similarly, the systemic causes of epistaxis are hematological diseases causing coagulopathy, cardiovascular diseases such as hypertension and vascular heart disease, liver disease, renal disease, and anticoagulant drugs. However in majority (80–90%) of patients no identifiable cause is found and is labeled as "idiopathic" [5]. Nose blowing habit, excessive coughing in chronic obstructive pulmonary disease (COPD), straining in constipation and benign prostatic hyperplasia (BPH), and lifting heavy objects are aggravating factors for the epistaxis.

Management of patient with epistaxis at any age group begins with resuscitating the patient, establishing the site of bleed, stopping the bleeding, and treatment of the underlying cause. There is no definite protocol for the management of epistaxis, although various treatment methods are available for the management ranging from local pressure, topical vasoconstrictor, nasal packing, cauterization (chemical/electric), to embolisation or ligation of vessels [6].

The aim of this study is to analyze the patients with epistaxis in terms of etiological factors and treatment methods who required hospitalization.

2. Materials and Methods

A retrospective study was carried out among the admitted patients with epistaxis who were managed in the Department of Otorhinolaryngology at Chitwan Medical College Teaching Hospital from May 2014 to April 2015. These patients were received from emergency room (ER), from outpatient department (OPD), or as a referral from other departments. Patients of all ages were included.

All the patients underwent routine investigations such as complete blood count, haemoglobin level, platelet count, random blood sugar, serum electrolytes, urea, creatinine, urine routine examination, and blood grouping. Coagulation profile such as prothrombin time, activated plasma thromboplastin time, and bleeding and clotting time was also performed. Computed tomography (CT) was done in selected cases to rule to neoplasms of nose and paranasal sinuses; and the nasopharynx. Additional investigations were ordered based on history and clinical examination about the possible etiology and comorbidity. Blood sample was also sent for crossmatch when indicated. Beside this, other investigations such as chest X-ray, electrocardiogram (ECG), and serological tests had to be performed for the fitness of procedures requiring general anesthesia, that is, conventional posterior nasal packing and surgical methods to control epistaxis.

Intravenous line was established in all patients with wide bore cannula. Management of the patient began with investigations and treatment side by side. Initially the patients were evaluated with anterior rhinoscopy to identify the site of bleeding. Patients who were brought to ER with complaint of recurrent episodes of excessive bleeding, on whom there was no active bleeding on arrival to the hospital and anterior rhinoscopy did not reveal bleeder, underwent nasal endoscopic examination to search the site of bleeding which might have been located more posteriorly. Treatment of the patients with epistaxis included conservative or nonsurgical treatment and surgical or interventional treatment. Nonsurgical treatment methods included application of topical vasoconstrictors such as oxymetazoline and xylometazoline nasal drop, chemical and electric cauterization of the bleeder, and anterior and posterior nasal packing. Surgical treatment methods were the endoscopic electrocauterization of the bleeder and the endoscopic SPA ligation. All the patients were initially treated conservatively and surgical treatment was considered only when conservative method failed to control the epistaxis. If the bleeder was accessible on anterior rhinoscopy then the patients were treated either with chemical cauterization with silver nitrate with concentration of 75% or with bipolar electrocautery depending on the surgeon's preference. When the bleeder was found to be located more posteriorly on nasal endoscopic examination bipolar electrocautery was used to

TABLE 1: Etiology of epistaxis ($n = 84$).

Causes	Number of patients	Percentage
Idiopathic cause	32	38.09%
Hypertension	23	27.38%
Trauma	13	15.47%
Coagulopathy	7	8.33%
Tumor (benign/malignant)	5	5.95%
Infection	4	4.76%

seal the vessel. If there was diffuse bleeding or when the bleeder could not be located then the patients used to receive anterior nasal packing. Patients with bleeding disorders were packed with absorbable gelatin sponge (Abgel); the rest of the patients received conventional anterior nasal packing with ribbon gauze. Posterior nasal packing was considered in the case of rebleed in a patient who had anterior nasal pack in situ. Surgical methods were the last resort to control bleeding in patients who had recurrent bleed or whose bleeding could not be controlled with those noninterventional methods.

Medical records of those patients were collected and evaluated for the demographics, cause of epistaxis, anatomical location of bleeding site, and the treatment methods provided. Analysis of data was done using SPSS computer software version 16.

3. Results

During the study period 84 patients with epistaxis were admitted to this hospital with age ranging from 5 to 86 years. Out of these patients 52 were males and 32 were females. Among these patients 60 (71.42%) presented through ER, 18 (21.42%) presented in OPD, and 6 (7.14%) were received from other departments. According to the type of epistaxis based on site of origin 54 (64.28%) patients had anterior epistaxis and 30 (35.71%) patients had posterior type of epistaxis.

Regarding the etiology, exact cause of epistaxis could not be ascertained in 32 (38.09%) patients, that is, idiopathic. Next common cause was hypertension (23; 27.38%) followed by trauma (13; 15.47%) and coagulopathy (7; 8.33%) (Table 1).

Regarding treatment modalities, conservative/nonsurgical method was sufficient to control epistaxis in most (79; 94.04%) of our patients (Table 2). Among the conservative methods, observation alone without active intervention was carried out in 7 (8.33%) patients. However, 44 (52.38%) patients were treated with anterior nasal packing. Chemical cautery was performed in 12 (14.28%) patients and electrocautery in 2 (2.38%) patients and 14 (16.66%) patients underwent posterior nasal packing. Surgical measures to control epistaxis were carried out in 5 (5.95%) patients. Among these patients 2 (2.38%) underwent resection of tumor; another 2 patients (2.38%) required endoscopic cauterization of SPA while 1 (1.19%) patient required septoplasty to control the epistaxis. Blood transfusion was required in 5 (5.95%) of our patients. None of our patients died due to epistaxis during the study period.

TABLE 2: Treatment methods for patients with epistaxis ($n = 84$).

Types of treatment	Number of patients	Percentage
Nonsurgical/noninterventional treatment	79	94.04%
Observation with topical vasoconstrictor only	7	8.33%
Chemical cauterization	12	14.28%
Electrocauterization	2	2.38%
Anterior nasal packing	44	52.38%
Posterior nasal packing	14	16.66%
Surgical/interventional treatment	5	5.95%
Endoscopic SPA ligation	2	2.38%
Excision of bleeding mass	2	2.38%
Septoplasty	1	1.19%

Anterior nasal pack was kept in situ for 48 hours while posterior nasal pack was removed after 72 hours. Broad spectrum antibiotic was used in patients with nasal packing to prevent infectious complications. Similarly, these patients also received antihistaminic and analgesic while the nasal pack was in situ. Antibiotic was also prescribed to the patients who underwent cauterization (chemical or electric) and surgical treatments. Besides these the patients on posterior nasal pack received mild sedation with oral alprazolam to relieve anxiety and pain. All the patients underwent nasal endoscopic examination before their discharge from hospital. Patients were advised to avoid the habits of nose picking and nose blowing if present, to prevent recurrent epistaxis. Patients were discharged from the hospital on oral antibiotic, topical antiseptic cream, and nasal decongestants and were advised to follow up after 1 week.

4. Discussion

Patient presenting with epistaxis is frequently encountered in our daily practices. It is common in people of all ages. According to the site epistaxis may be divided into anterior and posterior. Anterior epistaxis occurs more frequently in children and young adults. It is rarely serious as the bleeding point is anteriorly located and is easily identified. Its origin is usually arterial (kiesselbach's plexus) or occasionally venous (retrocolumellar vein). Posterior epistaxis occurs predominantly in the elderly and the site of bleeding is difficult to access as the site of origin is located more posteriorly so it poses a great challenge to arrest bleeding. Age related and cardiovascular diseases related angiopathy changes are probably responsible for the prolonged duration of bleeding. In our study, the age range of the patients varied from 5 to 86 years. Epistaxis was found to be more common in children younger than 10 years (18; 21.42%) and elderly people above 60 years of age (24; 28.57%) which is similar to the results of Pallin et al. [5]. Males were affected more often than females with a ratio of 1.6. Similar findings have been noted in other studies [7, 8]. This may be because the males are more frequently involved in outdoor activities such as sports and interpersonal violence. The higher prevalence of epistaxis in younger children is probably due to their habit of

nose picking which causes injury to the kiesselbach's plexus in the anteroinferior part of the nasal septum, that results into anterior epistaxis. Similarly the elderly people commonly have comorbidities such as hypertension and diabetes mellitus which cause degenerative changes in blood vessels making them more fragile which bleed easily on abrupt pressure changes such as straining during micturition and defecation in BPH and constipation respectively; excessive coughing in COPD; and lifting heavy objects. Rhinosinusitis, nasal allergy, temperature changes, and dry heat produce hyperemic nasal mucosa which can bleed while blowing nose or picking nose or with trivial trauma leading to anterior epistaxis [9].

Patient presenting with epistaxis should be thoroughly examined and history should be properly taken to identify the site and cause of bleeding. Most of our patients (32; 38.09%) with epistaxis did not have an identifiable cause which is similar to the study by Christensen et al. [10]. Hypertension was the second most common cause of the epistaxis in our patients which is similar to study by Varshney and Saxena [11]. Nowadays it is said that hypertension is not the cause of epistaxis but it prolongs the bleeding once it starts because in patients with hypertension there is arterial muscle degeneration that leads to defective muscle layer lacking the power to contract resulting in persistence rather than initiation of bleeding. However, the causative factor that might be responsible for the rupture of vessel is still unknown [11]. Some of our hypertensive patients with epistaxis were found to have uncontrolled hypertension due to cessation of antihypertensive medications and inadequate drug therapy because of infrequent check-up; hence the need of regular blood pressure check-up and compliance to the antihypertensive medications should be emphasized. Patients with epistaxis are anxious which might lead to transient hypertension, as the blood pressure was found to be higher in most patients on arrival to hospital. Other causes of epistaxis in our study were trauma (13; 15.47%), coagulopathy (7; 8.33%), infection (4; 4.76%), and tumor (5; 5.95%). The severity of trauma varied from trivial injury such as digital trauma to nasal bone fracture resulting from road traffic accident, physical assault, and sports. Comorbidities found in some of our patients were cardiovascular diseases, diabetes mellitus, and liver and renal diseases. Similarly the aggravating factors found to be associated with epistaxis were COPD, BPH, and constipation.

A variety of treatment methods have been used to control epistaxis which range from nose pinching to ligation of vessels. Method of treatment for epistaxis depends on site, severity, and etiology of bleeding. Treatment modalities can be broadly divided into nonsurgical and surgical approaches. The nonsurgical/conservative modalities include digital nasal compression, topical vasoconstrictor, local cauterization (chemical or electric), and nasal packing (anterior or posterior). If the bleeding point is visible the bleeding site may be sealed either with chemical cautery using silver nitrate, chromic acid, or trichloroacetic acid or with electrocautery using bipolar diathermy. We routinely use silver nitrate for chemical cautery at our institution. Similarly, for electrocauterization bipolar diathermy was used as the monopolar diathermy was associated with risk of optic or oculomotor nerve damage when used in or close to the orbit [12, 13]. Electrocautery can be performed under local anaesthesia in OPD also especially for minor anterior bleed. But for posterior bleed it is better to use electrocautery under general anaesthesia while searching for bleeding point. Nowadays bipolar cautery device with integrated suction tip has also been available. With this single instrument clots can be removed with suctioning which will localize bleeder that can be cauterized easily. Ahmed and Woolford reported 89% success rate with endoscopic electrocautery in patients with epistaxis [14]. If bleeding is not controlled by digital compression and cauterization then anterior nasal packing is done. Anterior nasal packing can be done with nasal tampons such as Merocel and rapid rhino, ribbon gauze, bismuth iodoform paraffin paste impregnated pack (BIPP), or "(absorbable nasal packing materials)." In a study done by Corbridge et al., Merocel nasal packing was found to be effective in 85% of cases, with no difference between the success rates when compared with conventional ribbon gauze [15]. If the bleeding is profuse and not controlled by anterior nasal packing, posterior nasal packing is done. It can be done either by using conventional pack made from gauze piece or Foley's catheter or by using commercially available balloon such as triluminal nasal balloon catheter (Invotec) and Epistat nasal catheter. Conventional posterior nasal packing should be done under general anaesthesia because this procedure is very painful and patient may not tolerate the procedure. Anterior nasal packing is also done once the posterior nasal packing is done. Nonsurgical treatment modalities were effective in most of our patients (79; 94.04%). Among the nonsurgical treatment modalities anterior nasal packing was the most common method followed by chemical cauterization. However, the failure rates of nasal packing in 33 to 40% compared to 3% failure rate of surgical treatment methods have been reported in literature [16]. We used medicated ribbon gauze in most of the patients and nasal tampon "Merocel" in few patients for anterior nasal packing. In our patients with coagulopathy "Abgel" was used to control the bleeding as there was diffuse bleeding from nasal mucosa. Posterior nasal packing was required in 16.66% (14) of our patients after failed anterior nasal packing, which was done either with ribbon gauze or with Foley's catheter followed by anterior nasal packing as well.

Surgical/interventional methods are usually the last resort for refractory epistaxis which does not stop after other means of conservative treatment such as posterior nasal packing. The surgical treatment options include selective arterial embolisation or arterial ligation. Angiographic embolisation uses coils, gel foam, or polyvinyl alcohol to embolise the bleeding vessel. This technique is found to have a success rate as high as 87% [17]. However, arterial embolisation has risk of complications such as cerebrovascular accident, hemiplegia, ophthalmoplegia, facial nerve palsy, and soft tissue necrosis [18]. None of our patients underwent embolisation of vessel. Various surgical techniques exist for ligation of vessels, that is, anterior/posterior ethmoidal artery ligation, internal maxillary artery, or external carotid artery ligation. Ligation of ethmoidal artery can be performed via the external ethmoidectomy incision. Transantral ligation of internal maxillary artery via the Caldwell-Luc approach was a common method to control epistaxis in the past. It was found to be effective in 87% of cases, which is similar to angiographic embolisation [19]. But it is rarely performed nowadays as this procedure is associated with various complications such as sinusitis, facial pain/swelling, oroantral fistula, and paresthesia [20]. Ligation of the external carotid artery has been historically described which is a nonspecific method of decreasing blood flow to the nose which also has frequent treatment failures thought to be due to collateral circulation from opposite external carotid artery [21]. Generally the ligation of external carotid artery is considered a last resort in uncontrolled bleeding when other interventional methods fail. Nowadays the surgical treatment method which has gained popularity among the rhinologists is endoscopic SPA ligation (with clip and electrocauterization or both), which is thought to be more ideal surgical treatment method, as it ligates a major arterial supply and therefore minimizes the risk of refractory epistaxis from collateral circulation. Success rate of 92% to 100% has been achieved with endoscopic SPA ligation [22]. This is a simple and effective method to control refractory epistaxis which also prevents the morbidity and complications of nasal packing. This technique is especially useful in systemically ill individuals who tolerate nasal packing poorly [23]. Failure of this technique is attributed to the failure to identify all the branches of sphenopalatine artery. Endoscopic SPA ligation with bipolar electrocauterization was required in 2.38% (2) of our patients.

There are other newer treatment methods for controlling bleeding such as fibrin glue, which is developed from human plasma cryoprecipitate that binds to the damaged vessels and arrests the bleeding. Randomized controlled trial has found that the local complications due to fibrin glue were lower than that of electrocautery, chemical cautery, and nasal packing. The rebleed rate of fibrin glue was 15% which is comparable to electrocautery [24]. Laser has also been introduced in the management of epistaxis that is found to be useful in cases of recurrent bleeds due to vascular abnormalities such as hereditary haemorrhagic telangiectasia [25].

5. Conclusion

Epistaxis is a common emergency condition in Otorhino-laryngology. People of all ages can be affected. Hypertension, trauma, and coagulopathy were the most common etiological/risk factors among the patients in whom etiology was found although in most of the patients etiology could not be found. Conservative or nonsurgical methods were effective to arrest epistaxis in most of the patients. Proper nasal packing is the effective method of controlling epistaxis. Surgical or interventional treatment is only required when epistaxis could not be controlled after nonsurgical treatment methods.

Conflict of Interests

The author declares that there is no conflict of interests regarding the publication of this paper.

References

[1] R. Douglas and P. J. Wormald, "Update on epistaxis," *Current Opinion in Otolaryngology and Head and Neck Surgery*, vol. 15, no. 3, pp. 180–183, 2007.

[2] M. Small, J. A. Murray, and A. G. Maran, "A study of patients with epistaxis requiring admission to hospital," *Health Bulletin*, vol. 40, no. 1, pp. 20–29, 1982.

[3] T. W. M. Walker, T. V. MacFarlane, and G. W. McGarry, "The epidemiology and chronobiology of epistaxis: an investigation of Scottish hospital admissions 1995–2004," *Clinical Otolaryngology*, vol. 32, no. 5, pp. 361–365, 2007.

[4] S. H. Ciaran and H. Owain, "Update on management of epistaxis," *West London Medical Journal*, vol. 1, pp. 33–41, 2009.

[5] D. J. Pallin, Y. M. Chng, M. P. McKay, J. A. Emond, A. J. Pelletier, and C. A. Camargo Jr., "Epidemiology of epistaxis in US emergency departments, 1992 to 2001," *Annals of Emergency Medicine*, vol. 46, no. 1, pp. 77–81, 2005.

[6] D. A. Klotz, M. R. Winkle, J. Richmon, and A. S. Hengerer, "Surgical management of posterior epistaxis: a changing paradigm," *Laryngoscope*, vol. 112, no. 9, pp. 1577–1582, 2002.

[7] N. C. Mgbor, "Epistaxis in Enugu: a 9 year review," *Nigerian Journal of Otorhinolaryngology*, vol. 1, no. 2, pp. 11–14, 2004.

[8] C. L. Huang and C. H. Shu, "Epistaxis: a review of hospitalized patients," *Chinese Medical Journal*, vol. 65, no. 2, pp. 74–78, 2002.

[9] D. A. Randall and S. B. Freeman, "Management of anterior and posterior epistaxis," *American Family Physician*, vol. 43, no. 6, pp. 2007–2014, 1991.

[10] N. P. Christensen, D. S. Smith, S. L. Barnwell, and M. K. Wax, "Arterial embolization in the management of posterior epistaxis," *The Otolaryngology—Head and Neck Surgery*, vol. 133, no. 5, pp. 748–753, 2005.

[11] S. Varshney and R. K. Saxena, "Epistaxis: a retrospective clinical study," *Indian Journal of Otolaryngology and Head and Neck Surgery*, vol. 57, no. 2, pp. 125–129, 2005.

[12] J. J. Schietroma and R. R. Tenzel, "The effects of cautery on the optic nerve," *Ophthalmic Plastic and Reconstructive Surgery*, vol. 6, no. 2, pp. 102–107, 1990.

[13] K. M. J. Green, T. Board, and L. J. O'Keeffe, "Oculomotor nerve palsy following submucosal diathermy to the inferior turbinates," *Journal of Laryngology and Otology*, vol. 114, no. 4, pp. 285–286, 2000.

[14] A. Ahmed and T. J. Woolford, "Endoscopic bipolar diathermy in the management of epistaxis: an effective and cost-efficient treatment," *Clinical Otolaryngology and Allied Sciences*, vol. 28, no. 3, pp. 273–275, 2003.

[15] R. J. Corbridge, B. Djazaeri, W. P. L. Hellier, and J. Hadley, "A prospective randomized controlled trial comparing the use of merocel nasal tampons and BIPP in the control of acute epistaxis," *Clinical Otolaryngology and Allied Sciences*, vol. 20, no. 4, pp. 305–307, 1995.

[16] M. B. Soyka, G. Nikolaou, K. Rufibach, and D. Holzmann, "On the effectiveness of treatment options in epistaxis: an analysis of 678 interventions," *Rhinology*, vol. 49, no. 4, pp. 474–478, 2011.

[17] J. J. Vitek, "Idiopathic intractable epistaxis: endovascular therapy," *Radiology*, vol. 181, no. 1, pp. 113–116, 1991.

[18] J. P. Bent III and B. P. Wood, "Complications resulting from treatment of severe posterior epistaxis," *Journal of Laryngology and Otology*, vol. 113, no. 3, pp. 252–254, 1999.

[19] E. B. Strong, D. A. Bell, L. P. Johnson, and J. M. Jacobs, "Intractable epistaxis: transantral ligation vs. embolization: efficacy review and cost analysis," *Otolaryngology—Head and Neck Surgery*, vol. 113, no. 6, pp. 674–678, 1995.

[20] S. E. Cooper and V. R. Ramakrishnan, "Direct cauterization of the nasal septal artery for epistaxis," *Laryngoscope*, vol. 122, no. 4, pp. 738–740, 2012.

[21] P. Spafford and J. S. Durham, "Epistaxis: efficacy of arterial ligation and long-term outcome," *Journal of Otolaryngology*, vol. 21, no. 4, pp. 252–256, 1992.

[22] S. Kumar, A. Shetty, J. Rockey, and E. Nilssen, "Contemporary surgical treatment of epistaxis. What is the evidence for sphenopalatine artery ligation?" *Clinical Otolaryngology and Allied Sciences*, vol. 28, no. 4, pp. 360–363, 2003.

[23] A. Thakar and C. J. Sharan, "Endoscopic sphenopalatine artery ligation for refractory posterior epistaxis," *Indian Journal of Otolaryngology and Head and Neck Surgery*, vol. 57, no. 3, pp. 215–218, 2005.

[24] M. Vaiman, S. Segal, and E. Eviatar, "Fibrin glue treatment for epistaxis," *Rhinology*, vol. 40, no. 2, pp. 88–91, 2002.

[25] J. A. Stankiewicz, "Nasal endoscopy and control of epistaxis," *Current Opinion in Otolaryngology and Head and Neck Surgery*, vol. 12, no. 1, pp. 43–45, 2004.

9

Impact of Educational Program on the Management of Chronic Suppurative Otitis Media among Children

Yousseria Elsayed Yousef,[1] Essam A. Abo El-Magd,[2] Osama M. El-Asheer,[3] and Safaa Kotb[4]

[1] *Department of Pediatric Nursing, Faculty of Nursing, Sohag University, Egypt*
[2] *ENT, Faculty of Medicine, Aswan University, Egypt*
[3] *Pediatrics, Faculty of Medicine, Assiut University, Egypt*
[4] *Public Health, Faculty of Nursing, Assiut University, Egypt*

Correspondence should be addressed to Essam A. Abo el-magd; esamali801@yahoo.com

Academic Editor: David W. Eisele

Background. Chronic suppurative otitis media (CSOM) remains one of the most common childhood chronic infectious diseases worldwide, affecting diverse racial and cultural groups in both developing and industrialized countries. *Aim of the Study.* This study aimed to assess the impact of educational program on the management of children with CSOM. *Subjects and Methods.* An experimental study design was used. This study included 100 children of both sexes of 2 years and less of age with CSOM. Those children were divided into 3 groups: group I: it involved 50 children with CSOM (naive) who received the designed educational program; control group: it involved 50 children who were under the traditional treatment and failed to respond; group II: those children in the control group were given the educational program and followed up in the same way as group I and considered as group II. *Tools of the Study.* Tool I is a structured questionnaire interview sheet for mothers. It consists of four parts: (1) personal and sociodemographic characteristics of child and (2) data about risk factors of otitis media (3) assessment of maternal practice about care of children with suppurative otitis medi (4) diagnostic criteria for suppurative otitis media. Tool II is the educational program: an educational program was developed by the researchers based on the knowledge and practices needs. This study was carried out through a period of 9 months starting from September 2013 to May 2014. The educational program was implemented for mothers of children with CSOM in the form of 5 scheduled sessions at the time of diagnosis, after one week, 1, 3, and 6 months. *Results.* There were significant differences between children who received the educational program and control group regarding the response to treatment after one and 3 months. The percentages of complete cure increased progressively 32%, 60%, and 84% after 1, 3, and 6 months in group I while they were 24%, 44%, and 64% in group II, respectively. Cure (dry perforation) was 64%, 36%, and 12% among children of group I after 1, 3, and 6 months while it was 64%, 44%, and 24% in group II, respectively. The percentages of compliance to the educational program improved with time in both groups: 44%, 64%, and 80% in group I and 32%, 48%, and 56% in group II after 1, 3, and 6 months, respectively. The percentages of cure were statistically significantly higher among children with complete compliance with the educational program in both groups in comparison to those with incomplete compliance ($P = 0.000$ for both). *Conclusions.* From this study we can conclude that the majority of children with CSOM had one or more risk factors for occurrence of the disease; the educational program is effective for management of CSOM (whether cure or complete cure); the higher the compliance of mothers with the program the higher the response rate; regular followup and explanation of the importance of the program played an important role in the compliance with the program.

1. Introduction

Chronic suppurative otitis media (CSOM) is defined as a chronic inflammation of the middle ear and mastoid cavity, which presents with recurrent ear discharges or otorrhoea through a tympanic perforation. The disease usually begins in childhood as a spontaneous tympanic perforation due to an acute infection of the middle ear, known as acute otitis media (AOM), or as a sequel of less severe forms of otitis media (e.g., secretory OM). The infection may occur during the first 6 years of a child's life, with a peak around 2 years [1–3]. It is the commonest childhood infectious disease worldwide

[4, 5]. The multifactorial nature of otitis media must be stressed. Inadequate antibiotic treatment, frequent upper respiratory tract infections, nasal disease, multiple episodes of AOM, being a member of a large family, and poor living conditions with poor access to medical care are related to the development of CSOM. Poor housing, hygiene, and nutrition are associated with higher prevalence rates. Bottle-feeding, passive exposure to smoking, attendance in congested centers such as day-care facilities, and a family history of otitis media are some of the risk factors for otitis media (Kenna, 1994) [6–9]. The World Health Organization (WHO) global estimate for disabling hearing impairment (degree of severity more than 40 dB) has more than doubled from 120 million people in 1995 to 278 million in 2005. A total of 364 million people have mild hearing impairment, while 624 million are estimated to have some level of hearing impairment and 80% of these live in low- and middle-income countries [10, 11]. Worldwide, there are between 65 and 330 million people affected, of whom 60% receive significant hearing loss. This burden falls disproportionately on children in developing countries [12]. Patients with CSOM respond more frequently to topical therapy than to systemic therapy. Successful topical therapy consists of 3 important components: selection of an appropriate antibiotic drop, regular aggressive aural toilet, and control of granulation tissue. Aural toilet is a critical process in the treatment of CSOM. For the best results, aural toilet should be performed 2-3 times per day just before the administration of topical antimicrobial agents. Failures of topical antimicrobial therapy are almost always failures of delivery [13].

2. Aim of the Study

This study aimed to assess the impact of educational program on the management of children with chronic suppurative otitis media.

2.1. Research Questions

(1) Is there an effect of the designed educational program on the cure of children with CSOM?

(2) Is there a difference between the response of naïve children with CSOM who received the program and those who received the program after failure of traditional treatment?

2.2. Significance. Worldwide, there are between 65 and 330 million people affected, of whom 60% receive significant hearing loss. This burden falls disproportionately on children in developing countries [12].

3. Subjects and Methods

3.1. Design. An experimental study design was used in carrying out this study.

3.2. Setting. This study was carried out in the outpatient clinics of the Departments of Pediatrics and ENT (Ear, Nose and Throat), Assiut University Hospital.

General objective of this program was to cure the children with chronic suppurative otitis media.

3.3. Patients. This study included 100 children of both sexes of 2 years and less of age with chronic suppurative otitis media according to the standard definition. Those children were divided into 3 groups.

(1) Group I: it involved 50 children with CSOM (naïve) who received the educational program.

(2) Control group: it involved 50 children who were selected from those attending the outpatient clinics under the traditional treatment and failed to respond.

(3) Group II: those children in the control group were given the educational program, followed up in the same way as group I, and considered as group II.

The history of the disease, follow-up visits, physician diagnosis, and assessment of the control group were taken from the child's mother and outpatient clinic follow-up card of the child.

3.4. Tools of the Study. The following tools were utilized to collect data pertinent to study. These were as follows.

3.4.1. Tool I: A Structured Questionnaire Interview Sheet for Mothers. It consists of four parts:

(1) personal and sociodemographic characteristics of child: they include age, sex, residence, birth order, maternal education and occupation, and number of family members;

(2) data about risk factors of otitis media: they include history of the disease, presence of dust, sources of vapors, using pacifier, type of feeding, and use of the ideal position for feeding;

(3) assessment of maternal practice about care of children with suppurative otitis media: this part was developed by the researcher to evaluate mother's practices given to child with suppurative otitis media;

(4) diagnostic criteria for suppurative otitis media: children who were diagnosed with suppurative otitis media were interviewed by the physician to evaluate the case, prescribe the appropriate treatment, and determine the schedule of followup (after one week and 1, 3, and 6 months).

3.4.2. Tool II: The Educational Program. An educational program was developed by the researchers based on the knowledge and practices needs in a form of printed Arabic booklet. It was also supplemented with information based on review of the relevant literature (nursing textbook, journals, internet resources, etc.) about care provided to children with CSOM. This was adopted from [13, 14]. Then, the program was reviewed by a panel of experts before its implementation.

The educational program included the following.

(1) Give the antibiotic regularly with the described dose.

(2) Clean the external ear from pus with cotton before adding ear drops.

(3) Put the ear drops with the correct way.

(4) Put a piece of cotton covered with Vaseline before bathing.

(5) Separate the infant away from dust, sources of steam and vapors, and those complaining of common cold.

(6) Stop using pacifier, sterilize the feeding bottle, and use the ideal position for feeding.

3.5. Program Evaluation. Evaluation of the program's success was based on the response of children with CSOM. This evaluation was done after the end of the program and followup (one week, one month, three months, and six months) using definition criteria for response (cure or failure). Complete cure means absence of otorrhoea and spontaneous closure of drum perforation. Cure (dry perforation) means absence of otorrhoea or presence of serous/mucous otorrhoea with negative microbiologic culture or presence of a perforation (hole) in the eardrum without any signs of discharge or fluid behind the eardrum. Failure means presence of purulent or mucopurulent otorrhoea irrespective of culture results or presence of serous/mucous otorrhoea with positive culture [15, 16].

3.6. Data Collection. Official approval letters were obtained from the heads of the departments of pediatrics and ENT to conduct the research.

Oral consent was taken from the mother to participate in the study after full explanation of the program and its benefits and hazards and complications of the disease. Those who accepted to participate were interviewed and the program of treatment was clearly explained where they were asked to share actively to achieve the full program. An Arabic translation of all study tools was done and was reviewed by experts in nursing and medicine to ascertain their content validity.

3.7. Field of the Work. This study was carried out through a period of 9 months starting from September to May. The educational program was implemented for mothers of children with CSOM in the form of 5 scheduled sessions at the time of diagnosis, after one week, 1, 3, and 6 months. The duration of each session was variable and ranged between 30 and 45 minutes. Each participant obtained a copy of the program booklet that included all the required instructions. The sessions were carried out in the waiting room after the physician observation. At the first visit, clear explanation of the nature of the disease and its possible complications was done by face-to-face interview of mothers of children with CSOM. The detailed items of the designed educational program were explained using a simple Arabic language. The educational program consisted of the following instructions.

(1) The antibiotic must be given regularly with the described dose.

(2) The mothers were trained to clean the external ear from pus and granulation tissue with pieces of cotton before adding ear drops.

(3) They were trained to put ear drops in the correct way in the supine position with the target ear facing the ceiling.

(4) Before bathing, a piece of cotton covered with Vaseline must be put in the external ear to keep the ear dry to avoid complications.

(5) They were instructed to separate the infant away from dust, sources of steam and vapors, and those complaining of common cold.

(6) They were advised to stop using pacifier, sterilize the feeding bottle, and use the ideal position for feeding (upright position when feeding).

In the next visits, the child was evaluated by the physician and clinical diagnosis was established. Then, the mothers were interviewed where the compliance with the items of the educational program was assessed to determine the adherence to the program.

3.8. Pilot Study. After developing the tools, a pilot study was implemented for purpose of testing clarity and completeness and to determine the time required for each case. According to the results of pilot, the needed modifications, omissions, and/or additions were done. A jury acceptance of the final forms was secured before actual study work and the reliability was assessed in a pilot study.

3.9. Ethical Consideration. An oral consent was taken from all participants in the study. The purpose and nature of the study were explained by the researcher through direct personal communication before starting the study. The data was confidential between mothers and the researchers and was used for the purpose of the research only.

Statistical analysis was done using SPSS-17 statistical software package and Excel for figures. Data were presented using descriptive statistics in the form of frequencies and percentages for qualitative variables and means and standard deviations for quantitative variables. Quantitative continuous data were compared by using Student's t-test in case of comparisons between the mean scores of the studied groups. Qualitative studied variables were compared using Chi-square test. Statistical significance was considered at P value < 0.05.

4. Results

In Table 1, both groups were matched regarding the demographic data except that family members more than 5 were significantly more common among control than study groups ($P = 0.016$).

In Table 2, regarding the possible risk factors for CSOM, children in the control group were significantly more exposed

TABLE 1: Demographic data of study and control groups.

	Group I ($n = 50$)		Control ($n = 50$)		P value
	Number	%	Number	%	
Age					0.224
6–12 months	18	36.0	24	48.0	
>12 months	32	64.0	26	52.0	
Mean ± SD (months)	15.44 ± 6.21		14.16 ± 5.60		0.282
Sex					0.420
Male	26	52.0	30	60.0	
Female	24	48.0	20	40.0	
Residence					0.532
Rural	34	68.0	31	62.0	
Urban	16	32.0	19	38.0	
Mother education					0.402
Illiterate	10	20.0	14	28.0	
Read and write	6	12.0	2	4.0	
Primary	6	12.0	10	20.0	
Preparatory	8	16.0	10	20.0	
Secondary	10	20.0	8	16.0	
University	10	20.0	6	12.0	
Mother job					0.629
Housewife	38	76.0	40	80.0	
Employer	12	24.0	10	20.0	

to passive smoking ($P = 0.035$), were more than the 3rd in the birth order ($P = 0.005$), and shared more than 2 children in one room in comparison to those in the study group. More than half of the children with CSOM in the study and control groups were more than the 3rd in the birth order, had more than 2 children in one room, and were exposed to vapors. In addition, more than two-thirds of them were bottle feeders, used pacifier, and were exposed to passive smoking.

In Table 3, when the response to treatment was compared among those who received the educational program (groups I and II) and those who received the traditional treatment (control group), there were significant differences especially after 1 and 3 months. The percentages of complete cure increased progressively, 32%, 60%, and 84% after 1, 3, and 6 months in group I and 24%, 44%, and 64% in group II, respectively. Cure (dry perforation) was 64%, 36%, and 12% among children of group I after 1, 3, and 6 months and 64%, 44%, and 24% in group II, respectively. On the other hand, no evidence of cure was found among control group. After one week of treatment, significant improvement was found among study and control groups in the form of absence of otorrhoea but no significant differences were found among groups. No differences were found between groups I and II regarding response to treatment after 1, 3, and 6 months. The total response to the educational program ranged from 88% in group II to 96% in group I (total response included complete cure and cure).

Table 4 shows that the percentages of compliance with the educational program improved with time in both groups, 44%, 64%, and 80% in group I and 32%, 48%, and 56% in group II after 1, 3, and 6 months, respectively. The percentages

of compliance with the educational program were higher among children of group I than group II after 1 and 3 months and the differences were statistically insignificant. After 6 months, the compliance was significantly higher among children of group I than group II ($P = 0.010$). Incomplete compliance after one month among children of group I: 8 (16%) achieved 60%–70% and 18 (36%) achieved 80%–90%. Incomplete compliance after one month among children of group II: 12 (24%) achieved 60%–70% and 6 (12%) achieved 80%–90%. Incomplete compliance after 3 months among children of group I: 14 (28%) achieved 70%–90% while 10 (20%) did in group II. Incomplete compliance after 6 months: 6 (12%) of each group achieved 70%–90%.

Table 5 shows the relation between the compliance with and the response to the educational program among children of both groups after one month. The percentages of cure were statistically significantly higher among children with complete compliance with the educational program in both groups in comparison to those with incomplete compliance ($P = 0.000$ for both).

In Table 6, after 3 months of treatment, the percentages of cure were 100% among those with complete compliance with the educational program among children of both groups. On the other hand, the percentages of cure were 28.6% and 17.6% among children of groups I and II, respectively, who achieved incomplete compliance with the educational program. The differences were statistically highly significant ($P = 0.000$ for both).

In Table 7, after 6 months of treatment, the percentages of cure were 100% among those with complete compliance with the educational program among children of both

TABLE 2: Possible risk factors for suppurative otitis media.

	Group I ($n = 50$)		Control ($n = 50$)		P value
	Number	%	Number	%	
Family members					0.016*
4-5 members	28	56.0	16	32.0	
>5 members	22	44.0	34	68.0	
Birth order					0.005*
2-3	30	60.0	16	32.0	
>3	20	40.0	34	68.0	
Children in one room					0.043*
1-2 children	26	52.0	16	32.0	
>2 children	24	48.0	34	68.0	
Breast feeding					0.218
Yes	46	92.0	42	84.0	
No	4	8.0	8	16.0	
Bottle					0.647
Yes	46	92.0	48	96.0	
No	4	8.0	2	4.0	
Pacifier					0.190
Yes	32	64.0	38	76.0	
No	18	36.0	12	24.0	
Father smoking					0.349
Yes	36	72.0	40	80.0	
No	14	28.0	10	20.0	
Baby passive smoking					0.035*
Yes	28	56.0	38	76.0	
No	22	44.0	12	24.0	
Source of vapor					0.102
Yes	26	52.0	34	68.0	
No	24	48.0	16	32.0	

groups. Although the compliance with the educational program among children of both groups was incomplete, the percentages of cure were 71.4% and 47.1% in groups I and II, respectively. However, the differences were statistically significant ($P = 0.019$ and 0.000, resp.).

5. Discussion

Chronic suppurative otitis media (CSOM) is a leading cause of mild to moderate conductive acquired hearing loss worldwide, especially in children, and particularly in developing countries [17–21]. It is characterized by long-standing ear discharge through a persistent perforation of the tympanic membrane. CSOM is believed to develop in early childhood, often following poorly managed acute otitis media, with potential of spilling over into adulthood, accounting for recurrent episodes of chronic discharging ears that can last for many years [22–26].

The current study included 100 children with CSOM. Fifty of them (naïve patients) once diagnosed were selected to receive educational program and followed up for 6 months (group I). The other 50 children were selected from those who received traditional treatment and failed to respond after 3 months (control group). The latter group of children were

given the educational program to assess its role after failure of traditional treatment and considered as a new group (group II).

More than half of children with CSOM in the study and control groups were more than the 3rd in the birth order, had more than 2 children in one room, and were exposed to vapors. In addition, more than two-thirds of them were breast and bottle feeders, used pacifier, and were exposed to passive smoking. This agrees with report of van der Veen et al. [27] and Parry et al. [9] who stated that the risk of developing CSOM increases with the following circumstances: multiple episodes of acute otitis media (AOM), living in crowded conditions, being a member of a large family, attending daycare, passive smoking, breast-feeding, socioeconomic status, and the annual number of upper respiratory tract infections.

Children who received the educational program (group I) showed complete cure (this means absence of otorrhoea and spontaneous closure of drum perforation) of 32%, 60%, and 84% after 1, 3, and 6 months in group I and 24%, 44%, and 64% in group II, respectively. The percentages of cure (presence of a perforation in the eardrum without any signs of discharge or fluid behind the eardrum) were 64%, 36%, and 12% among children of group I after 1, 3, and 6 months and 64%, 44%, and 24% in group II, respectively. These

TABLE 3: Comparison between study and control groups regarding the response to educational program.

	Group I ($n = 50$)		Group II ($n = 50$)		Control ($n = 50$)		P value[1]	P value[2]	P value[3]
	Number	%	Number	%	Number	%			
After 1 month							0.276	0.000*	0.000*
Complete cure	16	32.0	12	24.0	0	0.0			
Cure	32	64.0	32	64.0	0	0.0			
No response	2	4.0	6	12.0	50	100.0			
After 3 months							0.163	0.000*	0.000*
Complete cure	30	60.0	22	44.0	0	0.0			
Cure	18	36.0	22	44.0	0	0.0			
No response	2	4.0	6	12.0	50	100.0			
After 6 months							0.069	—	—
Complete cure	42	84.0	32	64.0	—	—			
Cure	6	12.0	12	24.0	—	—			
No response	2	4.0	6	12.0	—	—			

P value[1] between group I and group II, P value[2] between group I and control, and P value[3] between group II and control.

TABLE 4: Comparison between both study groups regarding the compliance with educational program.

	Group I ($n = 50$)		Group II ($n = 50$)		P value
	Number	%	Number	%	
After 1 month					0.216
Complete (100%)	22	44.0	16	32.0	
Incomplete (<100%)	28	56.0	34	68.0	
After 3 months					0.107
Complete (100%)	32	64.0	24	48.0	
Incomplete (<100%)	18	36.0	26	52.0	
After 6 months					0.010*
Complete (100%)	40	80.0	28	56.0	
Incomplete (<100%)	10	20.0	22	44.0	

results are supported by report of Roland et al. [13] who stated that, among children with CSOM, successful topical therapy consists of 3 important components: selection of an appropriate antibiotic drop, regular aggressive aural toilet, and control of granulation tissue. This is explained by the fact that the external auditory canal and tissues lateral to the infected middle ear are often covered with mucoid exudate or desquamated epithelium. Topically applied preparations cannot penetrate affected tissues until these interposing materials are removed. Failures of topical antimicrobial therapy are almost always failures of delivery. Specifically, failure of delivery describes the inability of an appropriate topical antibiotic to reach the specific site of infection within the middle ear [13]. The educational program included keeping the ear dry during swimming which is in agreement with the reports of Basu et al. [14] and Ball and Bindler [28] that patients with CSOM are usually advised to avoid swimming but if they swim they should put ear plugs and dry their ears afterwards.

After one month, the percentages of complete cure were significantly higher among children with complete compliance with the educational program in both groups in comparison to those with incomplete compliance ($P = 0.000$ for both). After 3 and 6 months of treatment, the percentages

of complete cure were 100% among those with complete compliance with the educational program among children of both groups. These results are in agreement with the results of Roland et al. [13] who reported that aural toilet is a critical process in the treatment of CSOM and it must be regular and aggressive. For best results, aural toilet should be performed 2-3 times per day just before the administration of topical antimicrobial agents.

The total response to the educational program ranged from 88% in group II to 96% in group I (total response included complete cure and cure). On the other hand, cure (dry ear) was found in 64% of children of both groups after one month of the program. These results agree with Verhoeff et al. [4, 5] who found that the overall success percentages (dry ear) of topical drops varied from 40% to 100% and concluded that treatment with antibiotic or antiseptic eardrops accompanied by aural toilet was more effective in resolving otorrhoea than no treatment.

6. Conclusions

From this study, we can conclude that the majority of children with CSOM had one or more risk factors for occurrence of the disease; the educational program is effective for

TABLE 5: Comparison of the response to and compliance with the educational program between both study groups after one month.

		Compliance with the program				P value
	Physician report	Complete		Incomplete		
		Number	%	Number	%	
Group I	Complete cure	14	63.6	2	7.1	
	Cure	8	36.4	24	85.7	0.000*
	No response	**0**	**0**	2	7.1	
	Total	**22**	**100.0**	**28**	**100.0**	
Group II	Complete cure	12	75.0	0	0.0	
	Cure	4	25.0	30	88.2	0.000*
	No response	**0**	**0**	4	**11.8**	
	Total	**16**	**100.0**	**34**	**100.0**	

TABLE 6: Comparison between the response to and compliance with the educational program in both study groups after 3 months.

		Compliance with the program				P value
	Physician report	Complete		Incomplete		
		Number	%	Number	%	
Group I	Complete cure	22	100.0	6	21.4	
	Cure	0	0.0	20	71.4	0.000*
	No response	**0**	**0**	2	7.1	
	Total	**22**	**100.0**	**28**	**100.0**	
Group II	Complete cure	16	100.0	6	17.6	
	Cure	0	0.0	22	64.7	0.000*
	No response	**0**	**0**	6	17.6	
	Total	**16**	**100.0**	**34**	**100.0**	

TABLE 7: Comparison between the response to and compliance with the educational program in both study groups after 6 months.

		Compliance with the program				P value
	Physician report	Complete		Incomplete		
		Number	%	Number	%	
Group I	Complete cure	22	100.0	20	71.4	
	Cure	0	0.0	6	21.4	0.019*
	No response	**0**	**0**	2	7.1	
	Total	**22**	**100.0**	**28**	**100.0**	
Group II	Complete cure	16	100.0	16	47.1	
	Cure	0	0.0	12	35.2	0.000*
	No response	**0**	**0**	6	17.6	
	Total	**16**	**100.0**	**34**	**100.0**	

management of CSOM whether cure or complete cure; the higher the compliance of mothers with the program, the higher the response rate; regular followup and explanation of the importance of the program played an important role in the compliance with the program.

7. Recommendations

This program should be applied to a wide scale to validate these results and evaluate its role in the prevention of CSOM especially hearing loss which could not be evaluated in the study.

Conflict of Interests

The authors declare that there is no conflict of interests regarding the publication of this paper.

References

[1] M. Tos, "Sequelae of secretory otitis media and the relationship to chronic suppurative otitis media," *Annals of Otology, Rhinology and Laryngology*, vol. 99, supplement 146, no. 4, pp. 18–19, 1990.

[2] K. A. Daly, L. L. Hunter, S. C. Levine, B. R. Lindgren, and G. S. Giebink, "Relationships between otitis media sequelae and age," *Laryngoscope*, vol. 108, no. 9, pp. 1306–1310, 1998.

[3] P. van Hasset, "Chronic supportive otitis media," *Community Ear and Hearing Health Journal*, vol. 4, no. 6, pp. 19–21, 2007.

[4] M. Verhoeff, E. L. van der Veen, M. M. Rovers, E. A. Sanders, and A. G. Schilder, "Chronic suppurative otitis media: a review," *International Journal of Pediatric Otorhinolaryngology*, vol. 70, no. 1, pp. 1–12, 2006.

[5] J. Acuin, A. Smith, and I. Mackenzie, "Interventions for chronic suppurative otitis media," *The Cochrane Database of Systematic Reviews*, no. 2, Article ID CD000473, 1998.

[6] World Health Organization, *Prevention of Hearing Impairment from Chronic Otitis Media. Report of a WHO/CIBA Foundation*, WHO, Geneva, Switzerland, 1998.

[7] C. E. Adair-Bischoff and R. S. Sauve, "Environmental tobacco smoke and middle ear disease in preschool-age children," *Archives of Pediatrics and Adolescent Medicine*, vol. 152, no. 2, pp. 127–133, 1998.

[8] A. O. Lasisi, O. A. Sulaiman, and O. A. Afolabi, "Socio-economic status and hearing loss in chronic suppurative otitis media in Nigeria," *Annals of Tropical Paediatrics*, vol. 27, no. 4, pp. 291–296, 2007.

[9] D. Parry et al., "Chronic Suppurative Otitis Media," Medscape, October 2011.

[10] B. O. Olusanya and V. E. Newton, "Global burden of childhood hearing impairment and disease control priorities for developing countries," *The Lancet*, vol. 369, no. 9569, pp. 1314–1317, 2007.

[11] A. W. Smith, "Update on burden of hearing impairment and progress of WHO/WWH hearing aids initiative," in *Proceedings of the WHO /WW Hearing 5th Workshop on the Provision of Hearing Aids and Services for Developing Countries*, Geneva, Switzerland, 2007.

[12] L. Monasta, L. Ronfani, F. Marchetti et al., "Burden of disease caused by otitis media: systematic review and global estimates," *PLoS ONE*, vol. 7, no. 4, Article ID e36226, 2012.

[13] P. S. Roland, B. Isaacson, and A. D. Meyers, *Chronic Suppurative Otitis Media Treatment & Management*, Medscape, 2013.

[14] S. Basu, C. Georgalas, P. Sen, and A. K. Bhattacharyya, "Water precautions and ear surgery: evidence and practice in the UK," *The Journal of Laryngology & Otology*, vol. 121, no. 1, pp. 9–14, 2007.

[15] N. Miró, "Controlled multicenter study on chronic suppurative otitis media treated with topical applications of ciprofloxacin 0.2% solution in single-dose containers or combination of polymyxin B, neomycin, and hydrocortisone suspension," *Otolaryngology—Head and Neck Surgery*, vol. 123, no. 5, pp. 617–623, 2000.

[16] *Otitis Media Model of Care. Perth: System Policy and Planning*, Department of Health, Perth, Western Australia, Australia, 2013.

[17] A. W. Smith, J. Hatcher, I. J. Mackenzie et al., "Randomised controlled trial of treatment of chronic suppurative otitis media in Kenyan schoolchildren," *The Lancet*, vol. 348, no. 9035, pp. 1128–1133, 1996.

[18] A. D. Olusesi, "Otitis media as a cause of significant hearing loss among Nigerians," *International Journal of Pediatric Otorhinolaryngology*, vol. 72, no. 6, pp. 787–792, 2008.

[19] M. A. Elemraid, B. J. Brabin, W. D. Fraser et al., "Characteristics of hearing impairment in Yemeni children with chronic suppurative otitis media: a case-control study," *International Journal of Pediatric Otorhinolaryngology*, vol. 74, no. 3, pp. 283–286, 2010.

[20] N. N. Nwokoye, L. O. Egwari, A. O. Coker, O. O. Olubi, E. O. Ugoji, and S. C. Nwachukwu, "Predisposing and bacteriological features of otitis media," *African Journal of Microbiology Research*, vol. 6, no. 3, pp. 520–525, 2012.

[21] R. Prakash, D. Juyal, V. Negi et al., "Microbiology of chronic suppurative otitis media in a tertiary care setup of Uttarakhand State, India," *North American Journal of Medical Sciences*, vol. 5, no. 4, pp. 282–287, 2013.

[22] M. A. Kenna, "Epidemiology and natural history of chronic suppurative otitis media," *Annals of Otology, Rhinology & Laryngology*, vol. 97, no. 8, 1988.

[23] C. D. Bluestone, "Epidemiology and pathogenesis of chronic suppurative otitis media: implications for prevention and treatment," *International Journal of Pediatric Otorhinolaryngology*, vol. 42, no. 3, pp. 207–223, 1998.

[24] S. M. Zakzouk and M. F. Hajjaj, "Epidemiology of chronic suppurative otitis media among Saudi children: a comparative study of two decades," *International Journal of Pediatric Otorhinolaryngology*, vol. 62, no. 3, pp. 215–218, 2002.

[25] F. E. Ologe and C. C. Nwawolo, "Chronic suppurative otitis media in school pupils in Nigeria," *East African Medical Journal*, vol. 80, no. 3, pp. 130–134, 2003.

[26] *Chronic Suppurative Otitis Media: Burden of Illness and Management Options*, WHO, Geneva, Switzerland, 2004.

[27] E. L. van der Veen, A. G. Schilder, N. van Heerbeek et al., "Predictors of chronic suppurative otitis media in children," *Archives of Otolaryngology—Head and Neck Surgery*, vol. 132, no. 10, pp. 1115–1118, 2006.

[28] J. W. Ball and C. Bindler, "Alterations in eye, ear, nose and throat function," in *Pediatric Nursing Care for Children*, J. W. Ball and C. Bindler, Eds., chapter 19, pp. 649–663, 4th edition.

10

Elicitation of the Acoustic Change Complex to Long-Duration Speech Stimuli in Four-Month-Old Infants

Ke Heng Chen and Susan A. Small

University of British Columbia, Vancouver, BC, Canada V6T 1Z3

Correspondence should be addressed to Susan A. Small; ssmall@audiospeech.ubc.ca

Academic Editor: Peter S. Roland

The acoustic change complex (ACC) is an auditory-evoked potential elicited to changes within an ongoing stimulus that indicates discrimination at the level of the auditory cortex. Only a few studies to date have attempted to record ACCs in young infants. The purpose of the present study was to investigate the elicitation of ACCs to long-duration speech stimuli in English-learning 4-month-old infants. ACCs were elicited to consonant contrasts made up of two concatenated speech tokens. The stimuli included native dental-dental /dada/ and dental-labial /daba/ contrasts and a nonnative Hindi dental-retroflex /daDa/ contrast. Each consonant-vowel speech token was 410 ms in duration. Slow cortical responses were recorded to the onset of the stimulus and to the acoustic change from /da/ to either /ba/ or /Da/ within the stimulus with significantly prolonged latencies compared with adults. ACCs were reliably elicited for all stimulus conditions with more robust morphology compared with our previous findings using stimuli that were shorter in duration. The P1 amplitudes elicited to the acoustic change in /daba/ and /daDa/ were significantly larger compared to /dada/ supporting that the brain discriminated between the speech tokens. These findings provide further evidence for the use of ACCs as an index of discrimination ability.

1. Introduction

One of the early steps for infants to learn a language is to recognize the phonetic distinctions and sound patterns of their native language. Infants with hearing loss are at risk for delays in speech and language development because they might not have access to important auditory cues during a period of rapid development in the first years of life. These early processes are complex and not fully understood in infants with normal hearing or limited auditory experience. One challenge in this area of research is the lack of a reliable, age-appropriate tool to assess an individual infant's capacity to detect and discriminate speech sounds. Such a tool would be invaluable in the clinic to assess hearing-aid benefit in infants in terms of ability to discriminate consonant and vowel contrasts. Because behavioural methods provide limited information about perceptual capacities and their underlying mechanisms, particularly in individual infants, cortical auditory-evoked potentials (CAEPs) offer a useful complement to behavioural measures. The slow cortical response, or P1-N1-P2, which is elicited to the onset of a stimulus has been studied extensively in adults and in some depth in infants to assess detection of speech sounds, although there are gaps in our understanding of these responses in infants, especially those with hearing loss who are aided. The acoustic change complex (ACC) which is elicited to a change in an ongoing stimulus has been a focus of recent research because it is thought to measure discrimination at the level of the auditory cortex which can provide insight into the brain's capacity to process the acoustic features of speech [1–3]. The ACC has also been well studied in adults but only a few studies to date have attempted to elicit the ACC in infants [4–7].

Research findings have suggested that the ACC may have the potential to be used as a clinical tool for assessing speech perception capacity. The ACC has been recorded in adults in response to speech stimuli such as consonant-vowel syllables, in which the acoustic change included frequency, amplitude, and periodicity cues similar to those found in normal conversational speech [1–3]. Ostroff et al. [3]

investigated cortical potentials in response to the naturally produced speech syllable /sei/ and a typical N1-P2 complex has been recorded to the acoustic change from /s/ to /ei/. The finding suggests that the ACC reflects changes of cortical activation caused by amplitude or spectral change at the transition from consonant to vowel and it may have the potential to demonstrate discrimination capacity. Changes from aperiodic to periodic stimulation have also produced changes in cortical activation that contribute to the observed response. The ACC has also been used to measure intensity discrimination [8] and frequency discrimination [9, 10] with results commensurate with behavioural findings. Another important feature of the ACC is that it has been shown to have excellent test-retest reliability in adults to natural speech stimuli [11]. The ACC was also shown to be efficacious in individuals with sensorineural hearing loss [12] and in those with cochlear implants [12]. Furthermore, when compared to other ERPs, such as the MMN, the ACC elicits responses with larger amplitudes and better signal-to-noise ratios, thus requiring less time and fewer stimulus presentations for recording [2]. These advantages can be very important for testing infants and other populations that are difficult to test.

Small and Werker [4] first recorded ACCs in infants in response to English and Hindi consonant contrasts. More recently, Martinez and colleagues [5] also recorded ACCs to vowel contrasts in a small number of young children with normal hearing and hearing loss (aided and unaided). Small and Werker [4] presented 4-month-old English-learning infants with speech contrasts generated from a synthetic place-of-articulation continuum: a native dental-dental contrast /dada/, a dental-labial contrast /daba/, and a nonnative Hindi dental-retroflex contrast /daDa/. These stimuli were the same as those used in a behavioural study by Werker and Lalonde [13] that showed that infants successfully discriminated native /daba/ and nonnative Hindi /daDa/ contrasts when they were under 6 months of age but not when they were 10 months of age, when their responses were similar to adults. These findings support the hypothesis that infants are born with a biological predisposition allowing them to discriminate the universal set of phonetic contrasts, then a decline or reorganization in this universal phonetic sensitivity takes place by the end of the first year as a function of linguistic experience of the ambient language [14]. Consistent with the behavioural data, Small and Werker [4] reported that robust ACCs were elicited in most infant participants to /daba/ with P1, N1, and P2 components, but fewer infants had the different components of the ACC present in their responses to /dada/ and /daDa/ and the morphology of these ACCs was more variable compared to /daba/. The ACC was recorded infrequently to English /dada/ presumably because no distinct acoustic change between the two speech tokens was detected. This study did not replicate the behavioural findings for nonnative stimuli (i.e., elicitation of the ACC to nonnative stimuli /daDa/ in the 4-month-old infants). One possible cause for the inconsistency between the ACC and behavioural findings posed by the authors was that the relatively short stimulus length might not have been long enough to accommodate the neural refractory periods in the immature brain in response to all stimuli.

Infant responses are frequently biphasic waveforms with a large positive peak and following negativity [15–18] due to immaturities in the underlying neurogenerators. The infant responses reported by Small and Werker [4] resemble the P1-N1-P2 complex recorded in adult participants in terms of the morphology of the waveforms but there are obvious differences in the relative prominence of the peaks and significantly prolonged latencies relative to the adults due to immaturity. These findings are similar to other studies that reported more complex waveforms in infants when the duration and complexity of the stimuli are increased and the stimulation rate is decreased [19–25]. There is some debate over which cortical components dominate at which age [26–32]. Some studies indicate that the large positive peak is the most predominant peak in early childhood (1–4 years) [33], and the negative trough that follows it becomes increasingly robust (3–6 years) and dominates the cortical response until adolescence. Some researchers claim that the earlier negative component (N1 in adults) can be recorded in addition to the negative trough from about three years of age with slow stimulation rate [34, 35], while others suggest that N1 can only be reliably evoked when children reach 9–13 years [29, 31]. It is also important to note that the labelling of the large positivity and following negativity in infant waveforms by different research groups is somewhat arbitrary. For example, some groups use the adult labels, P2 and N2, to describe these features [4, 17, 22]; others use P1 and N2 or N450 [5, 18, 36]. For the purposes of the present study, N1-P1-N1-P2 were used for convenience to describe the infant waveforms recorded.

Interstimulus interval (ISI) is thought to have substantial effects on the morphology, amplitude, and scalp distribution of the cortical response, particularly in immature auditory systems. For example, increasing the ISI up to at least 10 s results in larger amplitudes of N1 and P2 and their magnetic counterparts [35, 37]. When the ISI is decreased to less than 300 ms, the amplitude of N1 is usually diminished and may not be readily detected in some cases [38]. Some researchers suggest that an adult-like N1 component can only be recorded in children with ISIs longer than 1 s [19, 34]. An earlier study reported that a systematic decrease in the latency of the N1 component occurred with an increase in ISIs from 250 to 1000 ms for children aged 9–13 years, but not for adults [34]. Because the refractory properties of underlying neural components involved in N1 response may not have been fully developed in children, this finding may have resulted from prolonged N1 recovery cycles overlapping with robust P1 and N2 peaks.

Only a few studies have studied the effects of stimulus and presentation parameters on infant cortical responses. Golding et al. [18] recorded cortical responses dominated by a large positive peak (P1) when they presented /m/ and /t/ to 7-month-old infants using ISIs that varied from 750 to 1500 ms. They found a modest decrease in P1 amplitude and no change in latency with decreased ISI; Sharma et al. [36] found the same pattern of results for 10- and 20-week-old infants for ISIs of 910 to 4550 ms. Golding et al. [18] also investigated the effects of stimulus duration on infant cortical responses and found that decreasing stimulation duration from 31 to 79 ms resulted in a small decrease in amplitude but no change in latency.

Although the stimulus duration (282 ms for each speech token) and the ISI (2200 ms) used by Small and Werker [4] were adequate for eliciting the ACCs to the native speech contrast /daba/ in infants, the neural population in the infant brain may need a longer time to recover from the initial firing in a more challenging test condition (i.e., the nonnative /daDa/ condition). Linguistic experience with their ambient language may also have already played a role in the development of speech perception, such that the 4-month-old infant brain found it more difficult to discriminate the nonnative /daDa/, even though they were expected to discriminate the contrast behaviourally. A longer stimulus duration could potentially compensate for the longer refractory period needed by young infants and be more optimal for elicitation of an ACC.

The purpose of the present study was to investigate the effect of long-duration speech stimuli on the ACC elicited in young infants to native and nonnative consonant contrasts. By allowing more time for neural refractoriness, it is expected that ACCs will be recorded in response to the changes in both native and nonnative speech contrasts with better morphology than previously reported by Small and Werker (2012).

2. Materials and Methods

2.1. Participants. Ten adult (mean age: 29 years; range: 24 to 38 years) and 24 infant (mean age: 4 months; 11 days; range: 4 months; 0 days to 5 months; 15 days) participants with normal hearing were included in this study. Adults were recruited from the community; infants were recruited through a database managed by the Infant Studies Centre at the University of British Columbia. All adults were English-speaking and all infants were learning English as a first language and had no exposure to the Hindi language. Infant participants were screened for hearing using transient-evoked otoacoustic emission (TEOAE) with the Madsen AccuScreen Pro (GN Otometrics). One infant who did not pass the hearing screening was excluded from the study. Nine infant participants were also excluded because data collection was not completed due to crying, excessive movement, or technical problems.

2.2. Stimuli. The stimuli used in the present study were similar to those used by Small and Werker [4] and are shown in Figure 1. They were created from three speech tokens: English bilabial /ba/, dental /da/, and Hindi retroflex /Da/, which were selected from a synthetic voiced place-of-articulation continuum that was originally constructed to examine the perception of retroflex and dental-stop consonants in infants [13]. The three speech tokens were paired to form speech contrasts containing acoustic changes from /da/ to /ba/ and from /da/ to /Da/ (i.e., /daba/ and /daDa/) with no gap in between. Both speech contrasts started with the same token /da/ (denoted as S1), which was followed by one of the other two tokens /ba/ or /Da/ (denoted as S2). A third paring, /dada/, was also created to serve as a control condition

where there was no acoustic change between S1 and S2. Each stimulus was made by concatenating the two speech tokens using the Sound program in Compumedics Neuroscan Stim2.

Werker and Lalonde [13] created five formant stimuli and constructed a synthesized 16-step continuum by varying the starting frequency of F2 and F3 (second and third formants). The three speech tokens /ba/, /da/, and /Da/ selected in the present study represented equal step intervals across articulation locations and they were equivalent to the 3rd, 8th, and 13th tokens among the 16 steps, respectively. The fundamental frequency was 100 Hz for the first 100 ms then rose to 120 Hz. F1 rose from 250 to 500 Hz over a period of 50 ms while F4 and F5 remained constant at 3500 and 4000 Hz, respectively. The steady-state frequency was 1090 Hz for F2 and 2440 Hz for F3, and the transitions for both F2 and F3 lasted 50 ms. The starting frequency of F2 varied for /ba/, /da/, and /Da/, and they were 1000, 1250, and 1500 Hz, respectively. The starting frequency for F3 was 2384, 2528, and 2627 Hz for /ba/, /da/, and /Da/. Small and Werker [4] reported no significant differences in amplitudes and latencies of the P1, N1, P2, and N2 components elicited to /da/, /ba/, and /Da/ individually in adults except for N1 which had a larger amplitude to /da/ and /ba/ compared with /Da/.

In Small and Werker [4], S1S2 stimuli had a total duration of 564 ms (S1 and S2 were each 282 ms in duration) and were presented with an interstimulus interval (ISI) of 2200 ms. For the current study, the vowel portion for each of the original tokens was lengthened to a maximum 410 ms using Praat 5.3.23 software (vowel durations greater than 410 ms became distorted and sounded unnatural). The total stimulus duration for S1S2 in the present study was 816 ms (Figure 1). The longer S1S2 stimuli were presented with the same ISI as in the previous study; however, the onset-to-onset duration was necessarily increased.

The stimuli were presented at 86 dB peak SPL in the sound field. The stimuli were presented by Stim2 and then delivered to Tucker Davis Technologies PA5 and SM5 modules. The overall gain of the stimulus was reduced by 13 dB before routing it to the HB7 headphone driver which was connected to a loudspeaker placed one meter in front of the infant participant. A Larson Davis System 824 and Larson Davis Model 2559 0.5-inch random-incidence microphone placed at the approximate position of the infant's head were used to calibrate the speech stimulus in dB peak SPL.

2.3. Recordings. A four-channel electrode montage was used to record the ERPs in all participants. Individual gold-plated cup electrodes filled with electrode paste were placed at Cz, C3, M1, M2, and FPZ (International 10–20 system) and secured with tape. (Note: only the waveforms recorded at C3 that are presented as the responses at Cz were very similar.) M2 was chosen as the reference and the electrode located on the forehead served as ground. Eye-blink activity was monitored using bipolar electrodes pasted above and below the centre of the left eye. The Compumedics Neuroscan Synamps2 and SCAN 4.3 software were used to record the electroencephalograph (EEG). All interelectrode impedances were measured and kept below 5 kOhms with the SCAN 4.3 impedance routine.

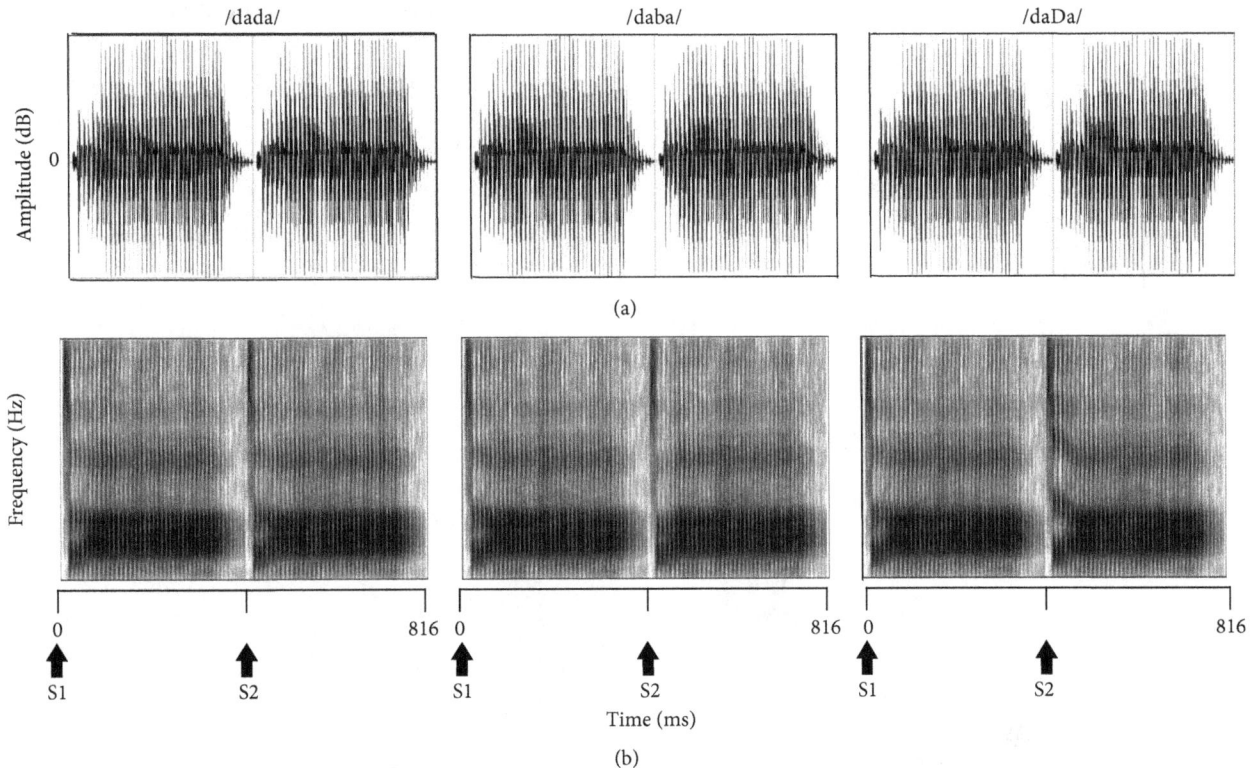

FIGURE 1: Stimuli used to elicit the acoustic change complex shown as waveforms in the time domain (a) and spectrograms (b). S1 and S2 indicate the time point where the first speech token /da/ and second speech tokens /da/, /ba/, and /Da/ begin.

During data acquisition, the EEG channels were filtered using a 30 Hz low-pass filter and a 1.0 Hz high-pass filter. The continuous EEG was amplified with a gain of 500 and converted using an analog-to-digital rate of 1000 Hz. The recording window consisted of a 100 ms prestimulus period and a 1400 ms poststimulus period. After acquisition, offline analysis used an epoch 900 ms in length (−100 prestimulus to 800 ms poststimulus). Single trials were baseline corrected across the entire sweep duration and an ocular artifact reduction was applied using an average of three epochs, which contained ocular movement greater than 250 ms epoched over −100 to 300 ms. Single trials were rejected automatically for adults when electrophysiological activity exceeded 75 μV in amplitude over a range of −100 to 800 ms; single trials were rejected manually by visual inspection for infants to optimize the number of accepted epochs in the final waveform. A minimum of 130 accepted epochs was required for each stimulus condition to be included in final data analysis based on pilot data for 4-month-old infants; fewer than 130 accepted epochs resulted in poorer morphology and replicability of averaged waveforms. The total number of recorded epochs ranged from 300 to 371 and from 260 to 483 for adults and infants, respectively. The average rejection rate was much lower for adults (5–8%) versus infants (43–48%) and resulted in 244–365 and 135–277 accepted epochs for adults and infants, respectively. A split-epoch method was used to generate two replications (i.e., odd- versus even-numbered epochs) for each condition tested. Figure 2 shows an example

of split-epoch average waveforms for each stimulus condition for individual infants.

2.4. Procedure. All tests were carried out in a double-walled sound-attenuated booth in the Pediatric Audiology Lab at the University of British Columbia. Adult participants were seated comfortably in an armed reclining chair and watched a movie with subtitles with no sound throughout testing. They were instructed to ignore the stimuli presented to them and to remain as quiet and still as possible. The infant participant was held by a parent who sat in a comfortable chair facing a loud speaker. An age-appropriate movie was played silently on a flat-screen monitor placed directly behind the loud speaker. An assistant also stayed in the booth to engage the infant's attention in order to minimize the head movement and reduce myogenic noise in the EEG.

Adults were required to complete all three stimulus conditions (i.e., /dada/, /daba/, and /daDa/) to be included in the study, while infants were required to complete at least one condition. The order of stimulus conditions was randomized for each participant. Only five infants completed more than one stimulus condition and none of them completed all three conditions. An experimenter observed the EEG during data acquisition to monitor the infant's state, muscle movement, and electrical artifact. Testing was stopped if the infant started to cry or vocalize continuously during the recording. Hearing screening was conducted in both ears at the end of the test session. The duration of the recording was approximately

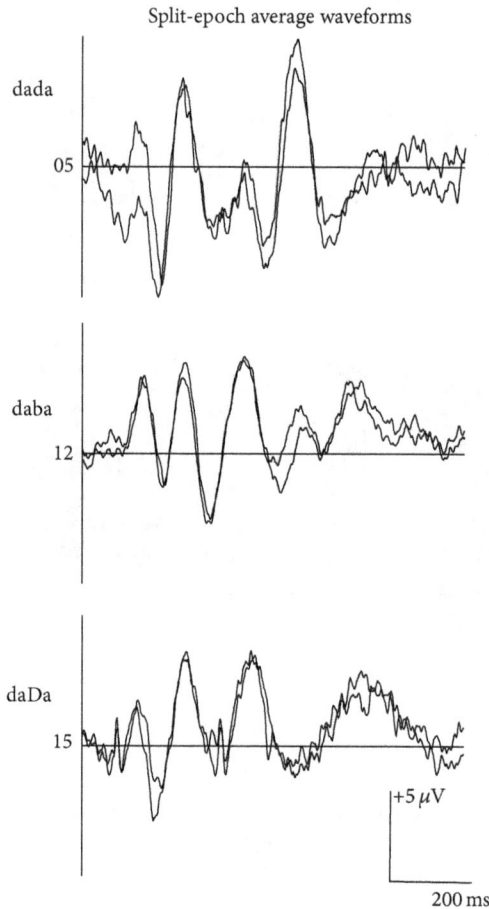

FIGURE 2: Split-epoch waveforms elicited to /dada/, /daba/, or /daDa/ for an individual infant participant for each stimulus condition.

FIGURE 3: Grand mean waveform elicited to /dada/, /daba/, and /daDa/ at C3 for 10 adult participants. The onset of the S1 and S2 portion of the S1S2 stimuli is shown at the bottom of the graph. The P1, N1, P2, and N2 components of the obligatory cortical response elicited to S1 are indicated on the graph.

1.5 hours for adults and 10 to 40 minutes for infants. After explaining the study to the adult participants and the parents of infant participants, written consent was obtained. An honorarium was given to the adult participants. A small honorarium and a gift were given to the parents and their infants at the end of the session.

2.5. *Data Analysis.* The morphology of ERP waveforms to /dada/, /daba/, and /daDa/ was compared qualitatively and the percentage of components present for each condition was calculated. The baseline-to-peak amplitude and latency of the largest peaks within each of the expected latency windows were also measured. Response latencies were measured for cortical components to S1 and S2 from the onset of S1 and the onset of S2, respectively. For amplitude measures, when the baseline was not at $0\,\mu V$ for the S2 conditions, the amplitude of P2 was measured from the negative trough preceding P2. Mean latency and amplitude values were calculated for each of the slow cortical components in response to the S1 and S2 portions of the stimulus. Peak-to-peak amplitudes for N1-P2 were also measured for adults and compared for responses elicited to S2 versus S1. Grand mean ERP waveforms to each

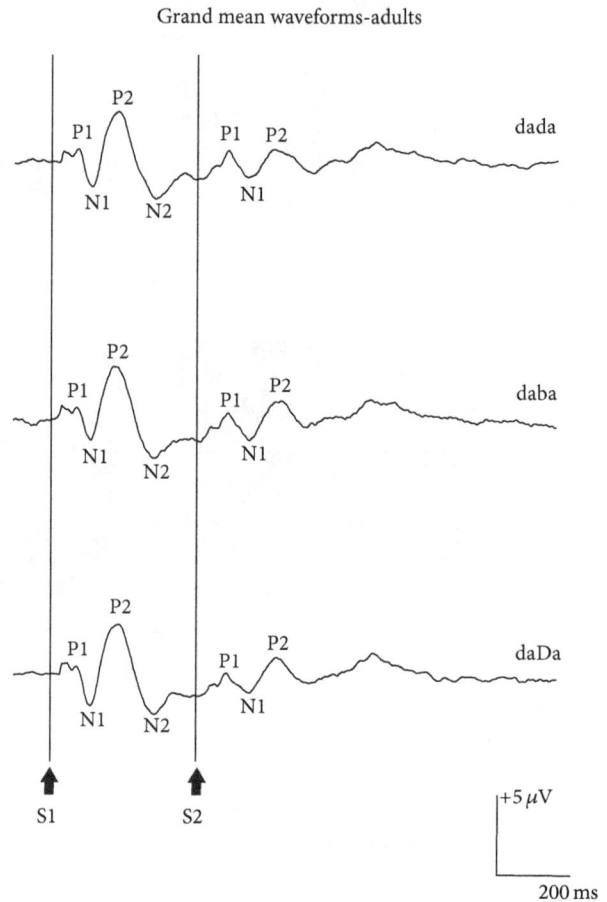

of the stimulus conditions were also compared in terms of morphology, amplitudes, and latencies.

For the adult group, two-way repeated-measures analyses of variance were carried out to compare (i) baseline-to-peak amplitudes and latencies of the P1, N1, and P2 components elicited to the S1 versus S2 portion of /dada/, /daba/, and /daDa/ and (ii) N1-P2 peak-to-peak amplitudes for S1 and S2 stimuli across stimulus conditions. For the infant group, two-way mixed-model analyses of variance were used to compare baseline-to-peak amplitudes and latencies of the P1 and N1 components evoked to the S1 versus S2 portion of /dada/, /daba/, and /daDa/. Newman-Keuls *post hoc* comparisons were performed for significant main effects. Results for all analyses were considered statistically significant if $p < 0.05$.

3. Results

3.1. Adults. As shown in Figure 3, robust P1, N1, and P2 components elicited to the onset of S1 were observed in all three conditions. A similar pattern with smaller amplitudes was also recorded for S2 and presumably in response to the acoustic change. As indicated in Table 1, clear P1 and N1

TABLE 1: Percentage of responses present for each stimulus condition for infant ($N = 8$) and adult ($N = 10$) participants. The terms "BP" and "BN" denoted "broad positive" and "broad negative" peaks, respectively.

	Token	Component	Stimulus condition		
			/dada/	/daba/	/daDa/
Infant	S1	P1	100	100	100
		N1	88	100	100
		P2	100	88	100
		N2	88	63	75
	S2	P1	100	88	100
		N1	75	75	88
		P2	75	50	38
		N2	25	38	13
		BP	0	13	38
		BN	38	13	25
Adult	S1	P1	90	100	100
		N1	90	90	90
		P2	100	100	100
		N2	100	100	100
	S2	P1	100	100	100
		N1	70	90	80
		P2	50	80	80
		N2	40	50	30

Grand mean waveforms-infants

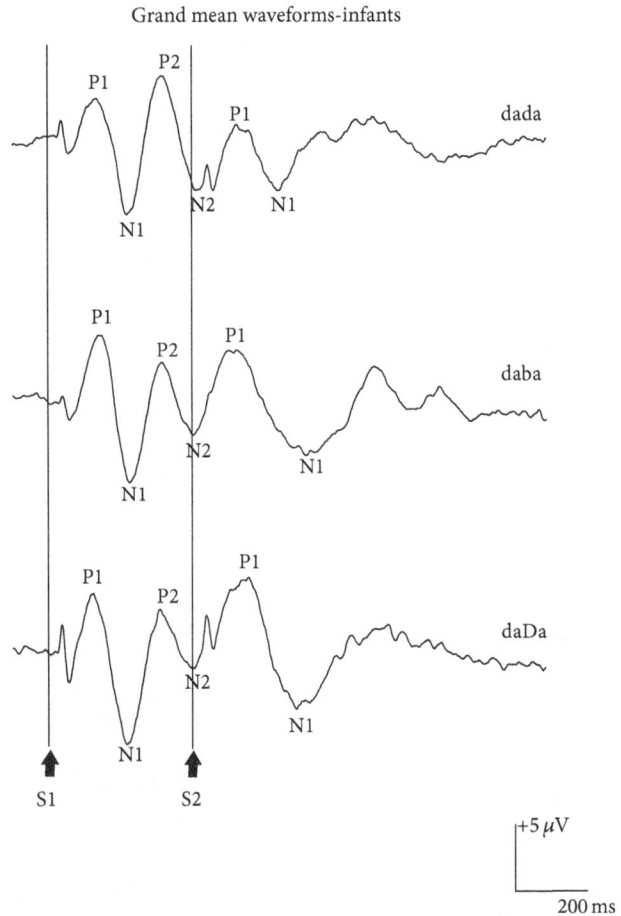

FIGURE 4: Grand mean waveform elicited to /dada/, /daba/, and /daDa/ at C3 for a total of 24 English-speaking 4-month-old infant participants with normal hearing. The onset of the S1 and S2 portion of the S1S2 stimuli is shown at the bottom of the graph. The P1, N1, P2, and N2 components of the obligatory cortical response elicited to S1 are indicated on the graph.

components were recorded in 90% of the adult participants, while P2 and N2 were present in all adults for S1 stimuli. Mean latencies elicited to S1 stimuli across stimulus conditions were 66, 110, 183, and 293 ms for P1, N1, P2, and N2, respectively, as indicated in Table 2. The mean baseline-to-peak amplitudes for the P1, N1, P2, and N2 components elicited to S1 stimuli across stimulus conditions were 1.92, −2.79, 5.34, and −3.67 μV, respectively.

The overall morphology of the waveforms recorded in response to the acoustic change from S1 to S2 (i.e., the ACC) was similar when compared across stimulus conditions /dada/, /daba/, and /daDa/ (Figure 3). For S2, the P1 component was present in all adult participants, while N1 was recorded in the majority of cases for /dada/, /daba/, and /daDa/; P2 was present in 80% of adults for /daba/ and /daDa/, but only half of the participants showed a clear P2 component for /dada/. N2 was absent in more than half of the adults. The mean latencies for S2 stimuli were on average 89, 168, and 254 ms for P1, N1, and P2, which were 23, 58, and 71 ms longer in comparison to the components evoked to S1. There were no statistically significant amplitude or latency effects for N1 or P2 with the exception that P2 amplitudes were larger and N1 latencies were longer for S2 versus S1 stimuli (Table 3). Comparisons of the peak-to-peak amplitudes for the N1-P2 complex for S1 versus S2 across stimulus conditions revealed that /daba/ was 11-12% larger compared to /dada/ and /daDa/, but this difference did not reach statistical significance [$F(2, 8) = 0.402$, $p = 0.682$]. Similar to the

pattern for individual components, the mean peak-to-peak amplitude of the N1-P2 elicited to S2 was smaller compared to S1 [$F(1, 4) = 8.251$, $p = 0.045$].

3.2. Infants. Waveform morphology was similar across conditions for the infant participants, as shown in Figure 4. Cortical responses from each of the 24 infants are shown in Figure 5. Similar to adults, cortical responses from most infant participants showed a P1-N1-P2 complex in response to the onset of the S1 stimuli; however, the P1 and N1 components were more prominent and the peak latencies were 26–222 ms later compared to the adult waveforms. A robust P1 was present in all cases and only 12% of the infants failed to show either a clear N1 in response to /dada/ or a clear P2 to /daba/. An N2 component was also found in 63–88% of the infants (Table 1). As shown in Table 4, mean amplitudes for the responses elicited to S1 were larger in comparison to adults and ranged from −9.30 to +7.46 μV; mean latencies across stimulus conditions for P1, N1, P2, and N2 were, on average, 132, 226, 320, and 415 ms, respectively.

TABLE 2: Adults: mean (1SD) baseline-to-peak amplitude and peak latency measurements for individual components of the waveform elicited to the S1 and S2 portion of the /dada/, /daba/, and /daDa/ stimulus conditions are shown. The latencies were measured from the onset of the S1 stimulus and from the onset of the change in the stimulus at S2. Mean (1SD) N1-P2 amplitudes are also indicated. Mean values that represent measurements from fewer than five responses are denoted with an asterisk (∗). The dashed line indicates that no responses were detected. The terms "BP" and "BN" denoted "broad positive" and "broad negative" peaks, respectively.

	Peak	Mean amplitude in μV (1SD)			Mean peak latency in ms (1SD)		
		/dada/	/daba/	/daDa/	/dada/	/daba/	/daDa/
S1	P1	1.86 (1.01)	2.08 (1.54)	1.82 (0.83)	68 (18)	64 (15)	65 (15)
	N1	−2.97 (1.29)	−2.30 (1.30)	−3.24 (2.50)	111 (7)	107 (15)	111 (7)
	P2	4.93 (2.65)	5.70 (2.70)	5.38 (2.58)	183 (14)	181 (19)	184 (18)
	N2	−3.43 (1.08)	−3.85 (1.73)	−3.74 (1.73)	291 (19)	299 (30)	294 (27)
	N1-P2	7.49 (3.42)	7.93 (3.20)	8.62 (4.10)			
S2	P1	1.45 (0.72)	1.40 (0.65)	2.56 (0.97)	86 (43)	65 (32)	136 (71)
	N1	−2.21 (0.40)	−2.16 (1.72)	−2.19 (0.53)	155 (63)	73 (20)	211 (103)
	P2	2.05 (1.05)	2.85 (1.29)	1.67 (1.23)	225 (18)	226 (17)	310 (124)
	N2	−0.90* (0.58)	−1.39* (1.07)	−0.71* (0.16)	291* (38)	297 (24)	309* (66)
	N1-P2	4.08 (1.63)	4.68 (1.84)	3.44 (0.79)			

TABLE 3: Adults: comparisons of amplitude and latencies for the P1 and N1 components of the slow cortical response to S1 versus S2 elicited by /dada/, /daba/, and /daDa/ using two-way repeated measures analyses of variance.

		Source	df	F	p
Amplitude	N1	Stimulus	2,8	0.888	0.339
		S1/S2	1,4	2.129	0.218
		Stimulus × S1/S2	2,8	0.633	0.555
Latency	N1	Stimulus	2,8	1.242	0.339
		S1/S2	1,4	12.38	0.025*
		Stimulus × S1/S2	2,8	1.242	0.339
Amplitude	P2	Stimulus	2,6	0.260	0.779
		S1/S2	1,3	16.197	0.028*
		Stimulus × S1/S2	2,6	1.509	0.295
Latency	P2	Stimulus	2,6	2.013	*0.214*
		S1/S2	1,3	7.137	0.076
		Stimulus × S1/S2	2,6	2.017	0.214

*Significant ($p < 0.05$).

TABLE 4: Infants: mean (1SD) baseline-to-peak amplitude and peak latency measurements for individual components of the waveform elicited to the S1 and S2 portion of the /dada/, /daba/, and /daDa/ stimulus conditions are shown. The latencies were measured from the onset of the S1 stimulus and from the onset of the change in the stimulus at S2. Mean (1SD) N1-P2 amplitudes are also indicated. Mean values that represent measurements from fewer than five responses are denoted with an asterisk (∗). The dashed line indicates that no responses were detected. The terms "BP" and "BN" denoted "broad positive" and "broad negative" peaks, respectively.

	Peak	Mean amplitude in μV (1SD)			Mean peak latency in ms (1SD)		
		/dada/	/daba/	/daDa/	/dada/	/daba/	/daDa/
S1	P1	5.25 (1.69)	6.69 (4.22)	6.19 (2.85)	133 (27)	139 (20)	124 (15)
	N1	−8.03 (4.48)	−9.13 (4.36)	−9.30 (3.69)	225 (16)	230 (24)	222 (28)
	P2	7.46 (3.46)	5.61 (2.67)	6.56 (4.04)	313 (14)	319 (29)	328 (55)
	N2	−5.81 (4.02)	−7.12 (2.37)	−3.37 (2.88)	430 (25)	432 (57)	384 (44)
	N1-P2	14.49 (6.77)	14.04 (3.64)	15.86 (6.21)			
S2	P1	3.99 (1.48)	7.81 (3.00)	9.62 (1.63)	136 (25)	134 (36)	142 (63)
	N1	−6.60 (3.22)	−10.05 (6.99)	−7.46 (3.62)	259 (48)	285 (58)	296 (31)
	P2	7.97 (5.43)	4.26* (2.58)	6.00* (5.08)	448 (69)	391* (97)	421* (34)
	N2	−4.28* (1.14)	−4.09* (3.92)	−3.71*	584* (206)	492* (124)	563*
	BP	—	4.81*	6.35* (1.24)	—	577*	518* (32)
	BN	−4.92* (0.94)	−10.09*	−5.69* (1.05)	537* (159)	319*	587* (26)
	N1-P2	14.57 (5.48)	13.69 (8.27)	17.50* (10.54)			

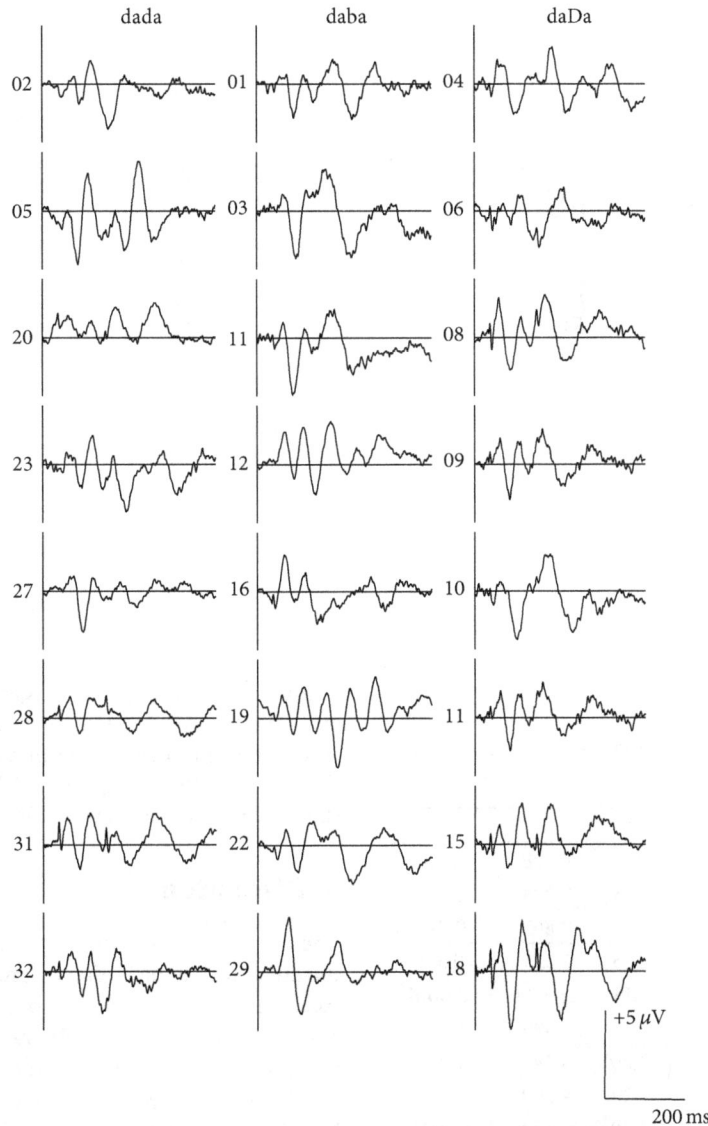

FIGURE 5: Individual waveform elicited to /dada/, /daba/, and /daDa/ at C3 for the 24 infants described in Figure 4.

The morphology of the grand mean waveform elicited to the acoustic change from S1/da/ to S2/da/, /ba/, or /Da/ resembled the morphology of the P1, N1, and P2 components of S1 responses (Figure 4); however, variability in the morphology and latency of the components was observed when the participants' waveforms were examined individually (Figure 5). All infant participants except one showed a robust P1 component and the mean peak latencies were 136, 134, and 142 ms for /dada/, /daba/, and /daDa/, respectively (Table 4). In contrast, the N1 component elicited to S2 was more variable. A clear N1 component was recorded in the majority of the participants (75–88%), but the grand mean waveform obscured some of the individual differences, resulting in later latencies and broader negative troughs for /daba/ and /daDa/ in comparison to /dada/. The mean peak latencies of N1 elicited to S2 were 259, 285, and 296 ms for /dada/, /daba/, and /daDa/ indicating that S2 responses occurred 34, 55, and 74 ms later compared with S1 responses. For each

of the stimulus conditions, the N1 component elicited to S2 either was absent or resembled a broad negative peak in 1-2 infants while the remaining infants had N1 peaks that varied in latency (more variability than what was observed for P1). A second positive peak that resembled P2 was also present in five out of eight infants for /dada/; however, P2 was present for fewer than half of the infants for /daba/ and /daDa/ and the latencies were more variable compared to /dada/. As a result, only /dada/ had a discernible S2 P2 peak in the grand mean waveform (Tables 1 and 4).

The results of a two-way mixed model ANOVA comparing the mean amplitudes of P1 and N1 elicited to S1 and S2 across the three stimulus conditions for infants are summarized in Table 5. There was a significant main effect of stimulus condition for P1 amplitudes, as shown in Figure 6, which was explained by a significantly smaller amplitude for /dada/ compared to /daba/ or /daDa/. The amplitude effect for S1 versus the S2 stimulus was marginally significant

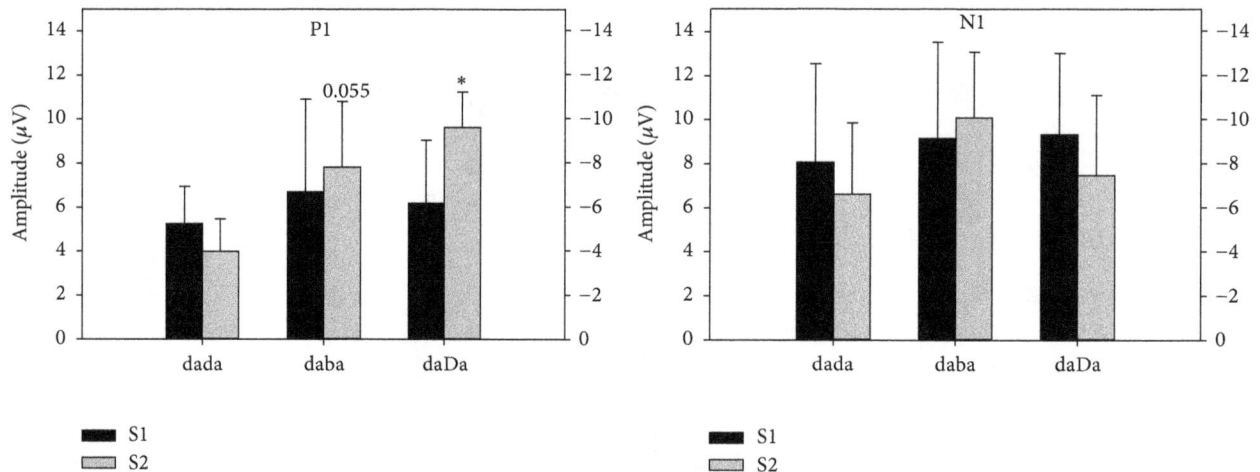

FIGURE 6: Infant: baseline-to-peak amplitude of the P1 and N1 components elicited to the S1 and S2 portion of the /dada/, /daba/, and /daDa/ stimulus conditions is shown. An asterisk (∗) denotes the statistical significance of results ($p < 0.05$); "0.055" denotes a p value that approached significance.

TABLE 5: Infants: comparisons of amplitude and latencies for the N1 and P1 components of the slow cortical response to S1 versus S2 elicited by /dada/, /daba/, and /daDa/ using two-way mixed-model measures analyses of variance.

		Source	df	F	p
Amplitude	N1	Stimulus	2,15	0.278	0.761
		S1/S2	1,15	0.924	0.352
		Stimulus × S1/S2	2,15	0.867	0.444
Latency	N1	Stimulus	2,15	1.035	0.379
		S1/S2	1,15	28.809	<0.0001∗
		Stimulus × S1/S2	2,15	2.599	0.107
Amplitude	P1	Stimulus	2,20	4.741	0.021∗
		S1/S2	1,20	4.309	0.051
		Stimulus × S1/S2	2,20	5.350	0.014∗
Latency	P1	Stimulus	2,20	0.020	0.980
		S1/S2	1,20	0.382	0.543
		Stimulus × S1/S2	2,20	0.566	0.577

∗Significant ($p < 0.05$).

and was explained by a larger mean P1 amplitude for the S2 condition. A significant interaction between S1 versus S2 and stimulus condition was also revealed for P1 amplitudes. The P1 amplitude elicited to S1 was larger than P1 elicited to S2 for /dada/, while the opposite pattern was found for /daba/ and /daDa/ (Figure 6). *Post hoc* comparisons using the Newman-Keuls test showed that the amplitudes of S2 P1 were significantly larger for /daDa/ versus /dada/ ($p = 0.003$) and marginally significantly larger for /daba/ versus /dada/ ($p = 0.055$). No statistically significant differences were revealed for P1 latencies.

In contrast to P1, N1 had the largest mean amplitudes elicited to both S1 and S2 across all stimulus conditions (Table 4), indicating its prominence in the morphology of the slow cortical responses recorded in infants. Although the

amplitude of S2 N1 was larger for /daba/ than for /dada/ and /daDa/ by visual inspection, a two-way mixed-model ANOVA did not reveal significant effects for N1 amplitudes. There were also no significant latency effects for N1 except that latencies were later for the responses to S2 versus S1.

4. Discussion

The results of the present study using a long stimulus duration for /dada/, /daba/, and /daDa/ resulted in similar ACC findings for adults and more robust ACCs in infants compared to Small and Werker [4]. In the present study, the differences in ACC magnitude across stimulus conditions for the adults were not statistically significant, although the N1-P2 grand mean ACC tended to be slightly larger for /daba/, similar to the findings of Small and Werker [4]. For infants, the morphology of the ACC was more complex for all three stimulus conditions. Robust P1 and N1 components were present in the majority of the participants, while fewer infants had a clear P2. For the /dada/ condition, most of the infant participants had the different components of the ACC, which were similar to the P1-N1-P2 complex recorded at the onset of the S1 token. Fewer infants had all three components of the ACC in response to /daba/ and /daDa/, and the morphology of the ACC elicited to these stimuli was more variable compared with ACCs to /dada/; in these cases, a broad negative peak or positive peak occurred at approximately 319 to 605 ms instead of distinct N1 and P2 peaks appearing earlier in the waveform between 179 and 510 ms. The amplitude of P1 elicited to the S2 token of the control condition /dada/ was significantly smaller compared with that of the S2 P1 to the experimental stimulus conditions /daba/ and /daDa/, suggesting that the brain discriminated between the control /da/ and the experimental S2 tokens.

Small and Werker [4] reported that only the infant ACC elicited to /daba/ consisted of P1, N1, and P2 components in their study, while the cortical response to the S2 of /dada/ and /daDa/ were comprised primarily of broad positive and negative peaks. The findings of the present study suggest that, by extending the stimulus length, allowing longer time to accommodate the longer neuronal refractory period for infants, better-defined components of the ACC can be recorded and the overall morphology of the grand mean waveforms are improved. Research has shown that age-related changes in myelination, synaptic refinement, and cortical fiber density underlie the maturation in latency, amplitude, and refractoriness of the cortical component [39, 40]. The formation of myelin along the axon increases the conduction velocity of a signal in transmission, and consequently affects the timing of subsequent signal propagation [41]. Because the latency and synchrony of the neuronal signal are affected by myelination, the evoked potential will have shorter latency, increased amplitude, and more defined waveform morphology with maturation [42]. Incomplete myelination and synaptogenesis will lead to longer neuronal refractory periods and lower cortical excitability in the immature central auditory system [32]. Despite these immaturities, Martin [6] and Martin et al. [7] found that it was more efficient to elicit an infant ACC to the vowel contrast /ui/ for an ISI of 250 ms compared to 500 and 1000 ms. They also found that presentation of a stimulus that continuously alternated was more efficient than an interrupted stimulus. However, they did not investigate separate components of the ACC or the effects of stimulus duration. Our results suggest that long-duration stimuli are needed to elicit robust ACCs with distinct components in infants (and possibly young children), at least for consonant contrasts.

Our findings support that the infant's brain can detect a change in the stimulus from /da/ to /da/, /ba/, and /Da/. Moreover, the larger P1 amplitudes recorded for /daba/ and /daDa/ may suggest that the brain has noticed that the acoustic change from /da/ to /da/ was smaller than the change from /da/ to /ba/ and from /da/ to /Da/. In our hypothesis, we had predicted that the ACC for both /daba/ and /daDa/ would have larger amplitudes and more distinct components compared with the ACC to /dada/ because behavioral studies had shown that English-learning infants under 6 months of age were able to discriminate the native /daba/ and nonnative /daDa/ contrasts [13, 43, 44]. Our findings revealed that the P1 amplitudes elicited to S2 of the experimental conditions /daba/ and /daDa/ were indeed significantly larger than that of the control condition /dada/, which supported our hypothesis. This result is consistent with other research findings, which have shown that speech tokens can evoke distinct neural response patterns; for example, synthesized voiced tokens have been reported to evoke responses that are larger in amplitude when compared with responses evoked by voiceless stimuli [11, 45].

Interestingly, our adult group did not show the same significant differences in the amplitudes of ACC components that we found for the infant group. We had expected a larger difference between the ACCs to /daba/ and the other two stimuli because both /dada/ and /daDa/ should have acted as "control" stimuli for the adults. A contributing factor might have been that the stimulus parameters that

were more optimal for infants were too long for adults. The speech stimulus used in the present study consisted of two consonant-vowel structures (CVCV), which was different from the typical CV (e.g., /da/) or VV (e.g., /ui/) stimulus used to elicit cortical responses. Although we only focused on the acoustic change between two CV syllables, the brief transition from consonant to vowel within a CV token may have also evoked cortical responses resulting in overlapping cortical waveforms thus affecting the overall morphology of the ACC [46]. Perhaps the longer duration of the CV syllable was not perceived as one syllable by the adults, so that cortical responses evoked by the brief change from the consonant to the vowel within a CV syllable affected the response to the change from /da/ to the other speech tokens.

There are some limitations to the current study. As mentioned above, the nonnative speech token might have reduced the impact of auditory experience. For example, a MMN study using similar Hindi speech contrasts reported that the magnitude of the MMN can be significantly affected by the order of stimulus presentation (i.e., the magnitude of the MMN is larger when /da/ is the standard stimuli and when /Da/ is the deviant) [47]. Therefore, there may be an order effect, that is, the amplitude of the ACC elicited to /daba/ may be different when compared to /bada/ which we did not assess. Also, we only investigated one set of consonant contrasts so we cannot rule out a stimulus effect; ACCs to a range of different contrasts should be assessed to confirm that this tool is an accurate index of discrimination capacity.

5. Conclusion

The most important finding of the present study is that an ACC to a change within a speech stimulus can be successfully recorded in young infants, and, by extending the stimulus length and allowing more time to accommodate the longer neuronal refractory period for infants, better-defined components of the ACC can be elicited. Our ACC results also suggest that distinct neural response patterns may be elicited to acoustic changes that vary in degree. In the present study, ACC components had larger amplitudes in response to a larger acoustic change within a stimulus. To confirm that the ACC is sensitive to a range of subtle acoustic changes in speech, more research is needed. As a technique in development, the ACC may hold promise for providing insight into the infant brain's capacity to discriminate the acoustic features of speech.

Disclosure

Portions of this paper were presented at the Academy Research Conference 2014, Audiology Now! Conference, (Orlando, USA, March 26, 2014), and the Hearing Across the Lifespan Conference 2014, (Cernobbio, Italy, June 5–7, 2014).

Conflict of Interests

The authors declare that there is no conflict of interests regarding the publication of this paper.

Acknowledgments

The authors thank Drs. Janet Werker and Priya Kandhadai for creating the stimuli for this study and Dr. Werker for her assistance with the recruitment of infants. The authors also thank the families who generously gave their time and patience to help with this research. This research was supported by Discovery Grants from the Natural Sciences and Engineering Research Council of Canada to Dr. Janet Werker (81103) and Dr. Susan Small (355927-09).

References

[1] E. Kaukoranta, R. Hari, and O. V. Lounasmaa, "Responses of the human auditory cortex to vowel onset after fricative consonants," *Experimental Brain Research*, vol. 69, no. 1, pp. 19–23, 1987.

[2] B. A. Martin and A. Boothroyd, "Cortical, auditory, event-related potentials in response to periodic and aperiodic stimuli with the same spectral envelope," *Ear and Hearing*, vol. 20, no. 1, pp. 33–44, 1999.

[3] J. M. Ostroff, B. A. Martin, and A. Boothroyd, "Cortical evoked response to acoustic change within a syllable," *Ear and Hearing*, vol. 19, no. 4, pp. 290–297, 1998.

[4] S. A. Small and J. F. Werker, "Does the ACC have potential as an index of early speech-discrimination ability? A preliminary study in 4-month-old infants with normal hearing," *Ear and Hearing*, vol. 33, no. 6, pp. e59–e59, 2012.

[5] A. S. Martinez, L. S. Eisenberg, and A. Boothroyd, "The acoustic change complex in young children with hearing loss: a preliminary study," *Seminars in Hearing*, vol. 34, no. 4, pp. 278–287, 2013.

[6] B. A. Martin, "The effects of stimulus alternation rate on the efficiency of the acoustic change complex in infants and toddlers," in *Proceedings of the 24th Biennial Symposium of the International Evoked Response Audiometry Study Group*, Busan, Republic of Korea, May 2015.

[7] B. A. Martin, L. S. Goldin, and R. M. Antony, "Efficient stimulus presentation strategies for eliciting the acoustic change complex in infants," in *Proceedings of the 24th Biennial Symposium of the International Evoked Response Audiometry Study Group*, Busan, Republic of Korea, May 2015.

[8] B. A. Martin and A. Boothroyd, "Cortical, auditory, evoked potentials in response to changes of spectrum and amplitude," *The Journal of the Acoustical Society of America*, vol. 107, article 2155, 2000.

[9] B. A. Martin, "Can the acoustic change complex be recorded in an individual with a cochlear implant? Separating neural responses from cochlear implant artifact," *Journal of the American Academy of Audiology*, vol. 18, no. 2, pp. 126–140, 2007.

[10] B. A. Martin, A. Boothroyd, D. Ali, and T. Leach-Berth, "Stimulus presentation strategies for eliciting the acoustic change complex: increasing efficiency," *Ear and Hearing*, vol. 31, no. 3, pp. 356–366, 2010.

[11] K. L. Tremblay, L. Friesen, B. A. Martin, and R. Wright, "Test-retest reliability of cortical evoked potentials using naturally produced speech sounds," *Ear and Hearing*, vol. 24, no. 3, pp. 225–232, 2003.

[12] L. M. Friesen and K. L. Tremblay, "Acoustic change complexes recorded in adult cochlear implant listeners," *Ear and Hearing*, vol. 27, no. 6, pp. 678–685, 2006.

[13] J. F. Werker and C. E. Lalonde, "Cross-language speech perception: initial capabilities and developmental change," *Developmental Psychology*, vol. 24, no. 5, pp. 672–683, 1988.

[14] P. D. Eimas, E. R. Siqueland, P. Jusczyk, and J. Vigorito, "Speech perception in infants," *Science*, vol. 171, no. 3968, pp. 303–306, 1971.

[15] V. M. Little, D. G. Thomas, and M. R. Letterman, "Single-trial analyses of developmental trends in infant auditory event-related potentials," *Developmental Neuropsychology*, vol. 16, no. 3, pp. 455–478, 1999.

[16] D. L. Molfese, "Predicting dyslexia at 8 years of age using neonatal brain responses," *Brain and Language*, vol. 72, no. 3, pp. 238–245, 2000.

[17] J. L. Wunderlich and B. K. Cone-Wesson, "Maturation of CAEP in infants and children: a review," *Hearing Research*, vol. 212, no. 1-2, pp. 212–223, 2006.

[18] M. Golding, S. C. Purdy, M. Sharma, and H. Dillon, "The effect of stimulus duration and inter-stimulus interval on cortical responses in infants," *Australian and New Zealand Journal of Audiology*, vol. 28, no. 2, pp. 122–136, 2006.

[19] R. Čeponienė, M. Cheour, and R. Näätänen, "Interstimulus interval and auditory event-related potentials in children: evidence for multiple generators," *Electroencephalography and Clinical Neurophysiology/Evoked Potentials Section*, vol. 108, no. 4, pp. 345–354, 1998.

[20] P. M. Gilley, A. Sharma, M. Dorman, and K. Martin, "Developmental changes in refractoriness of the cortical auditory evoked potential," *Clinical Neurophysiology*, vol. 116, no. 3, pp. 648–657, 2005.

[21] D. Kurtzberg, P. L. Hilpert, J. A. Kreuzer, and H. G. Vaughan Jr., "Differential maturation of cortical auditory evoked potentials to speech sounds in normal fullterm and very low-birthweight infants," *Developmental Medicine and Child Neurology*, vol. 26, no. 4, pp. 466–475, 1984.

[22] E. S. Orlrich, A. B. Barnet, I. P. Weiss, and B. L. Shanks, "Auditory evoked potential development in early childhood: a longitudinal study," *Electroencephalography and Clinical Neurophysiology*, vol. 44, no. 4, pp. 411–423, 1978.

[23] J. J. Rotteveel, E. J. Colon, D. F. Stegeman, and Y. M. Visco, "The maturation of the central auditory conduction in preterm infants until three months post term. IV. Composite group averages of the cortical auditory evoked responses (ACRs)," *Hearing Research*, vol. 27, no. 1, pp. 85–93, 1987.

[24] D. W. Shucard, J. L. Shucard, and D. G. Thomas, "Auditory event-related potentials in waking infants and adults: a developmental perspective," *Electroencephalography and Clinical Neurophysiology/ Evoked Potentials*, vol. 68, no. 4, pp. 303–310, 1987.

[25] J. L. Wunderlich, B. K. Cone-Wesson, and R. Shepherd, "Maturation of the cortical auditory evoked potential in infants and young children," *Hearing Research*, vol. 212, no. 1-2, pp. 185–202, 2006.

[26] R. Rita, T. Rinne, and R. Näätänen, "Maturation of cortical sound processing as indexed by event-related potentials," *Clinical Neurophysiology*, vol. 113, no. 6, pp. 870–882, 2002.

[27] J. J. Eggermont and C. W. Ponton, "Auditory-evoked potential studies of cortical maturation in normal hearing and implanted children: correlations with changes in structure and speech perception," *Acta Oto-Laryngologica*, vol. 123, no. 2, pp. 249–252, 2003.

[28] C. W. Ponton, M. Don, J. J. Eggermont, M. D. Waring, and A. Masuda, "Maturation of human cortical auditory function:

differences between normal-hearing children and children with cochlear implants," *Ear and Hearing*, vol. 17, no. 5, pp. 430–437, 1996.

[29] C. W. Ponton, J. J. Eggermont, B. Kwong, and M. Don, "Maturation of human central auditory system activity: evidence from multi-channel evoked potentials," *Clinical Neurophysiology*, vol. 111, no. 2, pp. 220–236, 2000.

[30] C. Ponton, J. J. Eggermont, D. Khosla, B. Kwong, and M. Don, "Maturation of human central auditory system activity: separating auditory evoked potentials by dipole source modeling," *Clinical Neurophysiology*, vol. 113, no. 3, pp. 407–420, 2002.

[31] A. Sharma, N. Kraus, T. J. McGee, and T. G. Nicol, "Developmental changes in P1 and N1 central auditory responses elicited by consonant-vowel syllables," *Electroencephalography and Clinical Neurophysiology/Evoked Potentials Section*, vol. 104, no. 6, pp. 540–545, 1997.

[32] W. W. Surwillo, "Recovery of the cortical evoked potential from auditory stimulation in children and adults," *Developmental Psychobiology*, vol. 14, no. 1, pp. 1–12, 1981.

[33] E. Kushnerenko, R. Eponiene, P. Balan, V. Fellman, M. Huotilainen, and R. Näätänen, "Maturation of the auditory event-related potentials during the first year of life," *NeuroReport*, vol. 13, no. 1, pp. 47–51, 2002.

[34] R. Paetau, A. Ahonen, O. Salonen, and M. Sams, "Auditory evoked magnetic fields to tones and pseudowords in healthy children and adults," *Journal of Clinical Neurophysiology*, vol. 12, no. 2, pp. 177–185, 1995.

[35] I. Czigler, G. Csibra, and A. Csontos, "Age and inter-stimulus interval effects on event-related potentials to frequent and infrequent auditory stimuli," *Biological Psychology*, vol. 33, no. 2-3, pp. 195–206, 1992.

[36] M. Sharma, P. K. H. Johnson, S. C. Purdy, and F. Norman, "Effect of interstimulus interval and age on cortical auditory evoked potentials in 10–22-week-old infants," *NeuroReport*, vol. 25, no. 4, pp. 248–254, 2014.

[37] T. W. Picton, D. L. Woods, and G. B. Proulx, "Human auditory sustained potentials. I. The nature of the response," *Electroencephalography and Clinical Neurophysiology*, vol. 45, no. 2, pp. 186–197, 1978.

[38] R. Näätänen and T. Picton, "The N1 wave of the human electric and magnetic response to sound: a review and an analysis of the component structure," *Psychophysiology*, vol. 24, no. 4, pp. 375–425, 1987.

[39] P. R. Huttenlocher and A. S. Dabholkar, "Regional differences in synaptogenesis in human cerebral cortex," *The Journal of Comparative Neurology*, vol. 387, no. 2, pp. 167–178, 1997.

[40] J. K. Moore and Y.-L. Guan, "Cytoarchitectural and axonal maturation in human auditory cortex," *Journal of the Association for Research in Otolaryngology*, vol. 2, no. 4, pp. 297–311, 2001.

[41] A. Salamy, "Commissural transmission: maturational changes in humans," *Science*, vol. 200, no. 4348, pp. 1409–1411, 1978.

[42] F. E. Musiek, S. B. Verkest, and K. M. Gollegly, "Effects of neuromaturation on auditory-evoked potentials," *Seminars in Hearing*, vol. 9, no. 1, pp. 1–13, 1988.

[43] J. F. Werker, J. H. Gilbert, K. Humphrey, and R. C. Tees, "Developmental aspects of cross-language speech perception," *Child Development*, vol. 52, no. 1, pp. 349–355, 1981.

[44] J. F. Werker and R. C. Tees, "Cross-language speech perception: evidence for perceptual reorganization during the first year of life," *Infant Behavior and Development*, vol. 7, no. 1, pp. 49–63, 1984.

[45] M. Steinschneider, I. O. Volkov, M. D. Noh, P. C. Garell, and M. A. Howard III, "Temporal encoding of the voice onset time phonetic parameter by field potentials recorded directly from human auditory cortex," *Journal of Neurophysiology*, vol. 82, no. 5, pp. 2346–2357, 1999.

[46] M. K. Ganapathy, V. K. Narne, M. K. Kalaiah, and P. Manjula, "Effect of pre-transition stimulus duration on acoustic change complex," *International Journal of Audiology*, vol. 52, no. 5, pp. 350–359, 2013.

[47] V. C. K. Tsui, *Mismatch negativity cortical event-related potential measures of cross-linguistic phoneme perception [M.Sc. thesis]*, Faculty of Graduate Studies (School of Audiology & Speech Sciences), University of British Columbia, Vancouver, Canada, 2000.

11

Gastric Decompression Decreases Postoperative Nausea and Vomiting in ENT Surgery

Kerem Erkalp,[1] **Nuran Kalekoglu Erkalp,**[2] **M. Salih Sevdi,**[1] **A. Yasemin Korkut,**[3]
Hacer Yeter,[1] **Sertuğ Sinan Ege,**[1] **Aysin Alagol,**[1] **and Veysel Erden**[4]

[1] *Istanbul Bagcilar Educational and Training Hospital, 34200 Istanbul, Turkey*
[2] *Ventigoo ENT and Balance Center, 34180 Istanbul, Turkey*
[3] *Istanbul Sisli Etfal Training Hospital, 34360 Istanbul, Turkey*
[4] *Istanbul Educational and Research Hospital, 34104 Istanbul, Turkey*

Correspondence should be addressed to Kerem Erkalp; keremerkalp@hotmail.com

Academic Editor: Charles Monroe Myer

There is a passive blood flow to the stomach during oral and nasal surgery. It may cause postoperative nausea and vomiting (PONV). We researched the relationship between gastric decompression (GD) and severity of PONV in ear, nose, and throat (ENT) surgery. 137 patients who have been into ENT surgery were included in the study. In Group I ($n = 70$), patients received GD after surgery before extubation; patients in Group II ($n = 67$) did not receive GD. In postoperative 2nd, 4th, 8th, and 12th hours, the number and ratio of patients demonstrating PONV were detected to be significantly more in Group II as compared to Group I. PONV was also significantly more severe in Group II as compared to Group I. In Group I, the PONV ratio in the 2nd hour was significantly more for those whose amounts of stomach content aspired were more than 10 mL as compared to those whose stomach content aspired was less than 10 mL. In the 4th, 8th, and 24th hours, there is no statistically significant difference between the stomach content aspired and PONV ratio. GD reduces the incidence and severity of PONV in ENT surgery.

1. Introduction

Postoperative nausea and vomiting (PONV) may develop due to risk factors associated with surgery as well as characteristics of patients [1]. General incidence of PONV is in the range of 20–30% while it increases up to 30–70% after ear, nose, and throat (ENT) surgery [2–4]. Risk factors may include early age, female sex, tobacco addiction, type of the surgery applied, history of PONV after surgical procedures previously applied, motion sickness, gastroparesis, obesity, and postoperative analgesic use of opioids [2, 3, 5].

PONV management includes single dose or multimodal antiemetic use, steroid treatment, and intravenous fluid support [6]. Additionally, it is suggested to reduce the use of opioid analgesics in postoperative pain control and it is preferred to use nonopioid analgesics [6]. Other treatment options are P-6 acupuncture point stimulation and perioperative gastric decompression (GD) practices [7, 8].

In ENT surgery, there is a passive blood flow to the stomach during the process [9, 10]. In literature, some studies demonstrate that removing swallowed blood through GD decreases PONV incidence, while there are also reports stating that it increases the incidence [9, 10].

In our study, we have researched the relationship between GD and PONV incidence and the correlation of the amount of contents aspired from the stomach with the severity of PONV.

2. Material and Method

Our study was conducted on 137 patients undergoing tonsillectomy, septoplasty, tympanoplasty, tympanomastoidectomy, adenoidectomy, adenotonsillectomy, microlaryngeal surgery, septorhinoplasty, dacryocystorhinostomy, functional endoscopic sinus surgery, neck dissection, thyroidectomy, septal concha radiofrequency application, and uvulopalatoplasty in an ENT surgery room, after obtaining an approval certificate from the hospital's local ethics committee and individual permissions from patients. In a six-month period (September 2010–April 2011), patients aged between 18 and 65 years and whose ASA risk condition is I/II/III were included in the study.

Patients with previous PONV history, motion sickness history, antiemetic drug allergy history, Meniere's disease, major cancer surgery, a hunger period shorter than 8 hours before elective surgery, kidney and liver disease, upper respiratory system pathology, a history of using antiemetic drugs, morbid obesity, and pregnancy were excluded from the study. Additionally, patients were excluded from the study in cases where major complications developed during surgery; surgery lasted for longer than 180 minutes and antiemetic drugs or steroids were used in the perioperative period.

All the cases were examined in terms of anesthesia one day before the operation. With the laboratory tests, all patients were controlled in terms of their blood count, coagulation parameters, electrolyte values, liver enzyme values (SGOT, SGPT), BUN, creatinine, and hunger blood glucose values.

The patients were separated into two groups by a nurse in the preparation room through a closed envelop method. While patients in Group I ($n = 70$) which is determined as study group received GD, the patients in Group II ($n = 67$) which is determined as control group did not receive GD.

Patients were taken to the operating room without receiving premedication. After tree-channel electrocardiogram (ECG), noninvasive blood pressure and peripheral oxygen saturation (SpO_2) monitoring were provided, the vascular access was opened with 22 gauge (G) intravenous cannula from the veins on the left hand, and Isolyte solution was infused with the pace of 8 mL/kg/hour. In anesthesia induction, 2-3 mg/kg propofol, 1 μg/kg fentanyl, and 0.6 mg/kg rocuronium for neuromuscular blockage were applied. After applying 6 L-100% oxygen for 3 minutes through the face mask, endotracheal intubation was performed. Ventilation was provided for all patients in volume-controlled ventilation mode as 50-50% air-O_2, 2 L/min. flow, and 1-2% sevoflurane (Datex-Ohmeda, S/5 Avance, GE Healthcare, USA). During ventilation, respiration frequency was adjusted to 12/min, inspiration and expiration rate was adjusted to be 1 : 2, and tidal volume was adjusted to be 8 mL kg^{-1}. The patients received 20 mg/kg iv paracetamol as postoperative analgesic. After the surgery finished, inhalation agents were closed and 100% oxygen was applied as 6 L/dk. The patients in Group I received CH14, 53 cm Mully suction catheter (Unomedical, ConvaTec Limited, UK), and GD process via oral access through airway (number 3). After the distal of the suction catheter was placed into the stomach, we waited for passive drainage of air. Then, the stomach contents were aspirated with a 50 mL feeding injector. Calculating the intraluminal volume of CH14, 53 cm suction catheter as 5 mL, the amount of stomach content suctioned with an injector was measured. After the drainage of stomach content through suction was finalized, the catheter was removed. The amount of stomach content aspirated during the period of GD process (minute) was recorded as "less than 10 mL" or "more than 10 mL."

Oral airway (number 3) was also placed to the patients in Group II but GD was not applied. After the spontaneous respiration began in patients, neuromuscular block, atropine as 0.01 mg/kg, and neostigmine as 0.05 mg/kg were recovered. When the spontaneous respiratory effort was enough, the patients were extubated. After extubation, patients were kept in a 30° head-up position and all patients received 6 L/min oxygen. PONV was evaluated as being present or absent as compared to the severity in the 1st, 4th, 8th, and 24th hours. In patients who demonstrated PONV, it was recorded as mild (mild nausea, vomiting once, and nausea through an outer stimulant [eating, drinking, and motion]), moderate (vomiting twice, mild nausea without an outer stimulant, and antiemetic medication need once), and severe (vomiting more than twice, severe nausea, antiemetic medication need more than once) [11]. Patients with moderate and severe PONV received 10 mg metoclopramide iv in antiemetic medication. Neither of the patient groups received opioid or antiemetic medication in intraoperative or postoperative periods.

Statistical Method. In supplementary statistics of the data, mean, standard deviation, ratio, and frequency values were used. The distribution of the variants was controlled through a Kolmogorov-Smirnov test. In analysis of quantitative data, an independent sampling t-test and Mann-Whitney U test were used. In analysis of the qualitative data, a chi-square test was used; when the conditions could not be obtained for a chi-square test, a Fischer test was used. $P < 0.05$ was considered to be statistically significant. The SPSS 20.0 program was used for analysis.

3. Results

Demographic data and anesthesia and surgery duration of patients in Group I and Group II were demonstrated in Table 1.

Average GD duration in Group I was 127.88 ± 45.54 seconds.

In postoperative 2nd, 4th, 8th, and 24th hours, the number and ratio of patients demonstrating PONV were detected to be significantly more in Group II as compared to Group I (Table 2). PONV was also significantly more severe in Group II as compared to Group I (Table 3).

In Group I, the PONV ratio in the 2nd hour was significantly more for those whose amounts of stomach content aspired was more than 10 mL as compared to those whose stomach content aspired was less than 10 mL. In the 4th, 8th, and 24th hours, there is no statistically significant difference between the stomach content aspired and PONV ratio (Table 4).

4. Discussion

PONV incidence may increase up to 70% in patients undergoing ENT surgery [1, 4]. In these patients, for whom inpatient surgery is quite common, PONV is an important

TABLE 1: Demographic data and anesthesia and surgery duration of patients in Group I and Group II.

	Group I Mean ± SD/n %		Group II Mean ± SD/n %		P
Age (year)		33.5 ± 14.0		34.2 ± 13.0	0.245
Gender					
Female	29	41.4%	31	46.3%	0.568
Male	41	58.6%	36	53.7%	
BMI (kg/m^2)		24.6 ± 4.2		23.6 ± 3.3	0.121
ASA					
I	58	82.9%	50	74.6%	
II	10	14.3%	16	23.9%	0.238
III	2	2.9%	1	1.5%	
Anesthesia duration (minute)		65.3 ± 38.6		71.2 ± 36.2	0.113
Surgery duration (minute)		52.4 ± 32.0		57.5 ± 35.0	0.065
Surgery type	Tonsillectomy $n = 5$ Septoplasty $n = 9$ Tympanoplasty $n = 3$ Tympanomastoidectomy $n = 2$ Adenoidectomy $n = 6$ Adenotonsillectomy $n = 5$ Microlaryngeal surgery $n = 4$ Septorhinoplasty $n = 6$ Dacryocystorhinostomy $n = 3$ Functional endoscopic sinus surgery $n = 7$ Neck dissection $n = 4$ Thyroidectomy $n = 3$ Septal concha radiofrequency application $n = 9$ Uvulopalatoplasty $n = 4$ ($n = \mathbf{70}$)		Tonsillectomy $n = 4$ Septoplasty $n = 11$ Tympanoplasty $n = 2$ Tympanomastoidectomy $n = 2$ Adenoidectomy $n = 5$ Adenotonsillectomy $n = 6$ Microlaryngeal surgery $n = 5$ Septorhinoplasty $n = 7$ Dacryocystorhinostomy $n = 2$ Functional endoscopic sinus surgery $n = 5$ Neck dissection $n = 4$ Thyroidectomy $n = 4$ Septal concha radiofrequency application $n = 7$ Uvulopalatoplasty $n = 3$ ($n = \mathbf{67}$)		0.216

indicator of patient satisfaction [12]. In addition to psychological effects, PONV may lead to airway obstruction, aspiration pneumonia, subcutaneous emphysema, bleeding, opening and latency of healing in incisions, increase of intracranial pressure, dehydration, electrolyte imbalance, malnutrition due to insufficiency of oral intake, lengthening in hospitalization period, and increased costs [1, 13, 14].

In patients undergoing ENT surgery, it is reported that the reason of PONV is blood flow to the stomach during the intraoperative and postoperative periods and surgical procedures applied in intraoperative period [6, 8, 15]. Direct stimulation of the chemoreceptor trigger zone through mucosal damage and accompanying pharyngeal edema is also effective in PONV formation [6, 8, 15]. Another reason for PONV is that oropharynx and stomach chemoreceptors and mechanoreceptors are activated when the trigeminal nerve is stimulated [6, 8, 15, 16]. The factors increasing PONV risk may include postoperative pain, anxiety, vertigo, early mobilization, early oral intake, and opioid analgesics [17, 18]. Additionally, it has been stated that PONV risk associated with gastric distension may increase in patients where the air pressure increases over 25 cm H_2O during ventilation with a mask [15].

Many methods have been used in order to decrease PONV incidence in ENT surgery. Prophylactic and treatment-purpose use of antiemetics is the most common [6,

18, 19]; it is frequently applied by anesthesiologists in gastric decompression. We are of the opinion that every anesthesiologist should apply GD to patients whether the patient is aware or not. The orogastric method is more easily, safely, and frequently used than the nasogastric method [8]. For this reason, we applied gastric decompression through the orogastric method in our study. We did not encounter any complications during or after application.

In literature, the number of studies searching for the effect of GD application in ENT surgery on PONV incidence is very low. Pasternak [20] reported that PONV and aspiration pneumonia risks can be eliminated by means of placing a gastric tube. Ferrari and Donlon [4] used prophylactic antiemetics in young patients undergoing tonsillectomy and applied GD in their studies and stated that the PONV incidence was 47% in the group where they used metoclopramide and 70% in the group where they did not use it. The PONV ratio in patients whom Ferrari applied prophylactic antiemetic together with GD is almost twice as much as the PONV ratio (21%) in patients to whom we applied only GD in this study. We can relate the low PONV rate to the patient group who underwent various ENT surgeries in our study. Trepanier and Isabel [15] reported the PONV ratio in 265 patients undergoing surgery in different branches as 55% in the group receiving GD and 48% in the control group and argued that GD has no effect on PONV incidence [15].

TABLE 2: The number and ratio of patients demonstrating PONV in postoperative 2nd, 4th, 8th, and 24th hours,.

		Group I		Group II		P
		n	%	n	%	
	First hour					
	None	63	90.0%	32	47.8%	
	PONV					
	Mild	3	4.3%	22	32.8%	
	Moderate	4	5.7%	8	11.9%	0.000*
	Severe	0	0.0%	5	7.5%	
	Fourth hour					
	None	57	81.4%	24	35.8%	
	PONV					
	Mild	9	12.9%	25	37.3%	
	Moderate	3	4.3%	14	20.9%	0.000*
PONV	Severe	1	1.4%	4	6.0%	
	Eighth hour					
	None	62	88.6%	24	35.8%	
	PONV					
	Mild	7	10.0%	35	52.2%	
	Moderate	1	1.4%	6	9.0%	0.000*
	Severe	0	0.0%	2	3.0%	
	24th hour					
	None	67	95.7%	50	74.6%	
	PONV					
	Mild	3	4.3%	16	23.9%	
	Moderate	0	0.0%	1	1.5%	0.000*
	Severe	0	0.0%	0	0.0%	

TABLE 3: Severity of the PONV in Groups I and II.

	Group I		Group II		P
	n	%	n	%	
PONV					
First hour	7	10.0%	35	52.2%	0.000*
Second hour	13	18.6%	22	64.2%	0.000*
Eighth hour	8	11.4%	8	64.2%	0.000*
24th hour	3	4.3%	5	25.4%	0.000*

However, in this study, it was stated that 35 patients had previous postoperative PONV histories and 21 patients had vertigo histories; these patients were not excluded from the study [15]. It was reported that in addition to the applied surgery type, use of opioids and nitrous oxide in anesthesia method also increases PONV incidence [3, 5, 15, 17]. PONV incidence is very variable in different ENT surgery types. For example, a 62–80% incidence of PONV following middle ear surgery has been reported [21]. The incidence of PONV was higher after middle ear surgery than tonsillectomy and the others [22, 23]. Our samples had been small heterogeneous surgery type about PONV incidence. Unfortunately it is the most limitation of recent study. Jones et al. [8] reported 85% PONV incidence in the group receiving GD and 74% PONV incidence in the control group in a study they conducted

TABLE 4: The amount of stomach content aspired during the period of GD process (minute) was recorded as "less than 10 mL" or "more than 10 mL." In Group I, the PONV ratio in the 2nd hour was significantly more for those whose amounts of stomach content aspired were more than 10 mL as compared to those whose stomach content aspired was less than 10 mL. In the 4th, 8th, and 24th hours, there is no statistically significant difference between the stomach content aspired and PONV ratio.

	The amount of stomach content				P
	Less than 10 mL		More than 10 mL		
	n	%	n	%	
PONV					
First hour	2	4.3%	5	21.7%	0.022*
Second hour	10	21.3%	3	13.0%	0.405
Eighth hour	6	12.8%	2	8.7%	0.615
24th hour	3	6.4%	0	0.0%	0.546

on 74 patients receiving adenotonsillectomy where they used 70% nitrous oxide and intravenous morphine sulfate through inhalation without using prophylactic antiemetic and steroid; they argued that GD application does not affect PONV incidence [8]. It was also stated that there is no correlation between gastric evacuation and PONV. Hovorka et al. [10] argued that GD application may be effective in reducing the frequency of PONV but cannot affect its severity. Burlacu et al. [2] reported that the need for postoperative antiemetic was 38.5% in the group receiving GD and 28.5% in the patients who did not receive GD, in 107 patients undergoing coronary artery bypass surgery using fentanyl and morphine sulfate. They argued that GD application does not have an effect on PONV incidence.

It is observed that the number of studies on this subject is low and there is no clear result on the effectiveness of GD. In our study, the PONV ratio was lower in the 4th and 24th hours in patients receiving GD. PONV incidence was lower, especially in the first 2 hours, in patients for whom the amount of content aspired from the stomach was lower than 10 mL as compared to those for whom the amount of content aspired from the stomach was more than 10 mL; namely, less stomach content means less PONV.

As a result, we can say that, in patients undergoing ENT surgery for whom we minimized PONV factors, GD applied just before extubation after the surgery reduces the incidence and severity of PONV. However, it should be noted that the more stomach content we aspire, the more frequently and severely PONV occurs. The number of studies pertaining to GD use should be increased in different surgeries, in different patient groups, and in different times and even in cases where risk factors are present. Since it is cheap and easily applicable, does not require special skills, and has a low complication rate, it can be preferred in adult ENT patients as an alternative for pharmacological treatment methods used today.

Conflict of Interests

The authors declare that there is no conflict of interests regarding the publication of this paper.

References

[1] D. J. Myklejord, L. Yao, H. Liang, and I. Glurich, "Consensus guideline adoption for managing postoperative nausea and vomiting," *Wisconsin Medical Journal*, vol. 111, no. 5, pp. 207–213, 2012.

[2] C. L. Burlacu, D. Healy, D. J. Buggy et al., "Continuous gastric decomposition for postoperative nausea and vomiting after coronary revascularization surgery," *Anesthesia & Analgesia*, vol. 100, no. 2, pp. 321–326, 2005.

[3] K. Leslie, P. S. Myles, M. T. Chan et al., "Risk factors for severe postoperative nausea and vomiting in a randomized trial of nitrous oxide-based vs nitrous oxide-free anaesthesia," *British Journal of Anaesthesia*, vol. 101, no. 4, pp. 498–505, 2008.

[4] L. R. Ferrari and J. V. Donlon, "Metoclopramide reduces the incidence of vomiting after tonsillectomy in children," *Anesthesia & Analgesia*, vol. 75, no. 3, pp. 351–354, 1992.

[5] C. A. M. Patti, J. E. Vieira, and F. E. M. Benseñor, "Incidence and prophylaxis of nausea and vomiting in post-anesthetic recovery in a tertiary teaching hospital," *Revista Brasileira de Anestesiologia*, vol. 58, no. 5, pp. 462–469, 2008.

[6] P. R. Bhandari, "Recent advances in pharmacotherapy of chemotherapy-induced nausea and vomiting," *Journal of Advanced Pharmaceutical Technology & Research*, vol. 3, no. 4, pp. 202–209, 2012.

[7] C. M. Bolton, P. S. Myles, T. Nolan, and J. A. Sterne, "Prophylaxis of postoperative vomiting in children undergoing tonsillectomy: a systematic review and meta-analysis," *British Journal of Anaesthesia*, vol. 97, no. 5, pp. 593–604, 2006.

[8] J. E. Jones, A. Tabaee, R. Glasgold, and M. C. Gomillion, "Efficacy of gastric aspiration in reducing posttonsillectomy vomiting," *Archives of Otolaryngology: Head and Neck Surgery*, vol. 127, no. 8, pp. 980–984, 2001.

[9] F. O. Yalcin, M. U. Yuksel, F. Korkulu, B. Dikmen, and O. Cuvas, "Effect of gastric decompression on postoperative nausea and vomiting," *Turkiye Klinikleri Journal of Anesthesiology Reanimation*, vol. 9, no. 1, pp. 20–26, 2011.

[10] J. Hovorka, K. Korttila, and O. Erkola, "Gastric aspiration at the end of anaesthesia does not decrease postoperative nausea and vomiting," *Anaesthesia and Intensive Care*, vol. 18, no. 1, pp. 58–61, 1990.

[11] K. T. Korttila and J. D. Jokinen, "Timing of administration of dolasetron affects dose necessary to prevent postoperative nausea and vomiting," *Journal of Clinical Anesthesia*, vol. 16, no. 5, pp. 364–370, 2004.

[12] A. Macario, M. Weinger, S. Carney, and A. Kim, "Which clinical anesthesia outcomes are important to avoid? The perspective of patients," *Anesthesia & Analgesia*, vol. 89, no. 3, pp. 652–658, 1999.

[13] S. Jolley, "Managing post-operative nausea and vomiting," *Nursing Standard*, vol. 15, no. 4, pp. 47–52, 2001.

[14] U. A. Pandit, S. Malviya, and I. H. Lewis, "Vomiting after outpatient tonsillectomy and adenoidectomy in children: the role of nitrous oxide," *Anesthesia & Analgesia*, vol. 80, no. 2, pp. 230–233, 1995.

[15] C. A. Trepanier and L. Isabel, "Perioperative gastric aspiration increases postoperative nausea and vomiting in outpatients," *Canadian Journal of Anaesthesia*, vol. 40, no. 4, pp. 325–328, 1993.

[16] J. Lerman, "Surgical and patient factors involved in postoperative nausea and vomiting," *British Journal of Anaesthesia*, vol. 69, no. 7, pp. 24–32, 1992.

[17] J. S. Carithers, D. E. Gebhart, and J. A. Williams, "Postoperative risks of pediatric tonsilloadenoidectomy," *The Laryngoscope*, vol. 97, no. 4, pp. 422–429, 1987.

[18] S. R. Furst and A. Rodarte, "Prophylactic antiemetic treatment with ondansetron in children undergoing tonsillectomy," *Anesthesiology*, vol. 81, no. 4, pp. 799–803, 1994.

[19] S. M. Barst, J. U. Leiderman, A. Markowitz, A. M. Rosen, A. L. Abramson, and R. S. Bienkowski, "Ondansetron with propofol reduces the incidence of emesis in children following tonsillectomy," *Canadian Journal of Anaesthesia*, vol. 46, no. 4, pp. 359–362, 1999.

[20] L. R. Pasternak, "Anesthetic considerations in otolaryngological and ophthalmological outpatient surgery," *International Anesthesiology Clinics*, vol. 28, no. 2, pp. 89–100, 1990.

[21] S. Mukhopadhyay, M. Niyogi, R. Ray, B. S. Mukhopadhyay, M. Dutta, and M. Mukherjee, "Betahistine as an add-on: the magic bullet for postoperative nausea, vomiting and dizziness after middle earsurgery?" *Journal of Anaesthesiology, Clinical Pharmacology*, vol. 29, no. 2, pp. 205–210, 2013.

[22] A. R. Mishra, U. Srivastava, D. Kumar et al., "Nausea and vomiting after ENT surgeries: a comparison between ondansetron, metoclopramide and small dose of propofol," *Indian Journal of Otolaryngology and Head & Neck Surgery*, vol. 62, no. 1, pp. 29–31, 2010.

[23] Y. Fujii, H. Tanaka, and N. Kobayashi, "Small doses of propofol, droperidol, and metoclopramide for the prevention of postoperative nausea and vomiting after thyroidectomy," *Otolaryngology: Head and Neck Surgery*, vol. 124, no. 3, pp. 266–269, 2001.

Pressure Flow Analysis in the Assessment of Preswallow Pharyngeal Bolus Presence in Dysphagia

Lara Ferris,[1,2] **Taher Omari,**[1,2] **Margot Selleslagh,**[3,4] **Eddy Dejaeger,**[5,6] **Jan Tack,**[3]
Dirk Vanbeckevoort,[6,7] **and Nathalie Rommel**[3,4]

[1]*Gastroenterology Unit, Child, Youth & Women's Health Service, Adelaide, SA, Australia*
[2]*School of Medicine, Flinders University, Adelaide, SA, Australia*
[3]*Translational Research Center for Gastrointestinal Disorders, KU Leuven, Leuven, Belgium*
[4]*ExpORL, Department of Neurosciences, KU Leuven, Leuven, Belgium*
[5]*Geriatric Medicine, University Hospital Leuven, Leuven, Belgium*
[6]*Center for Swallowing Disorders, University Hospital Leuven, Leuven, Belgium*
[7]*Radiology, University Hospital Leuven, Leuven, Belgium*

Correspondence should be addressed to Lara Ferris; lara.ferris@health.sa.gov.au

Academic Editor: Peter S. Roland

Objectives. Preswallow pharyngeal bolus presence is evident in patients with oropharyngeal dysphagia. Pressure flow analysis (PFA) using high resolution manometry with impedance (HRMI) with AIMplot software is a method for objective interpretation of pharyngeal and upper esophageal sphincter (UES) pressures and bolus flow patterns during swallowing. This study aimed to observe alterations in PFA metrics in the event of preswallow pharyngeal bolus presence as seen on videofluoroscopy (VFSS). *Methods.* Swallows from 40 broad dysphagia patients and 8 controls were recorded with a HRMI catheter during simultaneous VFSS. Evidence of bolus presence and level reached prior to pharyngeal swallow onset was recorded. AIMPlot software derived automated PFA functional metrics. *Results.* Patients with bolus movement to the pyriform sinuses had a higher SRI, indicating greater swallow dysfunction. Amongst individual metrics, TNadImp to PeakP was shorter and flow interval longer in patient groups compared to controls. A higher pharyngeal mean impedance and UES mean impedance differentiated the two patient groups. *Conclusions.* This pilot study identifies specific altered PFA metrics in patients demonstrating preswallow pharyngeal bolus presence to the pyriform sinuses. PFA metrics may be used to guide diagnosis and treatment of patients with oropharyngeal dysphagia and track changes in swallow function over time.

1. Introduction

Preswallow pharyngeal bolus presence is viewed on videofluoroscopic swallow study (VFSS) or fiberoptic endoscopic examination of swallowing (FEES) amongst many patients presenting with oropharyngeal dysphagia. There are two main causes for this presentation: poor oral bolus containment with premature bolus spillage and/or a delayed pharyngeal swallow trigger. Poor oral bolus containment results in passive or ineffective movement of a liquid or viscous bolus from the oral cavity into the pharynx prior to pharyngeal swallow onset [1]. By definition this occurs whilst the oral preparatory or oral stage of swallow is still underway [1],

that is, before or during lingual propulsion. Separately, a delay in the pharyngeal swallow trigger is defined by a failure of a coordinated and timely pharyngeal response following a purposeful transfer of the bolus into the pharynx [2]. Poor oral containment leading to premature bolus spillage can occur in isolation or in combination with a delayed pharyngeal swallow trigger [1–3]. Preswallow pharyngeal bolus presence puts a patient at risk of aspiration.

High resolution manometry with impedance (HRMI) with automated Pressure Flow Analysis (PFA) is a new method to diagnostically interpret pharyngeal and UES function. Pressure sensors detect activity of swallow musculature whilst impedance electrodes provide measures which indicate bolus flow. PFA derives a range of swallow metrics that indicate bolus flow timing, intrabolus pressure, contractile vigour, bolus presence, and UES luminal diameter, making it possible to measure and describe the function of different mechanical components of pharyngeal swallowing. A global swallow risk index (SRI) generated from PFA metrics as a means to amplify dysfunction has shown to correlate with the presence of aspiration and/or postswallow residue as seen on videofluoroscopy [4, 5]. Following on from this previous work, the purpose of this study was to use HRMI in combination with automated PFA to objectively describe pressure-flow patterns in the pharynx and UES in the event of *preswallow* pharyngeal bolus presence as seen on videofluoroscopy. We hypothesised that specific PFA metrics would be altered in patients with preswallow pharyngeal bolus presence compared to patients without preswallow pharyngeal bolus presence and controls. The aim of this study was to identify the altered PFA metrics which may provide a means to describe functional changes in the pharynx in the event of preswallow pharyngeal bolus presence.

2. Materials and Methods

2.1. Subjects. We analysed VFSS investigations performed in 40 adult patients with broad dysphagia (24 males, mean age 46 yrs, and age range 23–95 yrs) and 8 adult controls (3 males, mean age 38 yrs, and age range 24–47 yrs). At the time of initial investigation, all subjects were enrolled in study protocols that were approved by the Research Ethics Committee, University Hospital Leuven, Belgium. After understanding the study information, all subjects gave their consent freely. In patients with dysphagia, underlying diseases/conditions were identified through a review of medical records. Eighteen patients had a neurological history (10 patients were post stroke, 2 had Parkinson's disease, 1 Huntington's disease, 1 Multiple Sclerosis, 2 Dementia, 1 Spina Bifida and 1 post-neurosurgery). Of the remaining four patients 1 was post-cervical surgery, 1 Wegener disease, 1 postseptic shock, and 1 Diabetes. This database of patients with broad dysphagia has previously been reported on [4–9], and the diverse clinical presentations and dysphagia severity have been purposeful in order to concept-test PFA metrics in relation to radiological measures from VFSS. Previously this has included aspiration status, postswallow residue, UES opening, and in this case preswallow pharyngeal bolus presence.

2.2. Measurement Protocol. Studies were performed in the Radiology Department, University Hospital Leuven, with a 3.2 mm diameter solid state high resolution manometry and impedance catheter incorporating 25 1 cm-spaced pressure sensors and 12 adjoining impedance segments, each of 2 cm (Unisensor AG catheter, Attikon Switzerland). Subjects were intubated after topical anaesthesia (lignocaine spray) and the catheter was positioned with sensors straddling the entire pharyngoesophageal segment (velopharynx to proximal esophagus). Pressure and impedance data were acquired at 20 Hz (Solar GI acquisition system, MMS, Netherlands) with the subject sitting upright. Most subjects were tested

with at least 5 boluses in the lateral view: liquid (x3), semisolid (x1), and solid boluses (x1). A standard liquid contrast material (MicropaqueH) was given as liquid bolus and used with thickener (Thick & Easy) for semisolid boluses. A low osmotic hydrosoluble Iodium compound (UltravistH) was used when aspiration was suspected. The viscosity of the administered boluses was determined by a Rheomat 115 Viscometer. The Bingham viscosity of the liquid barium (MicropaqueH) was 0.22 Pascal seconds (PAs), 4.50 PAs for the semisolid bolus. All controls were given boluses of 10 mL volume while patients were given either 5 mL or 10 mL volumes as determined on clinical grounds by the attending specialist. Solid boluses consisted of a 4 cm² piece of bread soaked in the appropriate radiological marker which was chewed and swallowed. All swallows were prompted and the first swallow following bolus administration was marked for analysis. All bolus stock contained NaCl to enhance bolus conductivity, improving the impedance measurement.

2.3. Videofluoroscopic Assessments. Continuous videofluoroscopy sequences (25 frames/sec) of swallows were analysed by a speech pathologist (Author Lara Ferris) who was not present during acquisition and was blinded to study functional measures, patient history, and clinical reports. Only primary, lateral view swallows were analysed. Swallows with poor image quality were excluded from analysis. Each primary bolus swallow was reviewed to determine movement of the bolus and the level reached from the oral cavity into the distal pharynx prior to the onset of the pharyngeal swallow, defined by onset of rapid laryngeal excursion [1, 10, 11]. The levels reached were defined as follows: still in the oral cavity, base of tongue, valleculae, or pyriform sinuses. Discussions between authors ensured interrater agreeability before the analysis proceeded.

We applied conservative criteria to define clinically significant bolus presence. Bolus head location within the pyriform sinuses was used as the pathological benchmark.

Based on the results for all the analysed swallows patients were classified as follows:

(1) Group 1: patients who never demonstrated bolus movement to the pyriform sinuses prior to swallow onset.

(2) Group 2: patients who demonstrated bolus movement to the pyriform sinuses at least once prior to swallow onset.

Note: amongst controls, at swallow onset bolus movement was observed in the mouth or at the base of tongue for all swallows.

2.4. Pressure Flow Analysis. Pharyngeal PFA was performed using automated impedance manometry software (AIMplot) to calculate PFA metrics and two global indices which have been previously validated against VFSS, namely, the SRI, indicative of global dysfunction, and the integrated ratio of nadir impedance to impedance (iZn/Z), indicative of postswallow residue. The calculations used to derive PFA metrics have been previously described [4–9, 12]. In brief,

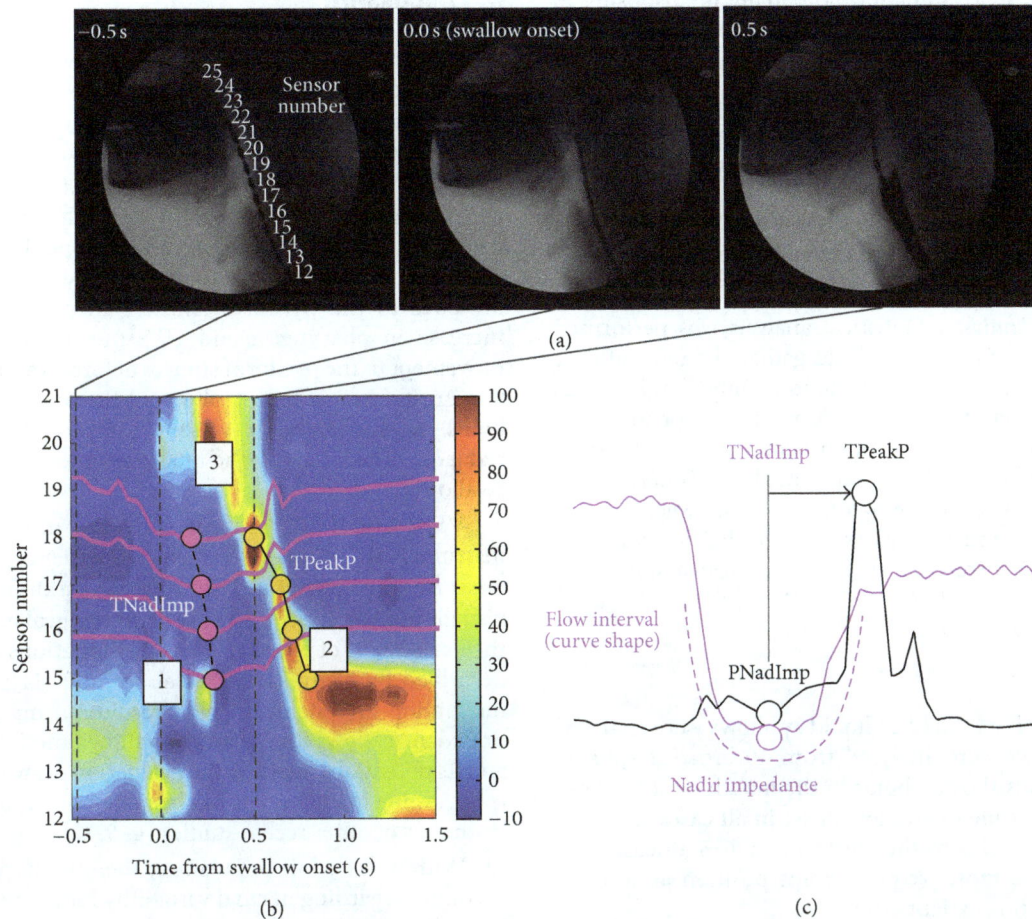

FIGURE 1: Pharyngeal HRMI and derivation of AIM analysis metrics. (a) Videofluoroscopic images of the catheter in situ in 43-year-old male subject. Consecutive images of a 10-liquid bolus swallow at 0.5 sec before swallow, at swallow onset, and at 0.5 ms after swallow onset. (b) A pressure topography plot of the swallow with impedance waveforms and an example of a PFA metric: PNadImp and PeakP superimposed on the plot. Landmarks defined for AIMplot analysis are marked (1: swallow onset time, 2: position of UES proximal margin post swallow, and 3: position of velopharynx). (c) An illustration showing calculation of the main PFA analysis metrics in the pharynx region. Note: a similar analysis was also applied to the UES region to derive UES Nadir Impedance.

pressure impedance recordings are displayed as pressure topography plots with embedded impedance recordings which show bolus flow movements, the pharyngeal stripping wave, and relaxation and movement of the UES pressure zone (Figure 1(b)). On selection of specific landmarks on the pressure topography space-time plot (with embedded impedance recordings), specific regions of interest (ROI) are mapped. The landmarks identified are (1) time of onset of pharyngeal swallow, (2) position of the UES proximal margin postswallow, and (3) position of the velopharynx during the swallow (numbered 1–3 in Figure 1(b)). There are three ROI encompassing (1) the pharynx, (2) distal pharynx, and (3) UES.

Within each of the ROI, PFA metrics were derived from pressure and impedance waveforms using automated algorithms. Specifically, identification of peak pressure defines the maximum contraction in space and time, the nadir impedance (NadImp) defines the centre of the swallowed bolus in space and time (Figures 1(b) and 1(c)), and the

pressure at nadir impedance (PNadImp, Figure 1(c)) defines pharyngeal intrabolus pressure. The time interval from nadir impedance to peak pressure (TNadImp to PeakP, Figure 1(c)) measures the time from bolus passage to pharyngeal contraction; the flow interval (FI) correlates with pharyngeal bolus transit time. The UES nadir impedance (UES NadImp) is measured as a correlate of UES opening diameter [7] and the UES intrabolus pressure (UES IBP) is measured using the established method of Ghosh et al., 2006 [13].

2.4.1. Global Assessment of Pharyngeal Dysfunction. The swallow risk index (SRI) was empirically derived and designed to amplify difference in swallow metrics previously shown to be altered in relation to swallow dysfunction and aspiration risk [4, 5]. These validation studies using concurrent VFSS showed that the SRI for liquid and viscous swallows is significantly higher in patients demonstrating penetration-aspiration compared to patients with no penetration or aspiration [4, 5]. Therefore the SRI quantifies the overall level of swallowing dysfunction potentially predisposing to aspiration risk [4, 5].

2.4.2. Impedance Based Detection of Post Swallow Residue. A postswallow residue score was designed using the integrated ratio of nadir impedance to impedance (iZn/Z ratio) which relates postswallow impedance to the impedance during bolus passage. This measure has shown to be significantly elevated in patients with postswallow residue [8].

2.5. Statistical Analyses. Statistical analysis was performed using IBM SPSS Statistics 22. Data gathered from multiple swallows were averaged for each subject. Only liquid boluses (5 or 10 mLs) were assessed. Volume was dependent on clinical decision. Data distribution across the study cohort was nonparametric and therefore medians (interquartile range) are presented. Mann-Whitney U tests were used to compare controls and patients grouped on VFSS assessment with Bonferroni correction for multiple comparisons, $P < 0.017$.

3. Results

Amongst controls a total of 24 liquid swallows were analysed and 102 swallows were analysed from 40 broad dysphagia patients. Controls showed bolus in the mouth or at the base of tongue at the time of swallow onset in all cases. 20 of 40 patients showed bolus to the pyriform sinuses at least once and this was the most frequent bolus position at swallow onset in 75% of this patient group.

As shown in Figure 2 using Mann-Whitney U tests, in this cohort of broad dysphagia patients the SRI, a global measure of swallowing dysfunction, was higher in relation to evidence of bolus to the pyriform sinuses prior to the pharyngeal swallow onset compared to controls ($P < 0.001$), and a trend was observed compared to patients who did not spill to the pyriform sinuses ($P = 0.02$).

The TNadImp-PeakP (poor ability for the bolus to be propelled ahead of the pharyngeal stripping wave) was shorter in both patient groups (group 1 $P < 0.002$ and group 2 $P < 0.001$) compared to controls; the flow interval (suggesting extended pharyngeal bolus dwell time) was longer in both patient groups (group 1 $P < 0.001$ and group 2 $P < 0.002$) compared to controls; and the iZn/Z (postswallow residue metric) was significantly higher in both patient groups (group 1 $P < 0.000$ and group 2 $P < 0.000$) compared to controls (Figure 2).

Two individual metrics in this data differentiate the patient groups: group 1: patients without preswallow bolus presence to the pyriform sinuses prior to swallow onset and group 2: patients with preswallow bolus presence to the pyriform sinuses prior to swallow onset. Pharyngeal mean impedance (correlating with reduced pharyngeal distension) was significantly higher ($P < 0.002$) in group 2 compared to group 1 and controls ($P < 0.001$) and the UES mean impedance (correlating with reduced UES opening) was higher ($P < 0.000$) in group 2 compared to group 1 and controls ($P < 0.001$).

4. Discussion

Collectively this pattern of pressure-flow differences is consistent with impairment of the mechanisms that drive bolus propulsion, pharyngeal distension, and relaxation and opening of the UES in accordance with laryngeal excursion. Inefficient bolus transfer into the esophagus is the net result.

As has been shown previously, a higher UES impedance recording correlates with reduced UES opening diameter [7] and therefore, in the case of preswallow pharyngeal bolus presence to the pyriform sinuses, an explanation for the increase in pharyngeal and UES mean impedance: bolus movement to the pyriform sinuses before swallow onset leads to a greater loss of bolus volume of the remaining propelled bolus. A smaller bolus volume for propulsion results in reduced distension of the pharynx and UES during the swallow.

VFSS and FEES are currently the most widely used instrumental swallow assessments; however differential diagnosis of oropharyngeal dysphagia can be difficult based on visualisation alone [10]. The use of pharyngeal manometry for the assessment of dysphagia has its limitations and has been described by Nativ-Zeltzer et al. in 2012 [14]; however the integration of concurrent high resolution manometry with impedance allows for dynamic swallow function assessment, and its potential to assist in the evaluation of swallow function is beginning to emerge, as has been demonstrated in this and a number of other recent studies [4–9, 12].

Within the adult population, there is discussion in the literature regarding normal variability for the presence of the bolus lower in the pharynx prior to swallow onset [15–19]. However, the spillage or propulsion of all or part of the bolus to the pyriform sinuses prior to pharyngeal swallow trigger is a pathological event [1–3, 20] suggesting markedly altered mechanics of bolus transport through the pharynx. The clinical relevance in detecting preswallow pharyngeal bolus presence lies in the fact that recognising the causes for bolus presence in the pharynx prior to pharyngeal swallow onset is important for treatment of oropharyngeal dysphagia. Our findings demonstrate how specific PFA metrics are altered in relation to a general pathological observation of preswallow pharyngeal bolus presence in dysphagia patients.

5. Conclusion

This pilot study presents specific pressure flow analysis metrics (using integrated high resolution manometry and impedance) which are significantly associated with a known pathological presentation of oropharyngeal dysphagia, that is, preswallow pharyngeal bolus presence to the pyriform sinuses. These results provide reason to further explore the potential differences in pressure flow analysis metrics that may distinguish the causes for preswallow pharyngeal bolus presence, that is, poor oral containment and/or delayed pharyngeal trigger. This will be the focus for future studies. Pressure flow analysis with AIMplot software deriving metrics and a global measure of dysfunction, the swallow risk index, have the potential to guide diagnosis and treatment of

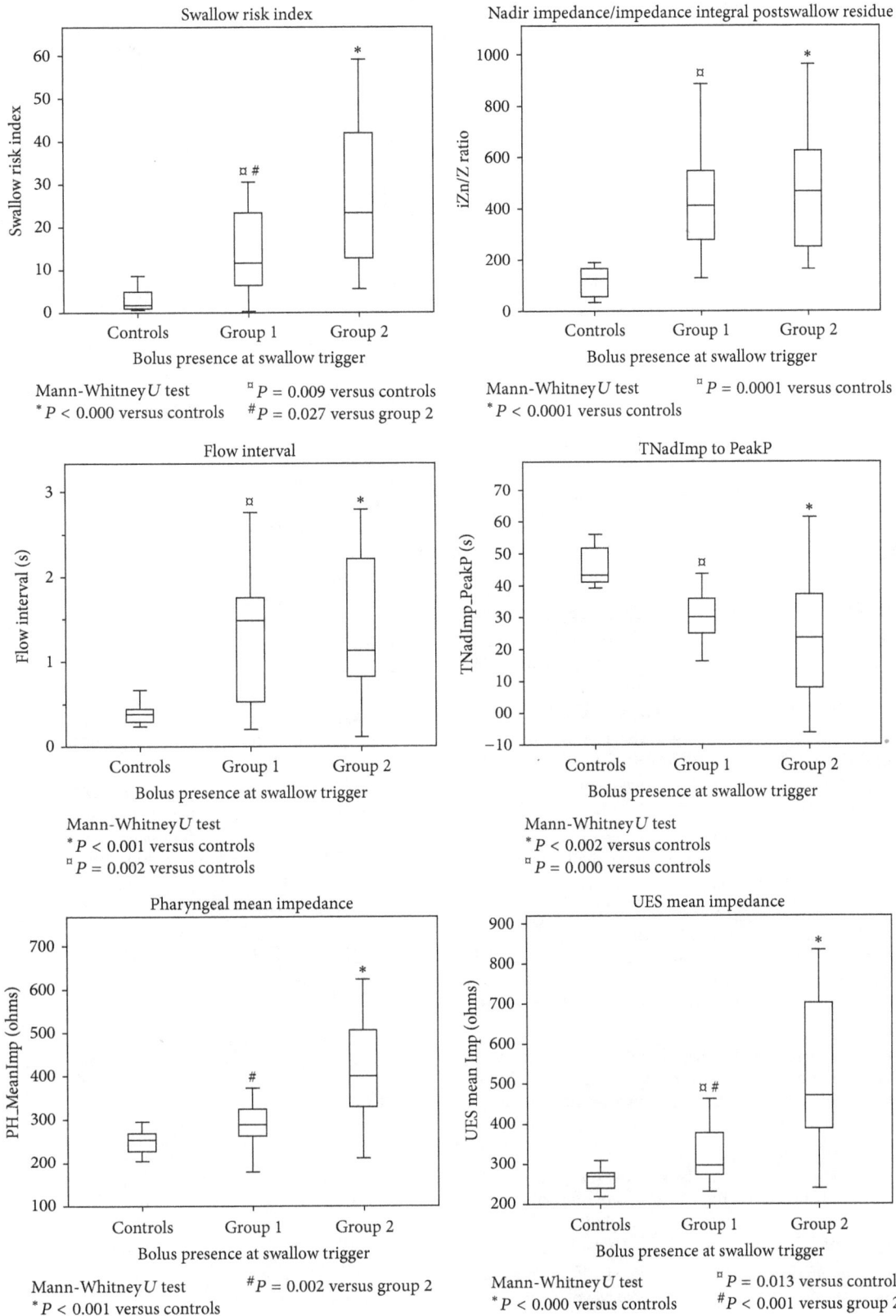

FIGURE 2: Pressure flow analysis metrics recorded in relation to bolus presence to the pyriform sinuses prior to swallow onset. Group 1: patients NEVER demonstrating bolus to the pyriform sinuses at the time of swallow onset. Group 2: patients demonstrating bolus to the pyriform sinuses AT LEAST ONCE at the time of swallow onset. Controls: in all cases bolus was in the mouth or at base of tongue at time of swallow onset. Data are median (IQR) for liquid swallows. P values are from Mann-Whitney U tests with Bonferroni correction for multiple comparisons, P < 0.017.

patients with oropharyngeal dysphagia and may be used to track patient changes in swallow function over time.

Conflict of Interests

Authors Nathalie Rommel and Taher Omari hold a patent on Pressure Flow Analysis, AIMplot methods. All other authors have no conflict of interests to declare.

Acknowledgments

This work was supported by project grants acquired by Taher Omari from the Thrasher Research Fund and the National Health & Medical Research Council.

References

[1] J. Logemann, *Evaluation and Treatment of Swallowing Disorders*, Pro-Ed, Austin, Tex, USA, 2nd edition, 1998.

[2] W. J. Dodds, E. T. Stewart, and J. A. Logemann, "Physiology and radiology of the normal oral and pharyngeal phases of swallowing," *American Journal of Roentgenology*, vol. 154, no. 5, pp. 953–963, 1990.

[3] R. A. Cassiani, C. M. Santos, L. C. Parreira, and R. O. Dantas, "The relationship between the oral and pharyngeal phases of swallowing," *Clinics*, vol. 66, no. 8, pp. 1385–1388, 2011.

[4] T. I. Omari, E. Dejaeger, D. van Beckevoort et al., "A method to objectively assess swallow function in adults with suspected aspiration," *Gastroenterology*, vol. 140, no. 5, pp. 1454–1463, 2011.

[5] T. I. Omari, E. Dejaeger, D. van Beckevoort et al., "A novel method for the nonradiological assessment of ineffective swallowing," *The American Journal of Gastroenterology*, vol. 106, no. 10, pp. 1796–1802, 2011.

[6] T. I. Omari, A. Papathanasopoulos, E. Dejaeger et al., "Reproducibility and agreement of pharyngeal automated impedance manometry with videofluoroscopy," *Clinical Gastroenterology and Hepatology*, vol. 9, no. 10, pp. 862–867, 2011.

[7] T. I. Omari, L. Ferris, E. Dejaeger, J. Tack, D. Vanbeckevoort, and N. Rommel, "Upper esophageal sphincter impedance as a marker of sphincter opening diameter," *American Journal of Physiology: Gastrointestinal and Liver Physiology*, vol. 302, no. 9, pp. G909–G913, 2012.

[8] T. I. Omari, E. Dejaeger, J. Tack, D. Vanbeckevoort, and N. Rommel, "An impedance-manometry based method for non-radiological detection of pharyngeal postswallow residue," *Neurogastroenterology & Motility*, vol. 24, no. 7, pp. e277–e284, 2012.

[9] T. I. Omari, E. Dejaeger, J. Tack, D. van Beckevoort, and N. Rommel, "Effect of bolus volume and viscosity on pharyngeal automated impedance manometry variables derived for broad dysphagia patients," *Dysphagia*, vol. 28, no. 2, pp. 146–152, 2013.

[10] T. Nishino, "The swallowing reflex and its significance as an airway defensive reflex," *Frontiers in Physiology*, vol. 3, no. 489, pp. 1–6, 2013.

[11] K. Matsuo, S. Kawase, N. Wakimoto, K. Iwatani, Y. Masuda, and T. Ogasawara, "Effect of viscosity on food transport and swallow initiation during eating of two-phase food in normal young adults: a pilot study," *Dysphagia*, vol. 28, no. 1, pp. 63–68, 2013.

[12] L. Noll, N. Rommel, G. P. Davidson, and T. I. Omari, "Pharyngeal flow interval: a novel impedance-based parameter correlating with aspiration," *Neurogastroenterology & Motility*, vol. 23, no. 6, pp. e551–e206, 2011.

[13] S. K. Ghosh, J. E. Pandolfino, Q. Zhang, A. Jarosz, and P. J. Kahrilas, "Deglutitive upper esophageal sphincter relaxation: a study of 75 volunteer subjects using solid-state high-resolution manometry," *American Journal of Physiology: Gastrointestinal and Liver Physiology*, vol. 291, no. 3, pp. G525–G531, 2006.

[14] N. Nativ-Zeltzer, P. J. Kahrilas, and J. A. Logemann, "Manofluorography in the evaluation of oropharyngeal dysphagia," *Dysphagia*, vol. 27, no. 2, pp. 151–161, 2012.

[15] S. Daniels and M. Huckabee, *Dysphagia Following Stroke: Plural Clinical Dysphagia Series*, Plural Publishing, San Diego, Calif, USA, 2008.

[16] J. R. Stephen, D. H. Taves, R. C. Smith, and R. E. Martin, "Bolus location at the initiation of the pharyngeal stage of swallowing in healthy older adults," *Dysphagia*, vol. 20, no. 4, pp. 266–272, 2005.

[17] B. Martin-Harris, M. B. Brodsky, Y. Michel, F.-S. Lee, and B. Walters, "Delayed initiation of the pharyngeal swallow: normal variability in adult swallows," *Journal of Speech, Language, and Hearing Research*, vol. 50, no. 3, pp. 585–594, 2007.

[18] B. R. Pauloski, A. W. Rademaker, C. Lazarus, G. Boeckxstaens, P. J. Kahrilas, and J. A. Logemann, "Relationship between manometric and videofluoroscopic measures of swallow function in healthy adults and patients treated for head and neck cancer with various modalities," *Dysphagia*, vol. 24, no. 2, pp. 196–203, 2009.

[19] H. Miyaji, T. Umezaki, K. Adachi et al., "Videofluoroscopic assessment of pharyngeal stage delay reflects pathophysiology after brain infarction," *The Laryngoscope*, vol. 122, no. 12, pp. 2793–2799, 2012.

[20] L. Flanagan, *The validity of a three-part criteria for differentiating between delayed pharyngeal swallow and premature spillage secondary to poor oro-lingual control on videofluoroscopy [M.S. thesis]*, UC Research Repository, 2007, http://ir.canterbury.ac.nz/handle/10092/1407.

Individual Optimization of the Insertion of a Preformed Cochlear Implant Electrode Array

Thomas S. Rau, Thomas Lenarz, and Omid Majdani

Department of Otolaryngology, Hannover Medical School, Carl-Neuberg-Straße 1, 30625 Hannover, Germany

Correspondence should be addressed to Thomas S. Rau; rau.thomas@mh-hannover.de

Academic Editor: Peter S. Roland

Purpose. The aim of this study was to show that individual adjustment of the curling behaviour of a preformed cochlear implant (CI) electrode array to the patient-specific shape of the cochlea can improve the insertion process in terms of reduced risk of insertion trauma. *Methods.* Geometry and curling behaviour of preformed, commercially available electrode arrays were modelled. Additionally, the anatomy of each small, medium-sized, and large human cochlea was modelled to consider anatomical variations. Finally, using a custom-made simulation tool, three different insertion strategies (conventional Advanced Off-Stylet (AOS) insertion technique, an automated implementation of the AOS technique, and a manually optimized insertion process) were simulated and compared with respect to the risk of insertion-related trauma. The risk of trauma was evaluated using a newly developed "trauma risk" rating scale. *Results.* Using this simulation-based approach, it was shown that an individually optimized insertion procedure is advantageous compared with the AOS insertion technique. *Conclusion.* This finding leads to the conclusion that, in general, consideration of the specific curling behaviour of a CI electrode array is beneficial in terms of less traumatic insertion. Therefore, these results highlight an entirely novel aspect of clinical application of preformed perimodiolar electrode arrays in general.

1. Introduction

An essential, but also risky, step in cochlear implantation is the insertion of the electrode array (EA) of a cochlear implant into the helically shaped scala tympani. The scala tympani is one of three tubular lumens inside the auditory portion (cochlea) of the inner ear. At one side, it is bordered by a fragile membranous structure, called the basilar membrane, which divides the cross section of the cochlea almost in the middle. The basilar membrane plays a crucial role in the biomechanics and hydrodynamics of the inner ear and, therefore, in the mechanism of sound sensation. Located on top of the basilar membrane is the organ of Corti, which includes the hair cells and forms the neural receptor for sound waves. Physical integrity of the basilar membrane is thus essential for acoustic hearing.

In hearing-impaired patients, the function of the hair cells, which convert acoustic signals into a neural response, is limited or completely absent. The latter case results in deafness. Otherwise, the degree of hearing loss depends on the amount of residual hearing and its usability for communication and environmental sound sensation. However, a useful and well-established surgical procedure—the implantation of an electronic device called a cochlear implant (CI, see Figure 1)—is available to treat deafness and profound to severe hearing loss.

Through electrical stimulation of the auditory nerve, a CI bypasses damaged portions of the ear and provides a sense of sound to the recipient. For this purpose, the CI system includes a component known as the electrode array (also referred to as the electrode carrier or simply the electrode), which is inserted into the cochlea (the terms "cochlea," "inner ear," and "scala tympani" are subsequently used synonymously; in all cases, what is meant is that the electrode array should be ideally inserted into the scala tympani, irrespective of the actually achieved outcome). This intracochlear portion is a thin, elongated silicone body incorporating embedded platinum contact electrodes. To achieve electrical stimulation of the auditory nerve, environmental sounds are recorded and converted into electrical signals by the CI system.

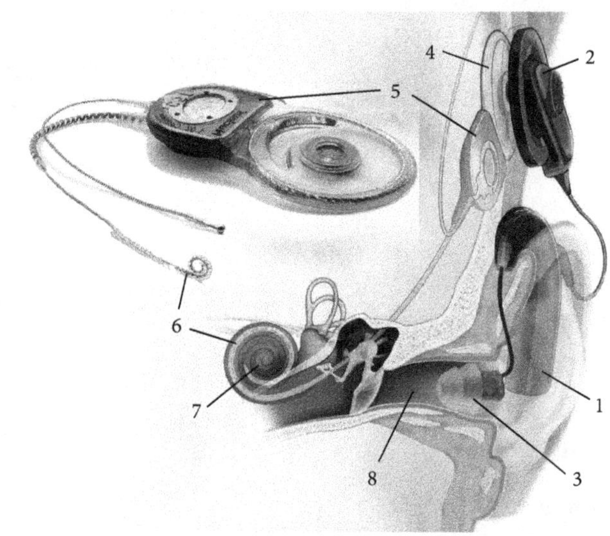

FIGURE 1: Cochlear implant system for hybrid stimulation. It consists of external (1–3) and internal (implanted) components (4–6). Sounds are captured and digitized by the external sound processor (1, including one or more microphones). Signals and energy are transcutaneously transferred to the implanted portions using an external (2) and an internal (4) coil. These signals are converted by the implant (5) into stimulus-correlated electrical pulses and transmitted to the electrode array (6) implanted into the cochlea (7). In this way, electric stimulation evokes neural responses in the intact auditory nerve. Additionally, low-frequency sound is amplified by the sound processor (1) and transmitted to the normal hearing pathway using an earmould (3) in the external auditory canal (8) (images by courtesy of Cochlear Ltd.).

Stimulus-correlated electrical signals are finally transferred to the electrode array; this in turn generates electrical fields in the surrounding tissue, including the fibres of the auditory nerve.

Historically, only deaf patients were considered to be candidates for CI treatment. In the present day, inclusion criteria are continuously being expanded, so that individuals with substantial residual hearing are now also getting implants. There are two main reasons why a CI is recommended to these patients. The first is that, in most cases, residual hearing is in the low-frequency range. In contrast, hearing at the high-frequency range (>1,000 Hz), including those frequencies essential for human speech, is not functional. These individuals are, therefore, excluded from day-to-day communication, a situation which cannot be improved by use of conventional hearing aids. The second reason is a strategy referred to as hybrid or electric acoustic stimulation (EAS). This involves the use of electrical stimulation via the CI to restore high-frequency hearing, with the residual hearing still being exploited and amplified for normal (acoustic) low-frequency hearing. A combination of both approaches to providing hearing sensation is known to deliver better hearing outcomes than electrical stimulation alone [1–7]. This is why EAS is currently one of the most important objectives in CI treatment and an important motivation for research. This leads us back to anatomical aspects of CI surgery,

as the integrity of the basilar membrane after electrode insertion is essential for residual hearing preservation and thus for electric acoustic stimulation.

In general, existing electrode arrays can be divided into two main groups: those straight in shape and those with a preformed, moulded silicone body. Numerous straight electrode arrays have been developed in recent years. High flexibility, reduced cross-sectional area, and limited insertion depth are considered as essential features to meet the requirements of atraumatic insertion, and hence preservation of residual hearing and electric acoustic simulation. The main disadvantage is the final position at the lateral wall of the cochlea, which is a large distance away from the neural tissue that is the target for stimulation.

In contrast, preformed electrode arrays are fabricated in a spiral configuration adjusted to the shape and size of an average human cochlea. As insertion into the cochlea initially requires a straight configuration, it is necessary to uncurl the electrode array and keep it straight prior to insertion. A commonly used mechanism is a thin but sufficiently stiff wire (stylet) inside the electrode array, which inhibits the curling forces of the spirally preformed and elastically deformed silicone body and the embedded platinum wires. During insertion this stiffening wire, the stylet is removed and the electrode array returns to its original helical shape.

Originally, these preformed electrode arrays were designed for intracochlear placement next to the modiolus, which is why they are known as perimodiolar implants. The modiolus is the central axis of the cochlea and contains the neural tissue that is the target for stimulation by the CI. Therefore, close proximity of the electrode contacts to the inner wall of the cochlea is beneficial for electric stimulation [8, 9]. Examples of this type of perimodiolar implant are the Contour Electrode, its successor the Contour Advance electrode, and the thinner Modiolus Research Array (MRA), all three of which are manufactured by Cochlear Ltd. (Sydney, Australia), and the HiFocus Helix electrode made by Advanced Bionics LLC (Valencia, CA, USA).

However, this perimodiolar design also has its drawbacks. In general, these electrode arrays have a larger diameter and (due to the stiffening wire) also exhibit greater overall stiffness than the thin and highly flexible straight models. Perimodiolar electrode arrays are thus associated with a higher risk of insertion trauma and are not normally used for patients with residual hearing. To overcome the disadvantages of additional stiffening elements (such as the stylet) with regard to residual hearing preservation, it would appear necessary to reduce the amount of contact between the implant and the intracochlear anatomical structures. One strategy could be to use robot assistance for insertion and to optimize its pose (position and orientation) with respect to the pose of the inner ear [10, 11]. Reduced contact implies reduced insertion forces, which are commonly accepted as being correlated to insertion trauma.

However, the integrated curling mechanism provides the opportunity to modify not only the pose but also the shape of the electrode array with regard to the individual anatomy. This entails the replacement of a uniform insertion technique (such as the Advanced Off-Stylet (AOS) technique; see Section 2.2.2 and Figure 2) by a patient-specific

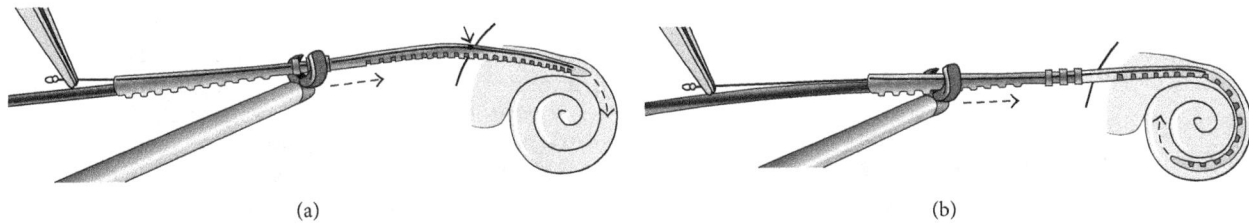

(a)   (b)

FIGURE 2: Schematic illustration of the Advanced Off-Stylet (AOS) technique. (a) The electrode array is inserted into the inner ear with the stylet inside until a marker is at the level of the cochleostomy site. (b) The stylet is kept stationary and the implant is advanced further into the cochlea until full insertion depth is achieved (image provided by courtesy of Karl STORZ, Tuttlingen, Germany).

one. This is, of course, possible only on a limited scale as the commercially available perimodiolar implants are not developed and designed for this purpose, and additional intraoperative surgical assistance devices are necessary because an individually optimized insertion process can no longer be performed manually. Nevertheless, thanks to recent advances in surgical master-slave systems [12], and especially in robot-assisted devices for CI surgery [13–18], as well as in automated insertion tools [11, 19–25], it seems to be only a question of time until accurate assistance devices can be used intraoperatively for electrode insertion.

Therefore, the aim of this study was to investigate whether, for the commercially available CA electrode array, an individually optimized insertion procedure is advantageous compared with the AOS insertion technique, which is recommended for all patients by the manufacturer, Cochlear Ltd. More generally, we wished to explore whether taking into account the curling behaviour of a CI electrode array is beneficial in terms of less traumatic insertion. In the light of this research question, we also investigated the situation when a minimally invasive approach to the cochlea is employed. This entails an alternative to the manually performed drilling of a large mastoid cavity (a procedure known as mastoidectomy, which involves the removal of parts of the temporal bone behind the ear to provide access to the inner ear). Instead, a single, straight drill hole should be used. This not only requires additional surgical assistance devices, which are currently under development by several research groups [13–15, 17, 18, 26–28]: a hole of such small size also means certain constraints in terms of electrode insertion, especially loss of several degrees of freedom.

Irrespective of the surgical approach chosen, the findings of this research on individually optimized electrode insertion are also of interest for other projects dealing with the functionalization of CI electrode arrays using different curling mechanisms. In recent years, there has been an increasing interest in "active" or "steerable" CI electrode arrays, which involves investigation of different actuator principles to bring about a controllable shape change. The following are examples of these mechanisms: use of an embedded actuation strand as described by Zhang et al. [24] and Zhang and Simaan [25], shape change of the silicone body by varying the pressure of an internal fluid as independently described by Arcand et al. [29] and Zentner [30], and the use of "smart materials" such as thermal shape-memory alloys. In

the latter, nickel-titanium (NiTi) alloys play a dominant role. One option is to use a single NiTi wire inside the electrode array, covering almost its entire length to provide a desired final shape [31, 32]. Alternatively, the integration of multiple, separately activatable actuators (in terms of an actuator array) is described [33, 34], the aim of which is to bring about a spatially resolved change in implant shape as, for example, via electrical resistance heating.

2. Materials and Methods

2.1. Hypothesis and General Approach. In contrast to manually controlled insertion, the automated insertion tool provides a means of adjusting the electrode's curling behaviour to the individual helical shape of the cochlea. The following working hypothesis was therefore proposed:

> *Individual adjustment of the curling behaviour of a preformed CI electrode array to the individual spiral shape of the cochlea can improve the insertion process in terms of reduced risk of insertion trauma.*

In order to test the hypothesis, a principle subject to general consensus in CI research was applied, according to which insertion forces are the main indicator of the risk of insertion trauma and are directly correlated to it. From a mechanical point of view, however, insertion forces are primarily a result of contact or constraining forces between the implant and the surrounding anatomy. Thus, the degree of contact between both "objects" allows a qualitative conclusion concerning the insertion forces and ultimately, therefore, concerning the risk of trauma. As a first step towards the substantiation of the working hypothesis, proof has to be provided that, by means of the controlled and continuous adjustment of the shape of the electrode array to that of the cochlea, the degree and severity of contact between them can be reduced. This enables a direct conclusion to be made concerning reduction of trauma risk.

For this purpose, the geometry and the curling behaviour of a commercially available CI electrode array were modelled, based on experimental data from a previous study [10]. Additionally, the anatomy of a representative number of human cochleae was modelled and brought together in a custom-made simulation tool called SimCInsert. Using this tool, the insertion process was simulated for the conventional manual procedure (both standard and minimally invasive access) and compared with full, manually optimized insertion. The risk of trauma was evaluated in all cases and discussed in the light of the working hypothesis.

2.2. Modelling the Preformed Electrode Array

2.2.1. Contour Advance Electrode Array.
The Contour Advance (CA) is a well-known and widely used preformed electrode array. Its silicone body is moulded in a precurved shape. Twenty-two half-banded platinum electrode contacts are embedded in it, each connected via a 25 μm thin platinum wire [35]. Therefore, the stiffness of the electrode array increases from the tip to the basal portion as the number of wires enclosed in the silicone increases. This stiffness gradient is reinforced by the decreasing diameter of the electrode array, which tapers from 0.8 mm down to 0.5 mm at the tip. The tip of the implant has a conical shape and was designed to reduce contact forces during insertion. This special feature of the CA is known as the Softip. A white marker between electrodes 10 and 11 (7.6 mm behind the tip) is a visual aid for the surgeon for estimating the insertion depth and was integrated to assist the execution of the Advance Off-Stylet (AOS) insertion technique. Finally, three silicone ribs at the end of the intra-cochlear portion indicate full insertion depth and facilitate sealing of the cochlea after insertion due to soft-tissue growth.

All electrode arrays employed in this study were provided by the manufacturer Cochlear Ltd. (Sydney, NSW, Australia). They were rejected during the production process owing to electrical defects. With respect to mechanical properties, which are of relevance for this study, these electrode arrays are, however, identical to commercially delivered and clinically used ones. They differ from the (also available) practice electrodes also provided by Cochlear Ltd. as, for example, part of surgical practice kits for teaching purposes and training courses. These practice electrodes are produced by a simpler manufacturing technique to be less expensive but therefore exhibit different curling behaviour than that of "real" implants. Practice electrodes were thus not usable for this kind of investigation [10].

2.2.2. AOS Technique.
Together with the new electrode array, the AOS insertion technique was introduced to standardize the manual insertion procedure and to provide the surgeon with a straightforward and reliable modus operandi. This launch of a "self-curling" electrode array [35], in conjunction with a special insertion technique, was therefore considered an important and valuable step conducive to decreasing the risk of soft-tissue trauma due to insertion. The AOS insertion technique involves keeping the CA electrode array straight and inserting it into the cochlea with the stylet inside until the white marker reaches the opening of the inner ear (cochleostomy). It is assumed that the white marker indicates that the tip of the implant reaches a central position within the basal turn of the cochlea. As a second step, the actual AOS phase, the stylet is kept stationary by the use of a small pair of tweezers and the electrode is advanced off it. Owing to internal bending stresses, the electrode array returns to its original shape and thus curls around the inner wall of the cochlea (modiolus).

2.2.3. Determination of Curling Behaviour.
The curling behaviour of several CA electrode arrays has already been determined in a former study [10]. Using a custom-made micromanipulator, the stylet was extracted in increments of 0.1 mm to 0.25 mm. After each step, the resulting shape of the CA electrode array was digitally documented using a reflected-light microscope (MZ 6, Leica Microsystems GmbH, Wetzlar, Germany, in conjunction with DS-L1, Nikon Cooperation, Tokyo, Japan). In this way, a series of images was generated which records the curling behaviour of each implant. For further processing of these images, a semi-automatic image-processing procedure was developed and applied to identify the centre of all 22 platinum contacts as well as the tip of the silicone body. The second step involved fitting a mathematical function, consisting of a logarithmic spiral and up to three straight segments, through the points. Hence, the actual shape of the electrode array (depending on the extent to which the stylet is removed) was finally modelled by a continuous curve. Figure 3 shows the visualization of one CA electrode array as a result of stylet extraction. After projection in the x-y plane, the movement of the electrode tip exhibits a typical sigmoidal curve (highlighted in blue in Figure 3(a)). This "curling profile" of each electrode array was used to compare the differences in the specific curling behaviour of different arrays.

To allow a representative investigation, four electrode arrays were selectively chosen from all measured implants referred to in [10], in order to cover the total range of known variability in curling behaviour. After determination of all curling profiles (the rigid gripping of the electrode array serving as the common reference), RE01 and RE08 were selected as examples of highly pronounced curling behaviour, measured as deflection of the tip from the straight configuration (see Figure 3(b)). RE06 was also chosen to represent a moderate curling profile and RE07 to represent the flattest curling profile.

2.2.4. Modelling the Electrode Array.
Based on these already existing data, the spatial dimensions of the electrode array in the curling plane were modelled. This was necessary for meaningful simulation of the intracochlear curling behaviour since, if the shape of the electrode array is represented only by a thin line, it is not sufficient to allow the interaction of the implant with the surrounding anatomical structures to be modelled. Therefore, the inner contour of the CA electrode array was modelled by drawing a second polyline at a constant distance of 0.15 mm to the fitted central path. The same applied to the outer contour of the electrode array, with decreasing distance between 0.65 mm and 0.45 mm to allow for the tapered shape of the silicone body. The tip was added to the outline by means of two straight lines. This approach to visualizing the changing geometry of the electrode array caused by stylet removal was verified by overlaying the original images with the drawn outline of the implant. Good agreement between the calculated shape of the electrode array and the experimental images was obtained, as shown in Figure 4.

(a) 2D visualization of curling behaviour

—— RE01	—— RE07
—•— RE02	—•— RE08
—•— RE05	—▲— RE09
—•— RE06	

(b) Curling profiles

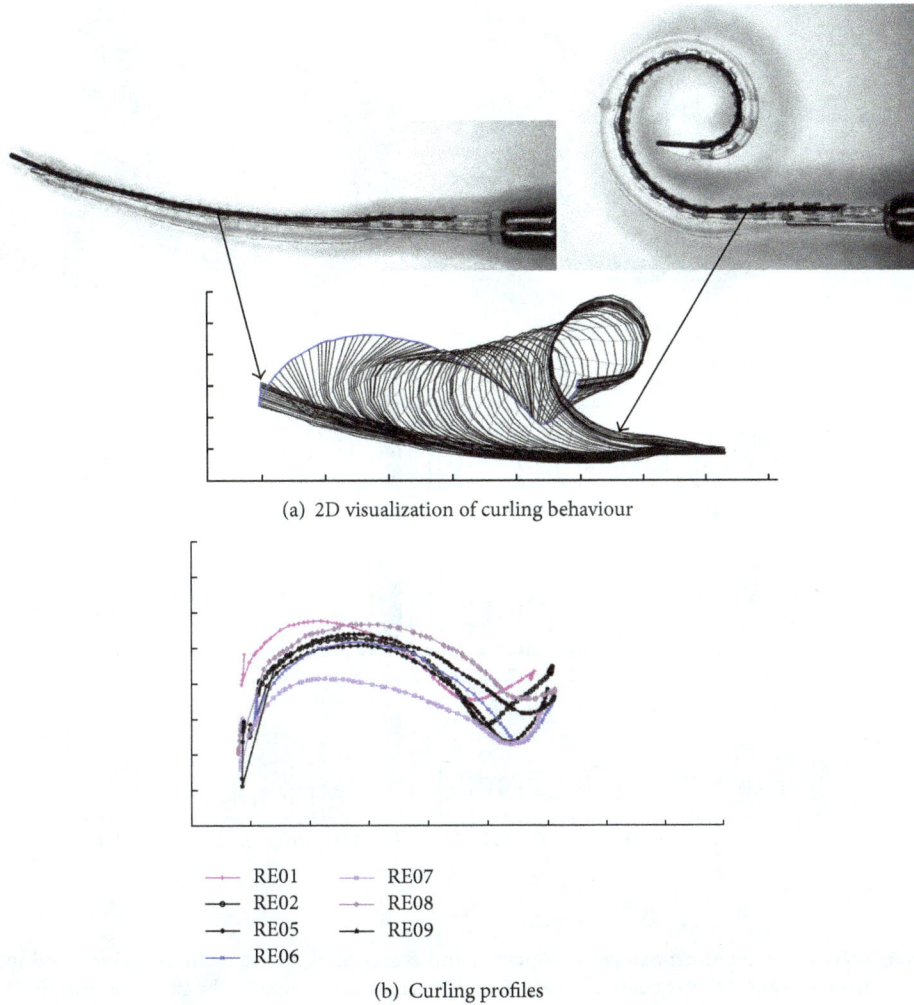

FIGURE 3: (a) Visualization of the curling behaviour of a preformed Contour Advance electrode array (RE06) using the 22 detected platinum contacts and the location of the Softip. The start configuration (on the left side) with stylet inside is characterized by a nearly straight configuration (compared with Figure 2(a)). Due to stylet extraction, the electrode array returns into its preformed spiral shape (right). By tracking the complete range of curling behaviour, the movement of the tip of the implant shows a typically sigmoidal curve. This curve is indicated using a bold blue line and is referred to as the curling profile of the electrode array (here RE06). Scale marks indicate 1 mm. (b) After determination of all curling profiles, four electrode arrays were selected and used in this study, which together cover the full range of curling behaviour investigated. RE01 and RE08 represent electrode arrays with a highly pronounced curling behaviour, measured as deflection of the tip from the straight configuration. RE06 was chosen to represent a moderate curling profile and RE07 to represent the flattest one.

2.3. Modelling the Inner Ear

2.3.1. Imaging and Segmentation.
Image data and segmentations of 23 human temporal bone specimens were available from former studies. These data were acquired using flat-panel-based volume computed tomography (fpVCT, GE Global Research Center, Niskayuna, NY, USA) [37, 38] at the Department of Diagnostic Radiology, Goettingen University Hospital (Goettingen, Germany). This experimental device allows higher resolution (approximately 200 μm, isometric) than does customary, clinically available computed tomography (CT) scanners. Using a threshold-based segmentation algorithm and manual refinement (iPlan 2.6 ENT, BrainLAB AG, Feldkirchen, Germany), 3D models of the human inner

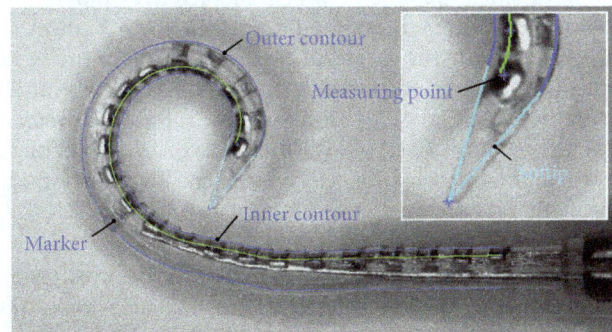

FIGURE 4: Overlay of an original image of the electrode array and its modelled shape.

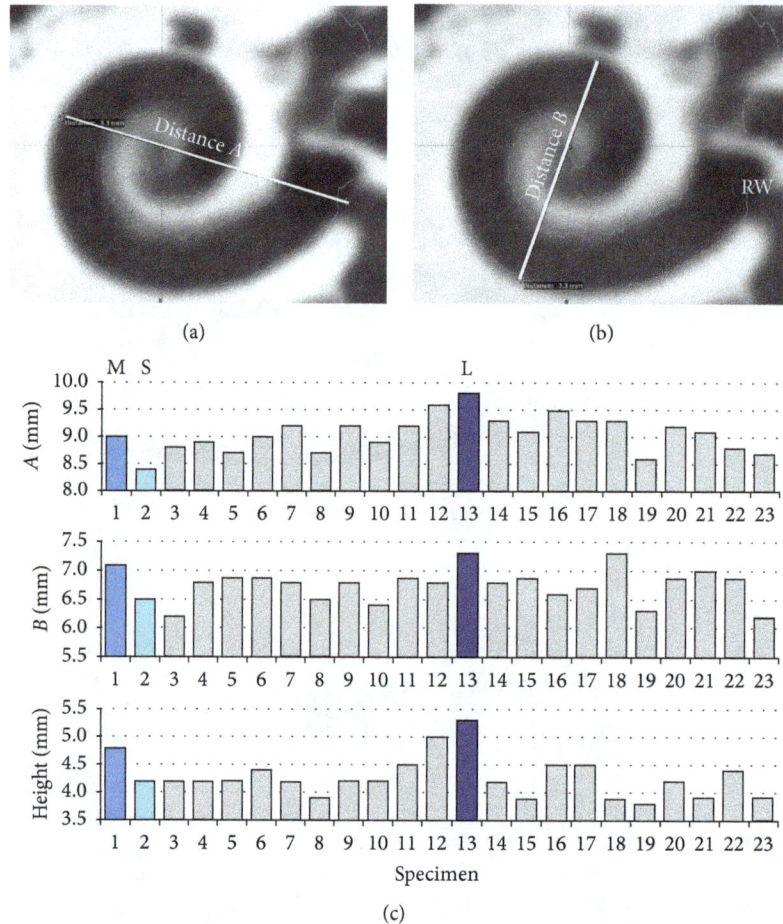

FIGURE 5: (a, b) Example images showing the measured distances *A* and *B* according to the metrological method introduced by Escudé et al. [36]. RW: round window membrane. (c) Bar chart showing *A* and *B* values and height of the inner ear for all 23 investigated cochleae. Distance *A* was used to distinguish the smallest, largest, and medium-sized cochlea.

ear had been generated. Segmentation covered the entire bone-embedded spiral canal of the cochlea and not merely the scala tympani, as the basilar membrane is not visible in X-ray-based imaging. Each 3D model of the inner ear had been saved as STL files (Standard Tessellation Language, a popular data format for 3D surface models).

The present study is designed to take into consideration the anatomical variability of the human inner ear. In order to have a single parameter which characterizes differences in size, a measurement method introduced by Escudé et al. [36] was applied. The greatest lateral dimension of the basal turn was measured (distance "A") in accordance with their description (see Figure 5). Based on these values, the smallest (CS), the medium-sized (CM), and the largest (CL) cochleae were chosen and used for the subsequent investigations as representatives of inherent anatomical variability.

2.3.2. Transformation into 2D.
The CA electrode investigated shows planar (two-dimensional, 2D) curling behaviour. This is common in perimodiolar cochlear implants for reasons of cost-effectiveness, as 3D curling behaviour requires separate products for left and right ears. The modelling of insertion

behaviour was, therefore, initially also considered as a 2D problem. This leads to the necessity of transferring the 3D volume data for the three selected cochleae into a 2D representation of their geometry. For this purpose, custom-made software was employed (courtesy of Mr. A. Hussong, Institute of Mechatronic Systems, Leibniz University of Hannover), which was developed using C++ in Visual Studio (Microsoft Corporation, Redmond, WA, USA) and VTK (Kitware Inc., Clifton Park, NY, USA). This program enabled the following steps:

(1) A segmented cochlea was loaded as an STL file.

(2) A rotation axis through the modiolus was manually determined. It was employed to calculate a cutting plane which provides a cross-sectional view of the cochlea.

(3) This cutting plane can be rotated in equal steps (here, 5° steps were used), starting with a plane which passes through the round window niche.

(4) Two points were manually selected for each resulting cross-sectional view. One marked the outer and the other the inner contour of the cochlea.

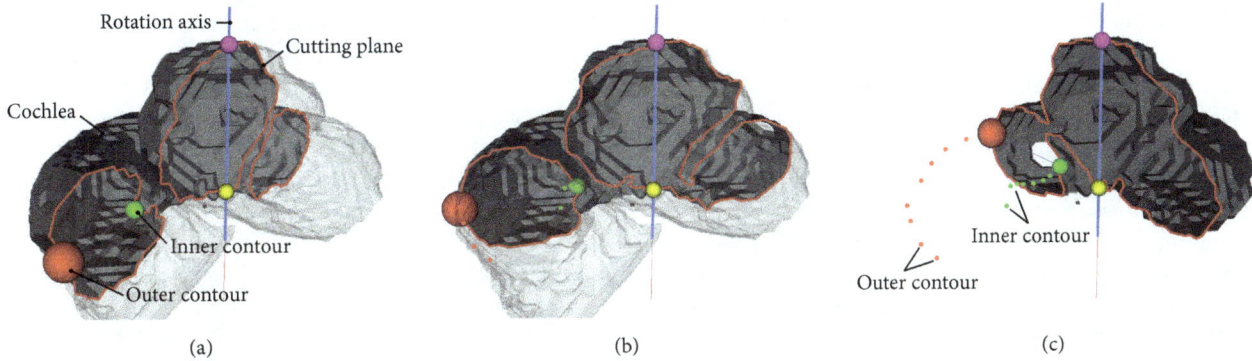

FIGURE 6: Principal procedure involved in transforming the three-dimensional geometric model of the cochlea into a two-dimensional one. A cutting plane, rotated around the central axis (modiolus), provides stepwise visualization of the cross sections. In each cross section, a point on the outer contour (red) and a second one on the inner contour (green) were manually marked. After perpendicular projection onto a common plane, the points in their totality described the geometry of the inner ear in a 2D manner.

By repeating steps (3) and (4), the spatial dimensions of the helical cochlear lumen were recorded as a 3D point cloud. Finally, these points were projected onto a plane (an orthogonal-distance regression plane) in order to obtain 2D curves describing the inner and outer contours of the cochlea (see Figure 6).

2.4. Modelling the Insertion Process

2.4.1. SimCInsert. Both in order to model intracochlear curling behaviour and for the intended optimization of the insertion process, a simulation tool called "SimCInsert" was developed using MATLAB (R2008b, MathWorks, Natick, MA, USA). The corresponding graphical user interface (GUI) is shown in Figure 7. The GUI allows loading of the prepared cochlear contours (see Section 2.3.2) which are visualized at a constant (fixed) position within the main window. In contrast, the visualization of the electrode array (also loaded via a task menu entry) is dynamic and based on the stored data on curling behaviour as a function both of stylet extraction and of interactively adjustable parameters for the position (Δx, Δy) and orientation ($\Delta \varphi$) relative to the cochlear contour. By using a slider at the bottom of the GUI, the user is able to control stylet retraction. The corresponding configuration of the electrode array is automatically loaded from the database (see Section 2.2.3). These "raw data" are transformed according to the manually chosen location parameters. As choosing the desired position and orientation of the electrode array relative to the cochlea's geometry involves a 2D task, there are displacements in both x and y directions, as well as one rotation around the cochleostomy. These "transformed data" are extended to the 2D representation of the electrode array as described in Section 2.2.4 and visualized in addition to the cochlear contour within the main window. Via translation in the negative x direction, for example, the feeding of the implant into the inner ear is simulated in SimCInsert (which is equal to insertion depth). In this way, SimCInsert provides a fairly simple means of simulating the conventional AOS technique, while also allowing manual optimization of the insertion process.

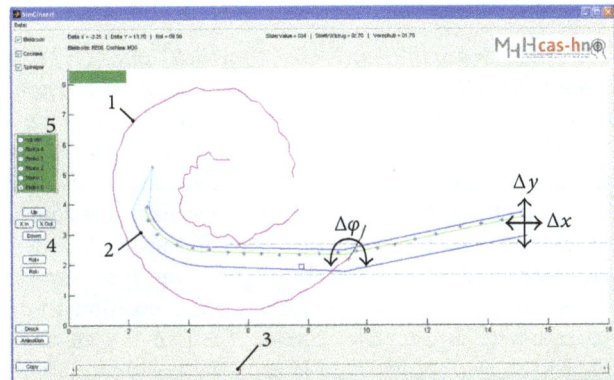

FIGURE 7: Graphical user interface (GUI) of the custom-made simulation tool "SimCInsert." It enables visualisation of both the geometrical data for the investigated inner ears (1, here: medium-sized) and the shape of the electrode arrays (2, here: RE06). Using the slider (3), the stylet (not visualized) can be virtually moved; that is, the array's shape is manipulated. Using six cursor buttons (4, two for each interactively adjustable parameter Δx, Δy, and $\Delta \varphi$), the location and orientation of the electrode array for each shape can be manipulated with respect to the cochlea plotted at the same (fixed) position. Use of both input options enables a complete insertion process to be simulated. Radio buttons (5) were included to interactively rate the risk of insertion trauma (see Section 2.5).

2.4.2. Simulation of the Manual AOS Technique (manAOS). The conventional, manually performed AOS insertion technique, as recommended by the CI manufacturer Cochlear Ltd., served as a reference for the subsequent optimization of the insertion process. In this case, only the second phase, with actual stylet extraction, was taken into account. However, the instructions for the AOS insertion technique are idealized. In reality, the CA electrode array shows a banana-shaped starting configuration, as opposed to a straight one, even where the stylet is fully plugged in. Therefore, a completely rectilinear/linear insertion into the basal turn (without contact with the cochlear walls) is in reality not possible.

Furthermore, each implant initially has a slightly different shape [10].

Thus, for the simulation of the manually performed AOS technique, it was assumed that the surgeon adjusts the insertion process (irrespective of whether this is done intuitively or in a controlled manner). Although there are no "hard data," this assumption is confirmed by observations in the operating theatre during cochlear implant (CI) surgery and the verbal reports of CI surgeons indicating that there is a slight compensatory movement when the initially curved electrode array is passed through the cochleostomy or the round window access. This manual adjustment is made possible by use of visual information through the surgical microscope, as well as haptic feedback. During the simulation, this compensatory movement was represented by a rotation in the xy plane. In this paper, the simulation of the manually performed AOS insertion technique is subsequently referred to as "manAOS."

2.4.3. Simulation of the Automated Approach (autoAOS).

The situation modelled as a second scenario involved accessing the inner ear by means of automated insertion through a minimally invasive drill canal. In this case, the electrode array is gripped behind the last platinum contact and is advanced in a strongly linear fashion into the cochlea inside the guiding tube of the insertion tool. In terms of the modelling in SimCInsert, this means that throughout the remainder of the insertion process, values for both the position in the y direction (Δy) and the rotation ($\Delta\varphi$) of the electrode array had to be kept constant after initial positioning. Only movement in the x direction (Δx) was used to insert the electrode array into the cochlear contour to the same extent as the stylet extraction. For evaluation of minimally invasive access, two parallel grey dashed lines in the main window of SimCInsert represent the edge of the drill hole or the guiding tube of the insertion tool.

2.4.4. Optimization of the Insertion Process (optIns).

Finally, the insertion of the CA electrode array was manually optimized and tailored to the three different sizes of cochleae, representing the anatomical variation in human individuals. All insertion parameters could, therefore, be modified in order to optimize the location of the electrode array within the cochlea. In particular, it was no longer necessary to maintain the strong linear relationship between stylet extraction and implant feed as specified by the AOS technique.

According to the initial working hypothesis, the aim of the optimization was to optimally tailor the curling of the implant to the individual anatomy of the inner ear at each stage of the overall insertion process. An optimum location within the cochlea was indicated by minimal overlap between the contour of the electrode array and the contours of the inner ear. A small amount of overlap was considered as equivalent to low contact forces (and hence low forces pertaining to insertion trauma) and vice versa.

This manual optimization was repeated for each stored configuration of the electrode array, that is, for all steps of stylet removal. Additional constraints were monotonic increase of implant feed (which means Δx), full insertion with complete stylet removal, and avoidance of abrupt changes in all insertion parameters. The latter was to ensure a well-adjusted and continuous insertion process which could be implemented by using, for example, an automated insertion tool and its programmable linear drives [19, 39]. Subsequently in this paper, the abbreviation "optIns" is used to refer to optimized insertion.

2.5. Trauma Risk: A Rating Scale for Risk of Insertion Trauma.

To allow comparative evaluation of these three different scenarios, especially comparison between individually optimized insertion and the conventional approach, a useful assessment procedure needed to be developed. Although it is known that "objective" measurement methods are generally considered to be more reliable than "subjective" ones, in this special case, a subjective rating scale was (on the strength of various arguments) introduced and preferred (discussed in detail in Section 4.3). The main argument is that there is a lack of computational structural mechanics. This means that deformation of the electrode array due to direct contact with the boundary of the inner ear cannot be simulated and correctly visualized. The main advantage of the new rating scale designated "trauma risk," explained below, is that the user is able, to a certain extent, to compensate for this lack of deformation simulation by their mechanical expertise. This allows holistic assessment of the insertion-related risk of trauma to the inner ear.

After Eshraghi et al. [40], a rating scale was introduced, known as "trauma risk," which extends between the grades 0 (no contact between implant and inner ear) and IV (extensive contour damage). Details can be found in Table 1. The classification was chosen based on the assumption that trauma risk of grades 0 and I has no negative influence on residual hearing preservation. Beginning with grade II, the risk of iatrogenic hearing loss or deafness increases, which is very likely at grade IV.

Using this risk-rating method for each step of the modelled insertions, the degree of conformity of the implants' shape and the shape of the inner ear was rated (see Figures 8 and 9). Ideally, the electrode array lies fully inside the contours of the cochlea without any intersection. This means contact-free insertion with no insertion forces and, therefore, no insertion trauma. Mechanical contact between the implant and the inner ear (resulting in contact forces and thus a corresponding risk of insertion trauma) is visualized as an intersection (damage) of the contour of the electrode array and the cochlear contour. The extent of contour damage allows a qualitative valuation of the corresponding risk of intracochlear trauma and therefore loss of residual hearing. However, the "trauma risk" rating scale introduced is not, unlike Eshraghi et al.'s [40] "trauma grade," a criterion for postexperimental evaluation. Rather, it is a method of estimating the risk of insertion trauma in advance (i.e., prospectively). Limitations of this evaluation method are discussed in detail in Section 4.3.

TABLE 1: Trauma risk: rating scale for evaluation of trauma risk, ranging from grade 0 to grade IV. Verbal description of the different criteria used for rating each step of electrode insertion.

Grade of "trauma risk"	Description and representation in the simulation
IV	(i) Extensive contour damage, secondary contact areas[†] due to electrode deformation and restraint[†] of the electrode array leading to high contact forces (ii) Electrode array is visualized far outside the cochlear contour
III	(i) Softip intersects with the cochlear contour by more than its total size (ii) Large-scale penetration of the silicone body by more than its total cross section (iii) Pronounced deformation[†] of the electrode array resulting in secondary contact areas[†] (iv) Involves additional contour damage[†], possibly including restraint[†] of the electrode array between inner and outer walls
II	(i) Softip intersects with the cochlear contour by more than half its size (ii) Orientation of the Softip contraindicates its yielding with low contact forces (iii) Large-scale penetration of the silicone body by more than a quarter of its cross section
I	(i) Slight contact between the Softip and the inner or outer contour (ii) Slight penetration of the silicone body up to 0.25 of the total cross section (iii) Intersection to such a small extent that it is assumed that the flexible Softip or the elastic electrode array results in (iv) no secondary contact owing to elastic deformations of the implant
0	(i) No contact between electrode array and cochlea.

[†]Not directly visualized but taken into consideration by the mechanically experienced user.

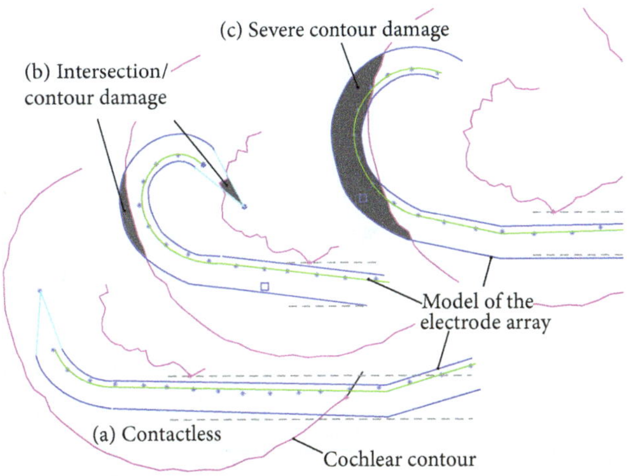

3. Results

In total, 36 insertions were modelled using three different cochleae (small, medium, and large) and four different electrode arrays in order to compare three different scenarios. As a reference, the manual procedure for inserting the Contour Advance (CA) electrode array using the Advance Off-Stylet technique (manAOS) was remodelled using SimCInsert. Applying the above-mentioned assumptions about the intuitive adjustment of the insertion process, the trauma risk of the insertion process is distributed as shown in Figure 10.

FIGURE 8: Examples of different kinds of contour damage/intersection. (a) Without contact between electrode array and cochlear contour (grade 0). (b) Trauma risk grade II with both penetration of the electrode tip into the inner wall and overlapping of the silicone body with the outer wall. In fact, both lead to relevant contact forces inside the inner ear. (c) Extensive contour damage which results in the highest risk of causing an insertion trauma (grade IV).

Irrespective of the specific electrode array and the size of the cochlea, a high proportion of the total process is characterized by a risk of trauma of grade ≥ II. More detailed information, using RE01 as an example, is provided in Figure 11. Differentiated according to the three different-sized cochleae, the trauma risk is plotted against stylet extraction (which is inversely proportional to insertion depth). Sample images from SimCInsert show the corresponding insertion depth as well as the contour damage. This schematic illustration demonstrates that insertion is initially less traumatic (in the basal turn of the cochlea) than with progressive insertion depth.

In contrast to the manual approach, the automated procedure is inadequate with regard to the necessary adjustable positioning and orientation, especially when using minimally invasive access to the inner ear. Simulation of the autoAOS scenario results in the trauma risk as shown in Figure 12. This figure clearly illustrates that a high proportion of phases are rated as high-risk (i.e., trauma risk ≥ III). For RE01 and RE08, the insertions were rated as potentially harmful in almost all cases. The RE07 electrode array is the exception; at least in some phases of the insertion process, the actual shape of the implant fits the anatomy of the cochlea, resulting in no or only minimal intersection of both contours.

Figure 13 provides detailed insight into the changing rating of the trauma risk with progressive insertion depth. For this purpose, the two extreme cases (RE01 and RE07) are plotted together in one figure to show the overall spectrum of the results and its correlation with the curling profile of the electrode array. While the insertion of RE01 is completely in the orange or red zone, the trauma risk using RE07 is at least reduced in the initial phase of insertion. It is striking that RE01 shows very pronounced deflection of the electrode tip from the ideal straight configuration, which means a marked

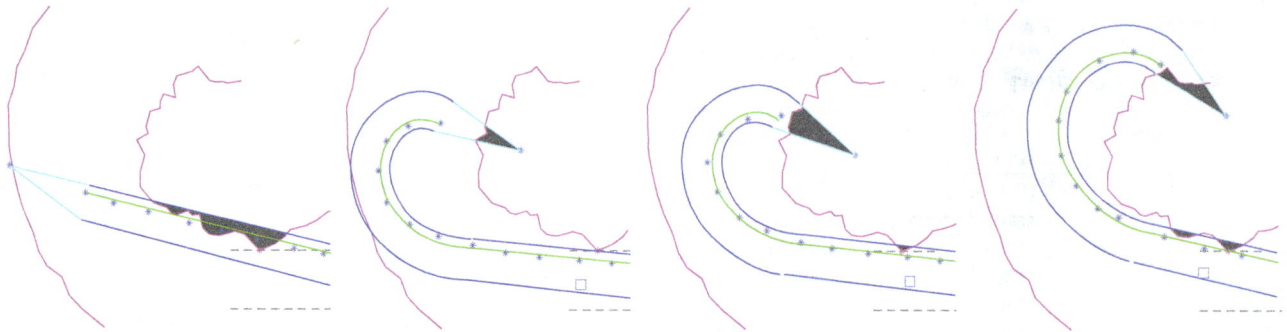

FIGURE 9: Examples of trauma risk grade II.

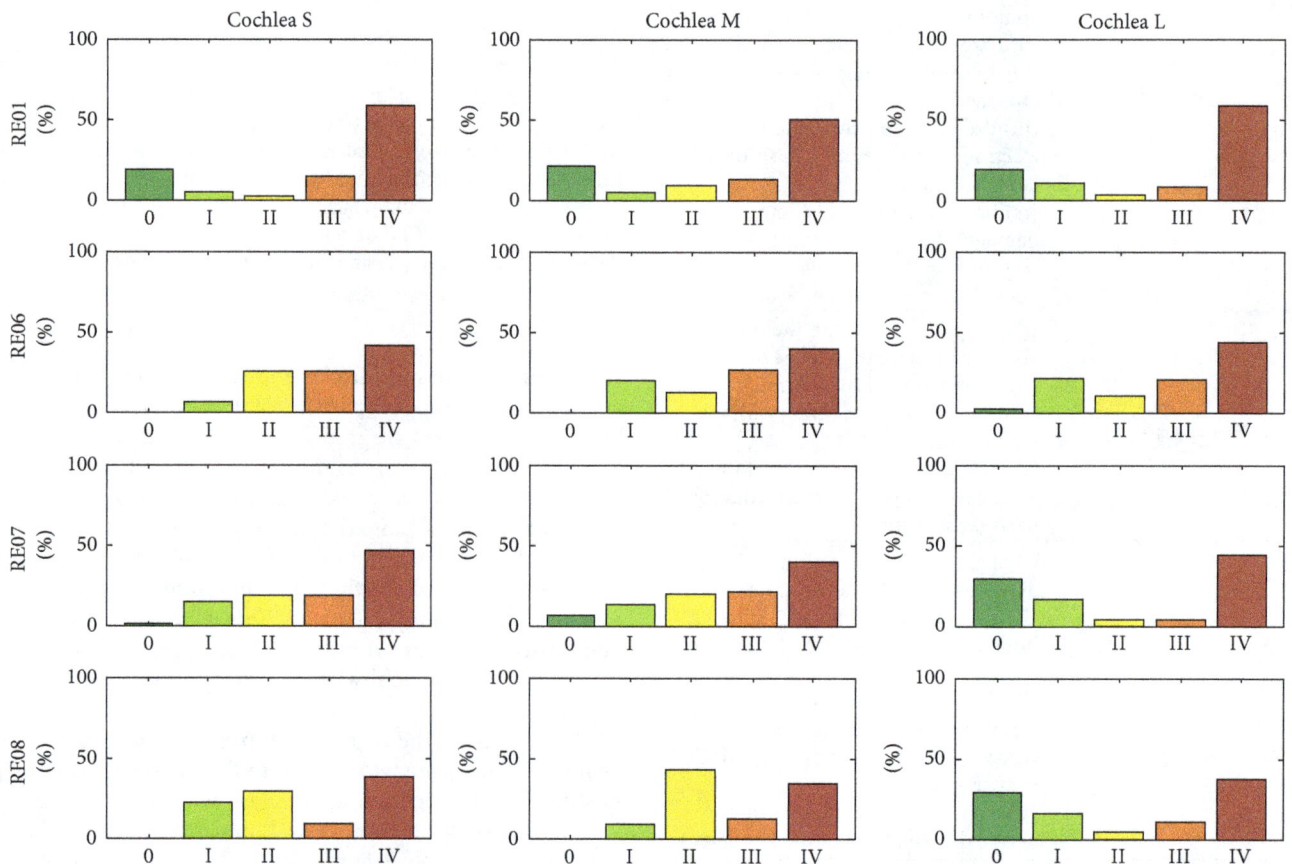

FIGURE 10: Histogram of the distribution (observation frequency) of the different trauma grades for each modelled insertion, where the procedure is performed manually (manAOS). To improve comparability, all results are normalized by reference to the total numbers of investigated steps in the insertion process.

initial curvature (starting configuration). In contrast, the profile for the curling behaviour of RE07 is very flat (see Figure 3). Based on this finding, it is concluded that the good straight starting curvature is causal and thus beneficial in terms of low trauma risk during the initial phase of the insertion process.

While insertion processes using the conventional AOS technique are mainly characterized by trauma risk grades III and IV, it is possible to reduce the risk of insertion trauma by means of the individual optimization strategy introduced. Figure 14 shows the percentage distribution of the trauma risk assessment for the optimized insertion

(optIns). In comparison with manAOS (see Figure 10) and minAOS (see Figure 12), it is evident that the overall insertion process is shifted toward less traumatic implantation. After optimization, by tailoring the specific curling behaviour of the electrode array to the individual anatomical constraints, the insertion process is chiefly characterized by trauma risk grade 0. In all 12 investigated cases (combinations of differing curling behaviour and cochlear anatomy), the rating of the trauma risk with grade 0 has the largest share.

The intracochlear curling caused by the stylet extraction and resulting from the individual optimization process is shown in Figure 15, with RE01 used as an example. As RE01 is

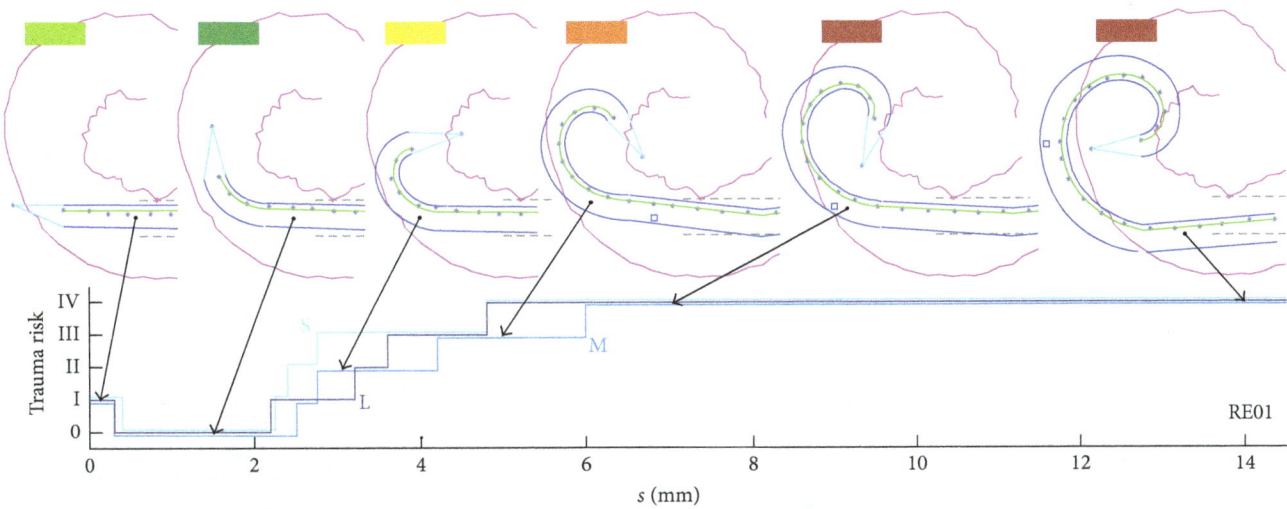

FIGURE 11: Change of trauma risk during the manually performed insertion process (manAOS), plotted for RE01 as an example, with corresponding screenshots from SimCInsert. Trauma risk is plotted against stylet extraction s.

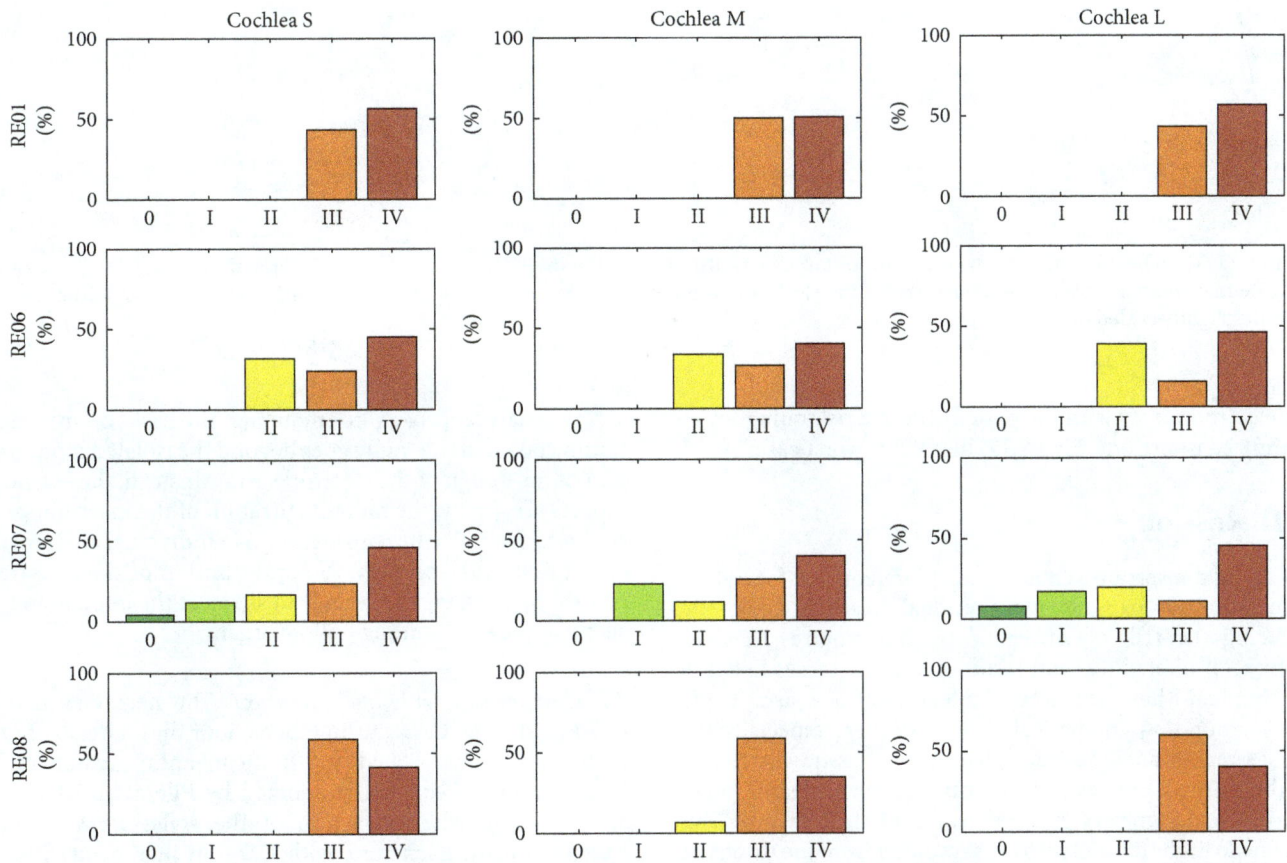

FIGURE 12: Histogram of the distribution (observation frequency) of the trauma risk where the procedure is performed in an automated manner. As no additional parameters could be adjusted to tailor the orientation of the electrode array, the simulation of the automated AOS technique (autoAOS) represents its most consistent implementation in this study. The histogram clearly shows the high portion of trauma risks III and IV on the insertion process. Only with RE07 is less trauma risk ($\leq$I) observed. Of the electrode arrays in the study, RE07 is the one with the flattest curling curve and pronounced straightening in the initial phase.

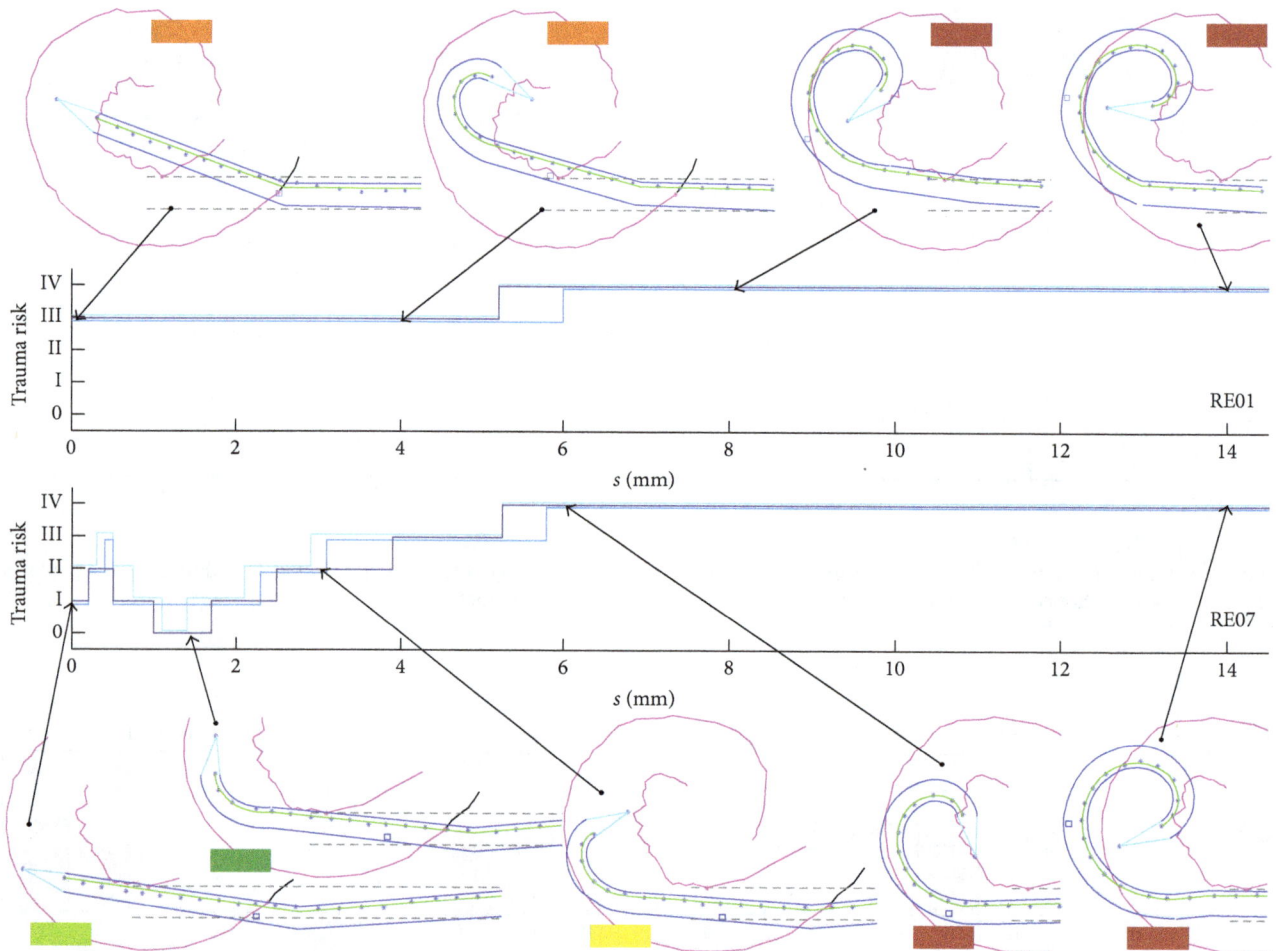

FIGURE 13: More detailed findings with regard to trauma risk throughout the insertion process for RE07 compared with RE01. The results indicate that where no additional adjustment of the electrode orientation is possible, a straight starting configuration is more advantageous than the slightly curled one.

the electrode array with the poorest trauma risk rating for all optimized insertions, Figure 15 shows the "worst case."

4. Discussion

Atraumatic insertion is a mandatory prerequisite for hybrid stimulation of patients with residual hearing. Generally, reducing the risk of iatrogenic trauma requires that the amount of interaction and resulting contact forces between the implant (here the intracochlear electrode array) and the surrounding anatomical structures (here especially the basilar membrane and other delicate soft-tissue structures) be diminished. One established strategy in cochlear implantation is to design very thin and flexible electrode arrays. This is done to limit the contact forces resulting from the extensive contact between these straight implants and the lateral wall of the cochlea. Another design strategy takes the shape of the inner ear into account: by producing helically preshaped electrode arrays, the aim from the outset was to reduce the amount of contact with the boundaries of the scala tympani. This was the purpose and motivation behind the introduction of the Contour Advance (CA) electrode.

The new approach to reducing the risk of insertion trauma taken in this study goes beyond the isolated modification of the design of the electrode array. Instead, the essential aspects are, firstly, the individualization of the insertion process, which entails the consideration of individual anatomical constraints and, secondly, the optimization of the insertion process by tailoring the change in shape of the implant to the shape of the surrounding hollow organ.

4.1. Comparison with the Literature. The necessary investigation of the CA's curling behaviour has already been performed and published [10]. In the meantime, comparable investigations have been conducted by Pile et al. [11], who also used stepwise extraction of the stylet from a fixed electrode array. Each step, with 1.27 mm increments (those in the present study being 0.1 mm to 0.25 mm), was digitally captured; the location both of the platinum contacts and of the electrode tip was manually marked and served as reference points for a curved line, that is, the mathematical shape model.

In contrast to the present study, their investigation was based on this line and did not consider the areal extent of

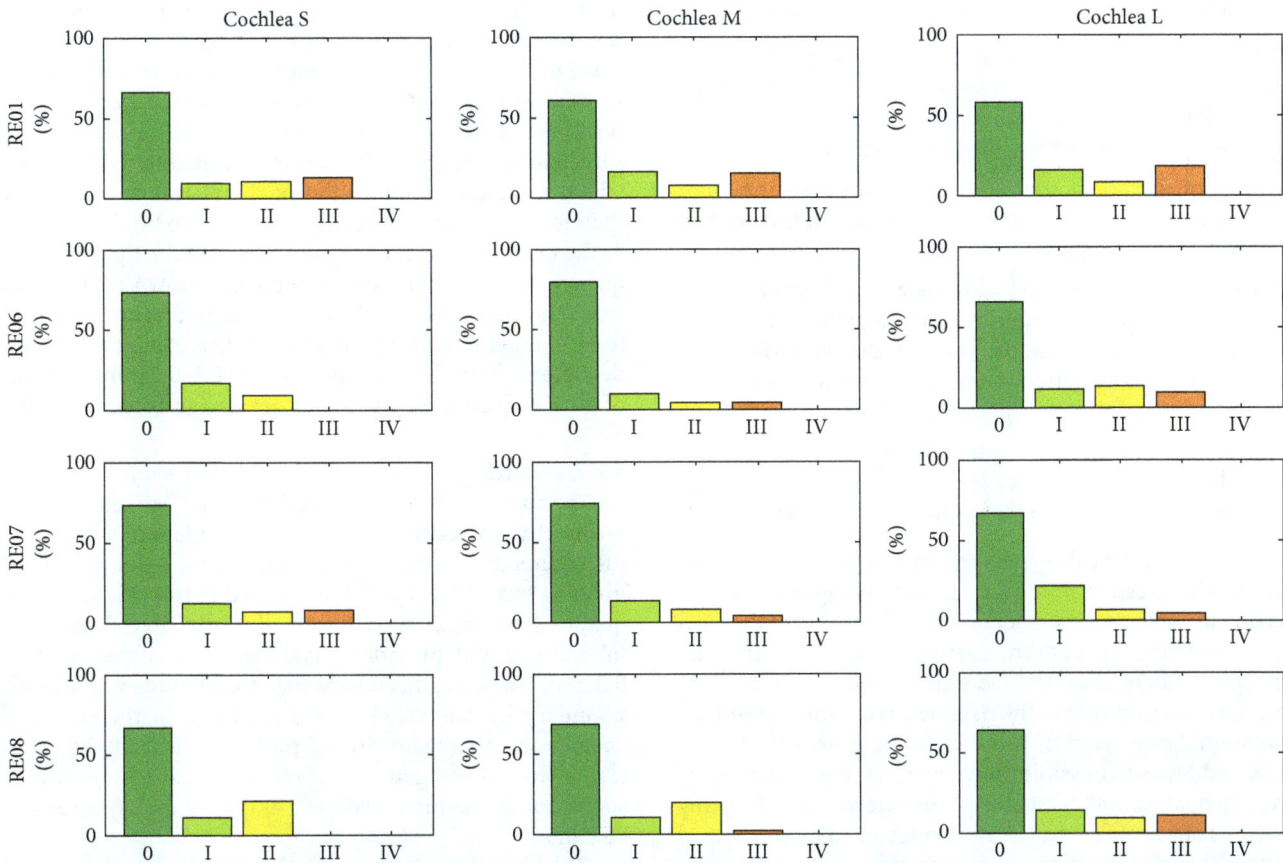

FIGURE 14: Histogram of the distribution (observation frequency) of the trauma risk after individual optimization of the complete insertion process (the AOS part). For all examined implants and inner ear geometries, it was possible to markedly reduce the risk of insertion trauma. Compare this figure with (optIns) Figure 10 (manAOS) and Figure 12 (autoAOS). The poorest outcomes are observed with RE01. However, after adjusting the curling of the electrode array to the surrounding anatomy, the insertion process is subject to trauma risk of grade 0 for all investigated cases.

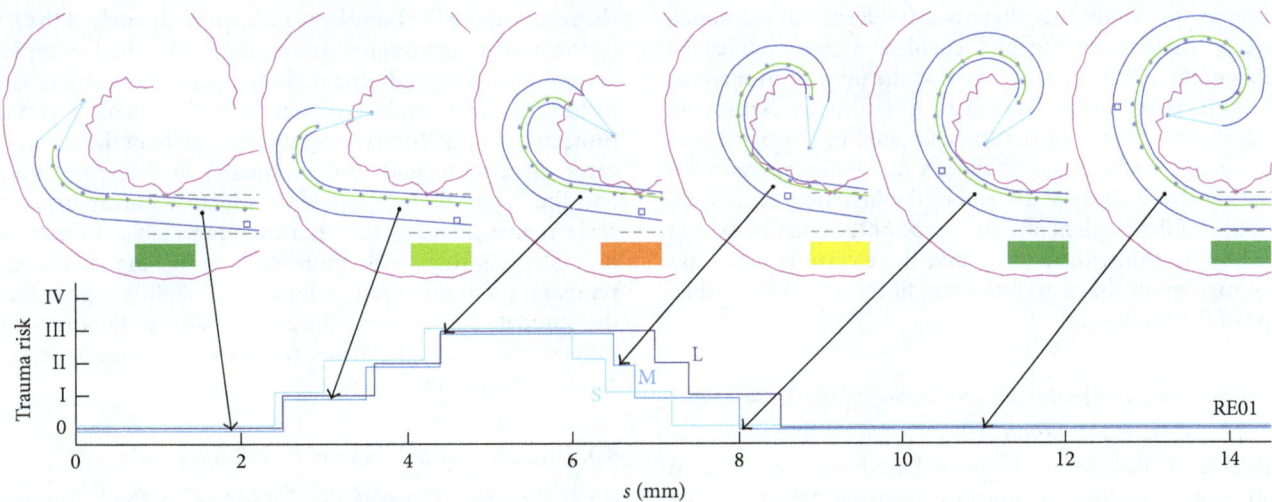

FIGURE 15: More detailed findings with regard to change in trauma risk during an optimized insertion. RE01 was chosen because, of all the optimizations, it represents the "worst case".

the implant. However, it is striking that both independent investigations lead to several similar results and conclusions:

(1) Comparison of different CA electrode arrays results in large variations. For optimized insertion, average values are less useful. Instead, the specific curling behaviour should be taken into consideration.

(2) Comparison of the curling behaviour of the same CA electrode array after repeated measurements produces fairly repeatable results.

(3) The shape of the CA electrode arrays does not fit the cochlear models employed. Instead, interference with the anatomical boundary can be observed. Therefore, a purely kinematic model cannot visualize the complex interaction as is possible with FEA.

(4) The optimization of controlled insertion of a movable electrode array is more effective if the array's orientation with respect to the cochlea can be changed.

In the context of their research on robot assistance for CI electrode insertion, Pile et al. [11] studied optimization of insertion by adjusting the orientation and location of the electrode array with respect to the cochlea. This means that their optimization algorithm covered four degrees of freedom, of which three correspond to the parameters Δx and Δy and the orientation $\Delta \varphi$ as used in this study. The fourth parameter was an additional possible movement in the x direction. This investigation was carried out using the measured curling behaviour of a set of seven CA electrodes and a mathematical cochlear model describing an average human scala tympani. Although the simulated robot-assisted insertion process was not compared with a conventional approach, their findings support the idea of automated insertion incorporating the specific "shape kinematic" (equivalent to what is referred to here as "curling behaviour"). The curling behaviour resulting from the Advanced Off-Stylet (AOS) technique was described as "incapable of not interfering to some degree with the inner wall of the scala tympani." This is in accordance with the finding in this study that there is a fundamental mismatch between implant curling and cochlear shape. While the curling of the electrode array starts at the tip with immediate and full recovery of the final shape due to stylet extraction, the electrode array is at that time located in the basal part of the cochlea, which is only slightly curved compared with the apical shape. Only at the end of the insertion process do the shape of the implant and the shape of the cochlea exhibit their best fit (notwithstanding that the electrode array has an average spiral shape and does not fit the actual individual shape of the inner ear).

4.2. Error Analysis: Quality and Reliability of the Modelling

4.2.1. Modelling the Contour Advance Electrode Array. The modelling of the electrode array based on the detected position of the platinum contact electrodes and the manually marked Softip proved to be useful [10]. Threshold-based segmentation algorithms had been tried out but did not provide usable results due to the weak contrast between the transparent silicone body and the background of the images.

In the two-dimensional (2D) model, the basal diameter is (at 0.8 mm) as specified by the manufacturer's data sheet. Toward the tip, however, the implant diameter modelled was, at 0.6 mm by 0.1 mm, larger than specified. This was the only way in which, for the vast majority of the images, it was possible to map the outer contour of the electrode array with sufficient accuracy. The reason is that the fitted central path, which represents the location of the platinum contacts and therefore the shape of the implant, tends to be shifted too far to the inside with increasing proximity to the tip. As a consequence, the inner contour is regularly drawn slightly offset from the true inner wall of the electrode array, which had to be compensated for by the larger diameter. However, total deviations are in the range of less than 0.1–0.2 mm. Modelling of the CA electrode array is thus deemed sufficiently accurate.

4.2.2. Modelling the Inner Ear. A similar value is estimated for the modelling error of the inner ear. Modelling quality is directly correlated with the segmentation which is, in turn, directly related to the quality and resolution of the imaging technique. FpVCT, employed in this study, is of high quality (compared with other clinically used X-ray-based modalities) and provides voxels with an isometric size of 0.2 mm. However, this means that a shift of the segmentation boundary by one voxel causes a change in the size of the cochlea model (again, by 0.2 mm). Additionally, there are errors due to the generation mesh, which triangulates the surface of the segmented object, as part of the export into the STL file.

The biggest shortcoming of the inner ear modelling is the absence of soft-tissue information (owing to the radiological imaging method). Therefore, the basilar membrane is not visible and the segmentation is not limited to the (actually crucial) scala tympani. Instead, the complete bony labyrinth of the inner ear is utilized for the measurement as described in Section 2.3.1. As a result, there is overestimation of the cross-sectional size of the scala tympani. The measurement procedure determines the maximum extension of the spiral-shaped cavity in the bony labyrinth approximately at the level of the basilar membrane. Assuming the implant occupies a central position inside the scala tympani, there is less space inside the "real" scala tympani than the cochlear contour projected in SimCInsert suggests. The extent of the associated error directly depends on the quality of the segmentation and the "vertical" location of the electrode array inside the scala tympani and is thus hardly quantifiable. In any case, it is obvious that, with more accurate sizing of the scala tympani, the trauma risk will be rated slightly higher for all the simulated insertions. The comparative evaluation of the different scenarios, however, remains unaffected by this, as do the conclusions drawn.

4.3. Discussion of the Trauma Risk-Rating Scale

4.3.1. Pros and Cons of the Subjective Method. The main disadvantage of the simplified modelling approach used in SimCInsert is the lack of computational structural mechanics. Instead of a "physical" simulation, as is possible with finite element analysis (FEA), the superposition of the interacting objects (electrode array and cochlear anatomy) is only visualized. Thus, the deformation of the flexible electrode array as a result of direct contact with the rigid cochlear walls is not calculated and therefore not displayed. Instead, the contact between both objects is visualized only as an intersection of both contours.

At an early stage of the project, an "objective" method of measurement was implemented in SimCInsert by calculating the depth of the intersection of the first contact area as the perpendicular distance between the farthest point of the contour of the electrode array and the cochlear contour. Although this method provided numerical values which were independent of the individual investigator, this approach was rejected because secondary contact of the implant inside the cochlea could not be taken into account. Thus, this measurement method is not suitable for assessing the overall intracochlear situation. Furthermore, numerical values misleadingly suggest accuracy. As there is no calculation of deformation, the correctness and validity of an "objective" measurement method of this nature are just as questionable as the preferred subjective rating method.

On the other hand, it is an advantage of the presented rating scale that users can benefit from their background knowledge about the flexible behaviour of the electrode array, as had been observed during insertion experiments on artificial cochlear models in the past [39]. Thus, the mechanical-deformation properties of the electrode array are taken more fully into account during the assessment of the contour damage than is possible with a strictly mathematical analysis of the simulation. The legitimacy of the subjective rating method is further strengthened by the fact that the introduced trauma risk is an assessment of the potential risk, that is, not a simulation of direct causal relationships. The direct prediction of real intracochlear damage is not possible with the SimCInsert tool because of the high complexity of the implant's interaction with the surrounding tissues. It is, therefore, of minor importance whether the trauma evaluation is carried out by a subjective assessment or an objective measurement. In both cases, the "trauma risk" allows only a qualitative statement about the likelihood ("very low" to "very high") that inner ear injury will occur.

4.3.2. Trauma Grade versus Trauma Risk.

It is important to bear in mind that the introduced "trauma risk" rating scale is usable only for estimating the potential risk, that is, for assessing the risk of insertion trauma in advance (prospective). In contrast to Eshragi's retrospective "trauma grade", it is not possible to rate or even to predict actual damage to intracochlear structures.

Therefore, it cannot be ruled out that a specific insertion, which is rated in the simulation with a high degree of "trauma risk," could be completely atraumatic in the (hypothetical) case of an identical real insertion. Conversely, some uncertainty remains concerning whether a simulated insertion rated with a low risk of intracochlear trauma could lead to significant hearing loss, if it has been possible to exactly experimentally reproduce the simulation. Of course, the already-mentioned complexity of the implant-tissue interaction, the necessary simplifications for SimCInsert, and,

finally, the fundamental limitations of the available analysis methods and technologies render such an experimental verification of the simulation results effectively impossible. To clarify the distinction regarding the actual trauma grade using Eshragi's rating scale, Roman numerals were used for the "trauma risk."

4.4. Validity of Simulation Results

4.4.1. manAOS. The simulation of the manually performed AOS insertion technique was based on the presumption that there is (intuitive) adjustment of the insertion process by the surgeon. This assumption was derived from observations, both directly in the operating theatre and using surgical videos. A compensation movement can be regularly observed, which is used by the surgeon to overcome the slight initial curvature of the electrode array when passing it through the incised round window membrane or the cochleostomy. Imperfect straightening of this kind can be found for all known perimodiolar electrode arrays and for certain straight ones (e.g., the Hybrid-L electrode, Cochlear Ltd.). Due to its extent (up to several millimetres), this movement is of relevance for the insertion process. After projection of the movement into the 2D simulation environment SimCInsert, it is equivalent to pivoting around the cochleostomy ($\Delta\varphi$). Taking this compensation movement into consideration for the modelling of the manual procedure is therefore justified and necessary if realistic results are to be obtained. In consequence, it was supposed that an ideal straight-line insertion (i.e., without rotational and translational motions of the implant which superimposes the feed) does not correspond to reality. The quantitative extent of this compensation movement has not, however, yet been measured and is, hence, an aspect that is potentially controversial. However, feasible measurement technologies that address this issue (e.g., stereooptical navigation systems) need to be very accurate, as well as small, lightweight, and inconspicuous, in order not to affect the surgeon's intuitive process. Thus, such technologies are currently not available.

4.4.2. autoAOS. The modelling of the AOS insertion technique as an automated process via minimally invasive access involved greater limitations. Here, the limits of the SimCInsert simulation tool were most clearly noticeable. A straightening effect of the surrounding guiding tube of an insertion tool (or, at least, of the bony wall of the drill canal) on the initial curved electrode array was not observed. Such an effect could only be (highly restrictively and indirectly) incorporated over the course of trauma risk assessment. In contrast, adequate consideration of a guiding tube in SimCInsert is possible only if separate series of measurements are available using mechanical guidance bars to limit the curling behaviour of the investigated electrode arrays during the measuring process. Alternatively, FE analysis is conceivable, which allows appropriate modelling of the restricted guidance of the tube (provided that reasonably accurate knowledge of the material parameters is available).

Of all three examined scenarios, the simulation of autoAOS represents the most consistent implementation of the AOS technique. Since stylet extraction and implant feed were the only two adjustable parameters (but directly linked by indirect proportionality), this is very much in accordance with the manufacturer's recommendations. It also corresponds to the situation when using an automated insertion tool and programs it according to the AOS standard. The integrated actuators will indeed implement the desired movements of implant and stylet in a precise but consistent manner. The insufficient initial straightening of the electrode array, combined with the lack of possibility of performing a compensation movement (owing to the absence of sensory feedback from an open, i.e., not closed, loop control), leads to a high frequency of ratings with grade III or even IV.

Individual results using autoAOS show the advantage of a straight starting configuration. The best outcomes were obtained with electrode array RE07. With the other electrode arrays, however, there are also phases of the insertion process without risk for hearing preservation (grades 0 and I). RE07 is characterized by the flattest curling profile and shows pronounced straightening in the initial phase. The shape of the "trauma risk" curve during insertion indicates that the process is less traumatic in the basal part of the cochlea than in the apical region (see Figure 13). These simulation-based results are confirmed by insertion experiments on transparent artificial cochlear models [39]. They support the conclusion that initial contact between the electrode array and the cochlear wall in the basal region can be prevented by a straight starting configuration. However, slightly bent electrode arrays touch the inner wall.

In practice, a major deficiency of preformed electrode arrays, namely, the insufficient initial straightening, can be compensated for by a guiding tube. This kind of mechanical straightening of the implants would have an impact on the intracochlear situation in the simulation with SimCInsert comparable to that of the adjustment of the intracochlear position of the electrode array toward a contactless midscala position using Δx and $\Delta \varphi$ for manAOS. It is therefore expected that, in practical implementation of autoAOS incorporating a guiding tube, the trauma risk for an insertion process of this kind (referred to as "minAOS") is in the same range as manAOS.

4.5. Individually Optimized Insertion: A Successful Approach

4.5.1. Benefit of Individually Optimized Insertion. Notwithstanding the inaccuracies involved in modelling of minAOS/autoAOS due to the insufficient consideration of the influence of a guiding tube, the results presented clearly demonstrate the advantages of individual optimization of the insertion process. Comparison of Figures 12, 10, and 14 clearly indicates that the entire insertion process is shifted toward a gentler procedure, which means a less traumatic and therefore less risky insertion process in terms of hearing preservation. This finding is highlighted by the contrasting juxtaposition, in Figures 16 and 17, of all three insertion strategies investigated. For the first strategy mentioned, the results of the risk rating for the different electrode arrays are shown in separate rows. The outcomes for the small, medium-sized, and large cochleae are summarized within each bar chart. In Figure 17, however,

the results are sorted by size of cochlea, with separate rows for CS, CM, and CL. The different electrode arrays are colour-coded in each bar chart. The shift in trauma risk toward lower values due to the increasing level of optimization is clearly visible in Figures 16 and 17: from autoAOS without adjustable insertion parameters, to manAOS with slightly adjustable orientation, and finally optIns representing holistic optimization.

It is noteworthy that the incidence of trauma risk grade IV is nearly equal in those cases with consistent (autoAOS) implementation and manual (manAOS) implementation of the AOS technique. This applies irrespectively of which electrode array (variations in curling behaviour) or which investigated cochlea (anatomical variations) is used. The "intuitively optimized," manual-insertion-only phases of the insertion process with grade ≤ III can be carried out in a more minimally traumatic manner. Only by considering information about both the individual anatomy and the specific curling behaviour of the inserted electrode array, as was carried out for optIns, is it possible to substantially reduce the risk of insertion trauma.

This remarkable improvement in insertion behaviour with optIns is evident in the high percentage of grade 0 outcomes. For optIns, this degree of risk rating accounts, in all cases, for the largest portion of the total insertion process. After optimization, by adjusting the specific intra-cochlear curling behaviour of the electrode array to the individual anatomical constraints, the insertion process is unquestionably less risky than without optimization. The working hypothesis is thus substantiated.

The summary of the results in Figures 16 and 17 highlights that the differences in the rating of trauma risk for the insertion of the same electrode array into different cochlea are comparatively low, whereas the outcomes for different arrays but the same cochlea vary far more. In Figure 17, the probability of trauma risk III in the case of an automated AOS insertion is illustrated. The marked grouped bar plots appear quite similar for all three cochleae, indicating that there is not much difference in trauma risk for different-sized cochleae. However, in each bar plot the results for different electrode arrays vary greatly. This finding is a strong indication that insertion behaviour (i.e., insertion forces and insertion trauma) is more dependent on the specific implant's curling characteristics than on the patient-specific anatomy of the inner ear. Hence, the variability of the curling behaviour has a higher impact on the achievable reduction of trauma risk within the optimization process than individual differences do in cochlear anatomy.

These findings are supported by a closer look at the insertion parameters, as provided in Figures 18 and 19. In both cases, subfigure (a) shows the optimized insertion parameters $\Delta \varphi$ and Δy in comparison with the AOS technique. In subfigure (b), the same graphs are colour-coded by cochlear size, and in subfigure (c) equal colors indicate the same electrode array. Only in the second case can regularities be found in the insertion process supporting the conclusion of a greater impact of curling behaviour on the quality of the insertion process. In a converse consideration, this means that only if the curling behaviour of the used implant

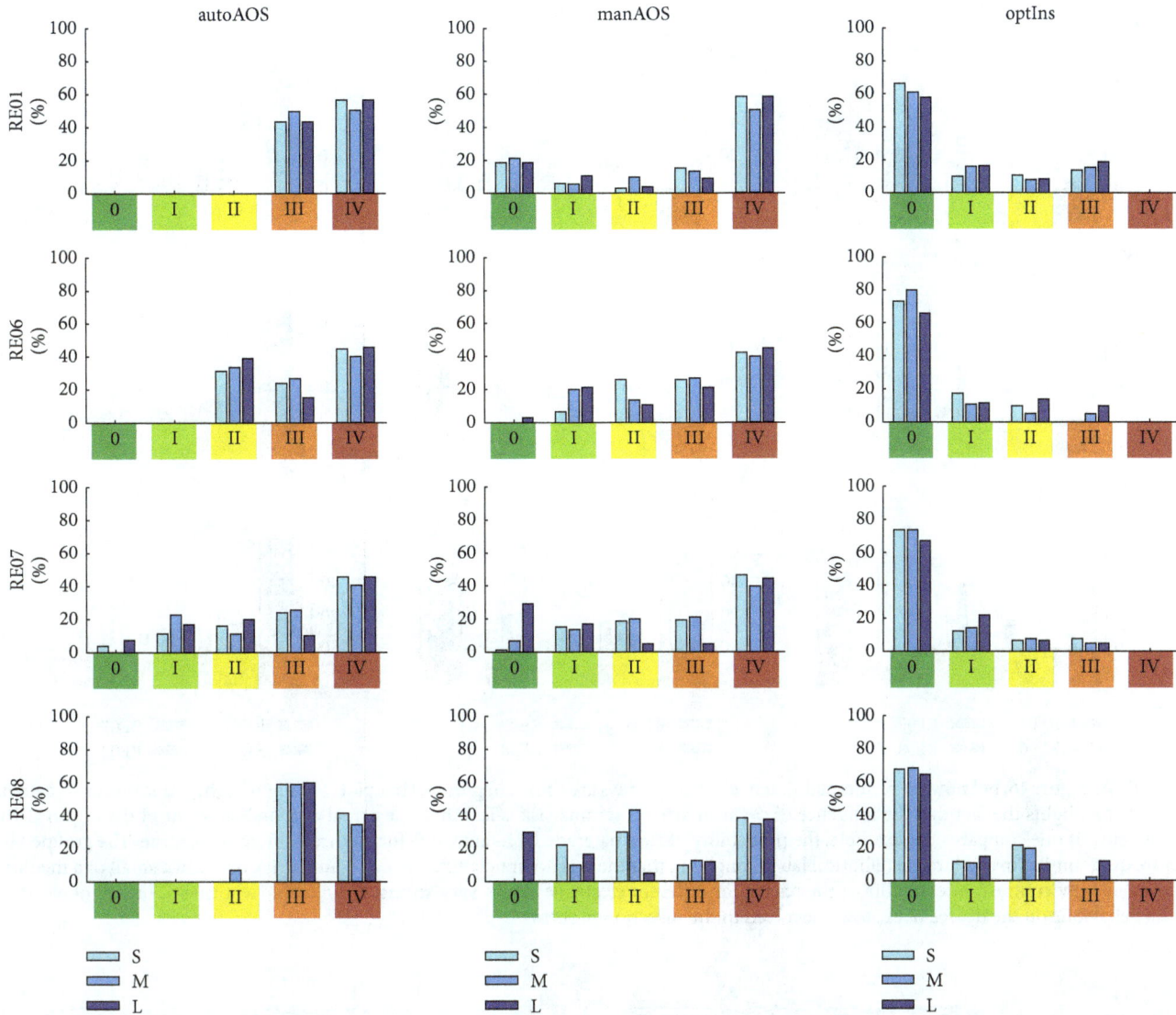

FIGURE 16: Comparison of results with respect to the electrode array investigated (rows of tabularly arranged histograms). Different cochlear size is indicated by different colours (cf. Figure 5) in the grouped bars of each plot.

is known during preoperative planning can the insertion process be significantly optimized. Knowledge only of the individual anatomy (shape of the cochlea) does not allow prediction of the most useful insertion parameters for gentle and therefore less traumatic insertion.

The converse implication of this finding is that improvements to the electrode arrays, such as more predictable curling behaviour, a straight starting configuration, or even steerable electrodes for truly controlled insertion, have strong potential to enhance the insertion process. This primary importance of curling behaviour with regard to an optimization process for electrode insertion is an encouraging outcome in terms of clinical implementation. Even with the available electrode arrays, and later with technical advances to the implants, improved insertion is possible. Only when this optimization potential is fully exploited is a detailed consideration of the individual anatomy necessary for further improvements. Thus, innovative, clinically approved,

high-resolution imaging methods to acquire detailed anatomical information on the patient are not absolutely essential in the short term. Improvement of the insertion process is already possible even before these become available. This is why optimization strategies regarding cochlear implant (CI) electrode insertion should address the implant's curling behaviour and curling mechanism.

4.5.2. Limitations. The outcomes of the optimization process also show that it was not possible in all cases to find a "contactless" shape and location for the electrode array inside the inner ear. There are two main reasons why individual optimization of the insertion process by using the CA electrode array is of only limited benefit. The first reason is related to the type of passive curling behaviour which can be found in that type of preformed electrode array. In consequence, that portion of the electrode array which is released from the stiffening effect of the stylet reverts immediately and

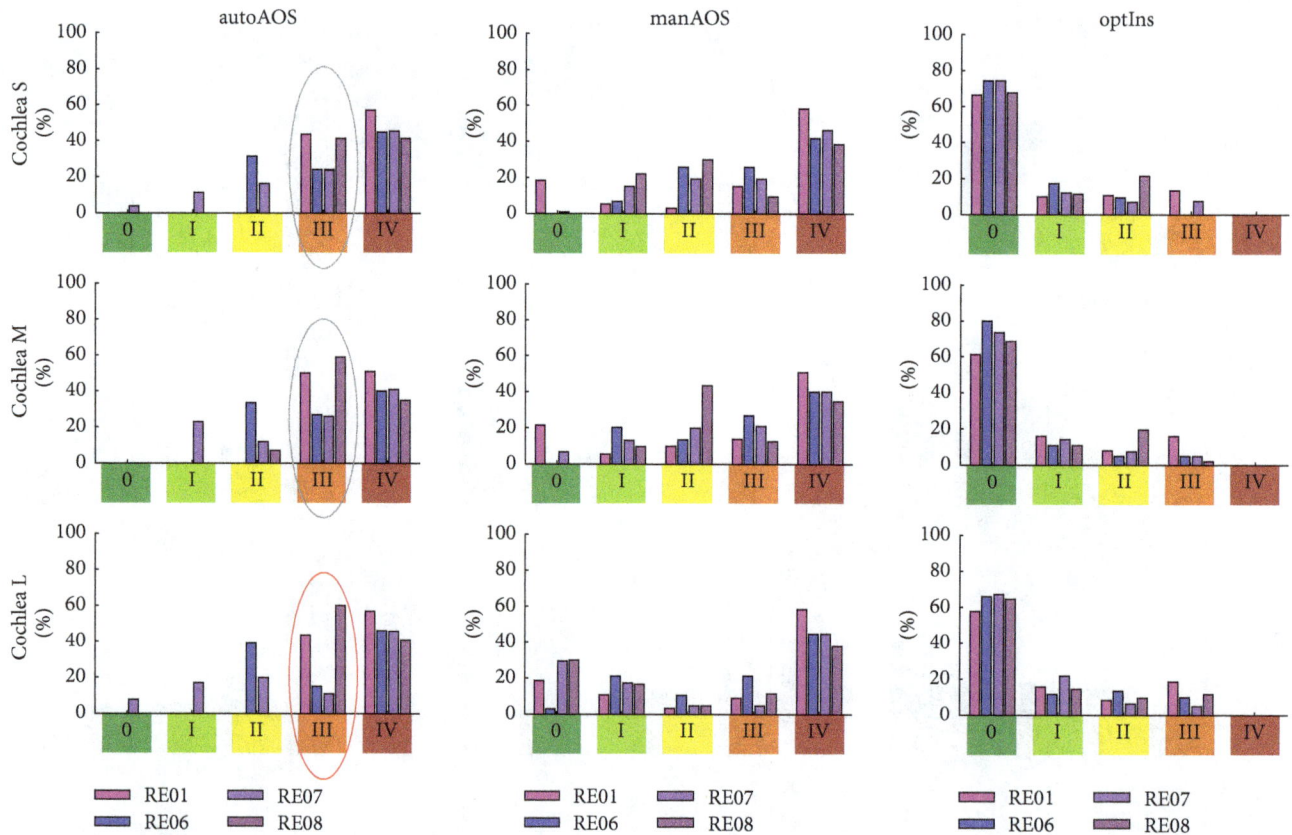

FIGURE 17: As Figure 16, but now the results of different electrode arrays are shown in grouped bar plots (cf. Figure 3(b)). This means visualizing the results highlights the fact that the influence of cochlear size on trauma risk is less than the actual curling behaviour of the implant. This becomes clear if one compares, for example, the probability of trauma grade III in autoAOS for all three different cochleae. The grouped bar plots are quite similar in appearance (elliptical label), implying that there is not much difference in trauma risk between a small or a medium-sized cochlea. By contrast, in each ellipse, the results for different electrode arrays vary strongly, indicating a strong influence of electrode curling behaviour on the degree of exposure involved in the insertion process.

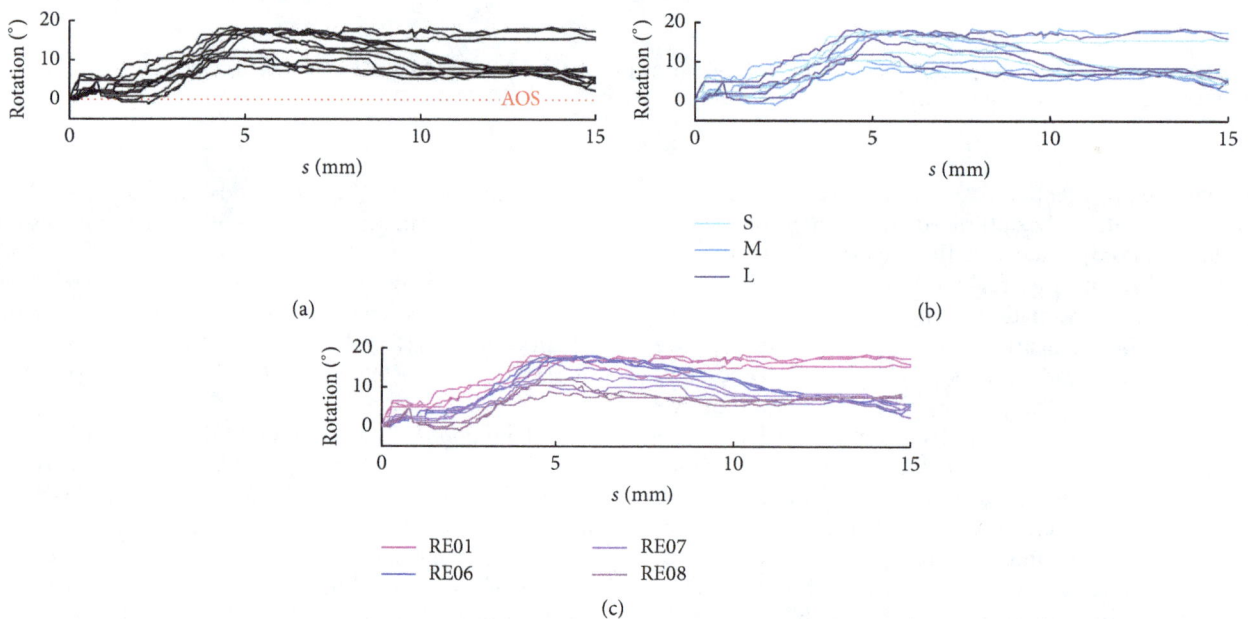

FIGURE 18: Process parameter $\Delta\varphi$ against stylet extraction s for all manually optimized insertions, normalized by the initial value at $s = 0$ mm. (a) All 12 optimized simulations compared with the AOS technique without rotation. (b) Different cochlear size is indicated by different colours. (c) Different electrode arrays are colour-coded.

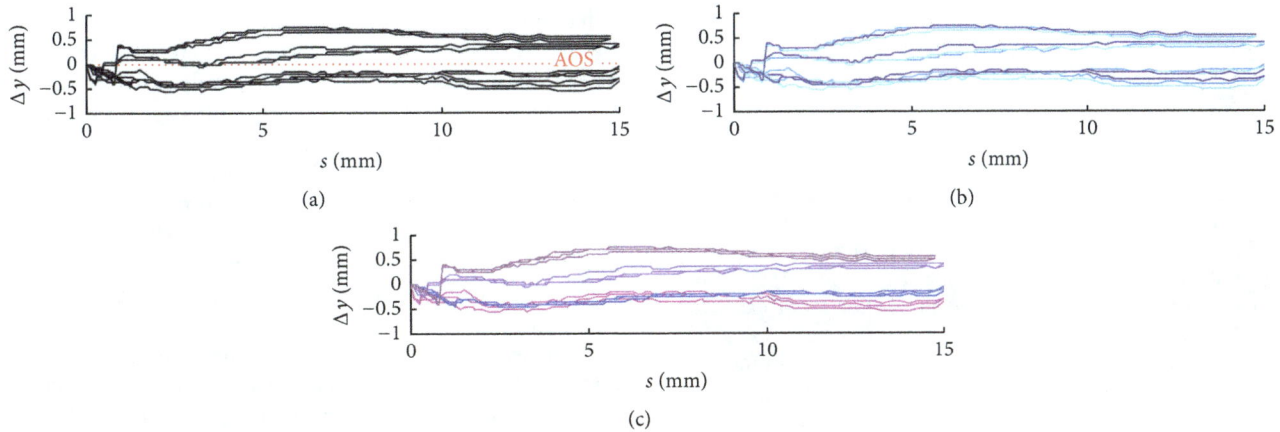

FIGURE 19: Process parameter Δy against stylet extraction s for all manually optimized insertions, normalized by the initial value at $s = 0$ mm. Refer to Figure 18 for legend.

completely into its manufactured shape. Thus, a characteristic aspect of curling behaviour in the CA electrode is the coiling which starts from the tip of the implant. However, this leads to a fundamental mismatch between the changes in the spiral shape of the electrode array and the spiral shape of the inner ear, one which cannot be overcome by the optimization process. While the electrode array is moved in the basal, and therefore only slightly curved, part of the inner ear, the electrode array already shows the final and maximum curvature in the tip region due to the onset of stylet extraction. Only with total insertion depth and in the final position shapes of the electrode array and the inner ear is there an ideal match.

However, this confirmation is also limited, which leads to the second of the above-mentioned reasons: the average spiral shape with which the CA electrode is produced. The shape of the electrode array is neither individually produced, nor is it possible to individualize the curling behaviour itself (as would be possible with an integrated microactuator array, as described by [34]). Instead, adjustment to the patient-specific shape of the inner ear is (as in the present study) indirectly possible only by tailoring the parameters of the insertion process.

4.6. Prospects for Clinical Implementation. The benefits of an individually optimized CI electrode insertion process will lead to noticeable and measurable advantages for the patient only if it can be transferred into clinical practice. As well as the challenges involved in enhancing the experimental prototypes of the automated insertion tool [21, 41] into an intraoperatively usable medical device, the use of the CA electrode array in the context of this new approach necessitates that certain issues be addressed. A central aspect is that the specific curling behaviour of the inserted electrode array must be known or calculable during a preoperative planning and optimization procedure. In other words, the designated electrode array, after removal from the sterile packaging, must show exactly the same curling behaviour in practice that was assumed during the virtual simulation process to achieve the best-possible optimization outcome.

Every deviation between the simulated and the actual curling profile reduces the benefits of the optimization process.

As this entails higher complexity and additional effort, it is appropriate to consider the least time-consuming approach in using average data. This could involve one-off measurements of a representative number of electrode arrays and calculation of an average curling profile. In the course of the preoperative, patient-specific optimization process, this average curling profile needs only to be combined with individual image data for the cochlea. Although both Rau et al. [10] and Pile et al. [11] showed that there is large variability between different CA electrode arrays, a closer look at the results of the present study reveals that even a simplified and limited approach of this nature provides advantages compared with a fully nonoptimized procedure. In particular, for robot-assisted and therefore automated insertion without sensory feedback (and intuitive adjustment, as with the manual approach), anatomy-specific planning would appear to be beneficial, and for several reasons:

(1) Although the white marker is a good and established indicator of initial insertion depth (the first step of the AOS technique), this can be improved by taking into account the individual length of the basal turn of the cochlea. As the length between electrode tip and white marker is not dependent on the curling profile, there are no relevant differences between different CA electrodes.

(2) A closer look at the relationship between implant feed and stylet extraction shows that there is uniform deviation from the original AOS technique after optimization. As Figure 20 shows, even if an averaged insertion profile (black line) is used, the trauma risk can be reduced. This applies especially to the last two-thirds of the insertion process.

(3) Where the AOS technique was employed for the simulation, excessively deep insertion was frequently observed resulting in a large degree of contour damage/intersection. As already mentioned in (2), average limitation of the insertion depth may be expected to reduce insertion forces.

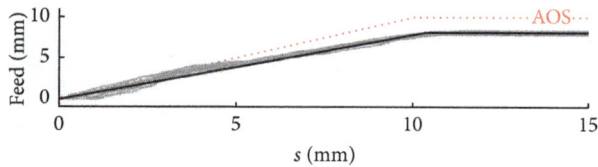

FIGURE 20: Comparison of the relationship between implant feed (*y* axis) and stylet extraction (*x* axis) for the AOS technique (red dotted line, strong linear relationship as recommended by the manufacturer) and for the optimized insertions (grey lines). The black line indicates an averaged profile for stylet extraction during the insertion process; even this small change appears to be advantageous compared with the conventional AOS technique.

However, the use of the CA electrode array in conjunction average values for curling behaviour has several drawbacks. It should not be forgotten that the CA was not originally designed for this concept. Two independently performed investigations showed high variability in curling behaviour, which limits the usefulness of previously experimentally determined average values. As a consequence, there would be large deviations between the planned and actually performed insertion with corresponding reductions in the benefit from a given optimization. For a comprehensively optimized insertion process, the determination of an averaged curling profile is not an option. In order that the advantages of individually optimized insertion can be fully exploited intraoperatively, it is necessary to compensate for the high amount of variability in curling behaviour. For this purpose, different strategies are under consideration which are listed below (sorted by increasing complexity):

(1) Individual determination of the curling behaviour of the electrode array.

(2) Design features:

 (a) Insertion tool with guiding tube.
 (b) Stiffer stylet for straighter starting configuration.

(3) New technologies to reduce variability.

 (a) Automated manufacturing processes (batch processing) for higher reproducibility of curling behaviour.
 (b) Active curling mechanism; steerable or controllable curling behaviour.

Clinical implementation in the near future can be achieved by individual determination of curling behaviour. This requires no changes in the design of the electrode array and only minor modifications of the certified manufacturing processes. As regards production, an assembling process already exists by which the stylet is integrated into the electrode array. The measurement can, therefore, be carried out by the CI manufacturer. After reloading of the stylet, the electrode array can be delivered together with the associated curling profile data. This approach is supported by two facts: first, the high degree of reproducibility of the curling

behaviour after repeated extraction of the stylet [10, 11] (if the implant is not affected by mechanical forces with plastic deformation) and, secondly, curling behaviour being strongly influenced by the starting configuration and initially exhibiting pronounced variations. After approximately 2 mm of stylet removal, the variation decreases substantially. Relative changes are between 0.1 and 0.2 mm [10] which allows mathematical prediction of subsequent curling. For practical purposes, this means that only the initial phase of curling behaviour needs to be measured, making it significantly easier to determine.

The second strategy to reduce the amount of variability between different electrode arrays is based on the finding that the starting configuration has a strong impact on it. Thus, use of a straightening tube will improve the predictability of curling behaviour and, therefore, the benefit of the optimization procedure. Comparable results could be achieved by use of a stiffer stylet which helps to overcome the slightly curved starting configuration with its (demonstrated and discussed) drawbacks regarding insertion behaviour.

A more forward-looking approach involves research activities in the field of CI electrode development which address how to obtain more controllable and steerable curling behaviour in order to perform a controllable insertion. Different curling mechanism or integrated actuators are currently under investigation, including embedded actuation strands [24, 25], fluidic actuators [29, 30], and the use of smart materials such as Nitinol [31, 32]. In the context of actuated CI electrode arrays, it is worth distinguishing between mechanisms which change curling behaviour in a global manner and those which allow for individual and spatially differentiated changes in implant shape. While the former types of development may provide curling behaviour with higher reproducibility and therefore improved predictability, only the use of multiple microactuators [33, 34], which are arranged inside the electrode array along its longitudinal axis, may allow an insertion which is genuinely individualized. However, this experimental research is at present far removed from clinical practice.

5. Conclusion

In this study, it was shown that the passive curling behaviour of clinically established cochlear implant (CI) electrode arrays holds potential for further optimization of the insertion process. By means of controlled, individualized tailoring of the movement and change in shape of the implant to the inner ear anatomy of a given patient, the insertion process can be optimized regarding a reduced risk of intracochlear damage. It is especially noteworthy that this improvement was achieved without any modifications or even development of new, active (i.e., steerable) electrode arrays with an integrated curling mechanism, but rather with a commercially available implant. Therefore, these findings highlight out an entirely novel aspect of clinical application of the Contour Advance (CA) in particular and preformed perimodiolar electrode arrays in general. Although this has not yet been investigated, it is self-evident that comparable improvement can also be achieved using other preformed CIs such as those incorporating MRA or HiFocus Helix electrodes.

Disclaimer

Responsibility for the contents of this publication lies with the authors.

Conflict of Interests

The authors declare that there is no conflict of interests regarding the publication of this paper.

Acknowledgments

The authors would like to thank Professor Hartmut Witte (head of Biomechatronics, Faculty of Mechanical Engineering, Ilmenau University of Technology) for helpful discussions concerning the optimization procedure and the rating of the simulation outcomes and Mr. A. Hussong (formerly of the Institute of Mechatronic Systems, Leibniz University of Hannover) for providing the software used in Section 2.3.2. The authors are also grateful to Mr. C. Richardson for paper proofreading. The project was funded by the German Federal Ministry of Education and Research (BMBF). The project numbers are 01EZ 0832 and 16SV 3943.

References

[1] A. Büchner, M. Schüssler, R. D. Battmer, T. Stöver, A. Lesinski-Schiedat, and T. Lenarz, "Impact of low-frequency hearing," *Audiology and Neurotology*, vol. 14, no. 1, pp. 8–13, 2009.

[2] P. Van De Heyning and A. K. Punte, "Electric acoustic stimulation: a new era in prosthetic hearing rehabilitation," *Advances in Oto-Rhino-Laryngology*, vol. 67, pp. 1–5, 2010.

[3] M. F. Dorman, A. J. Spahr, P. C. Loizou, C. J. Dana, and J. S. Schmidt, "Acoustic simulations of combined electric and acoustic hearing (EAS)," *Ear and Hearing*, vol. 26, no. 4, pp. 371–380, 2005.

[4] M. F. Dorman, R. Gifford, K. Lewis et al., "Word recognition following implantation of conventional and 10-mm hybrid electrodes," *Audiology and Neurotology*, vol. 14, no. 3, pp. 181–189, 2009.

[5] W. Gstoettner, J. Kiefer, W.-D. Baumgartner, S. Pok, S. Peters, and O. Adunka, "Hearing preservation in cochlear implantation for electric acoustic stimulation," *Acta Oto-Laryngologica*, vol. 124, no. 4, pp. 348–352, 2004.

[6] W. K. Gstoettner, P. van de Heyning, A. F. O'Connor et al., "Electric acoustic stimulation of the auditory system: results of a multi-centre investigation," *Acta Oto-Laryngologica*, vol. 128, no. 9, pp. 968–975, 2008.

[7] M. Jurawitz, A. Büchner, T. Harpel et al., "Hearing preservation outcomes with different cochlear implant electrodes: nucleus hybrid L24 and nucleus freedom CI422," *Audiology and Neurotology*, vol. 19, no. 5, pp. 293–309, 2014.

[8] S.-M. Cords, G. Reuter, P. R. Issing, A. Sommer, J. Kuzma, and T. Lenarz, "A silastic positioner for a modiolus-hugging position of intracochlear electrodes: electrophysiologic effects," *American Journal of Otology*, vol. 21, no. 2, pp. 212–217, 2000.

[9] E. Von Wallenberg and R. Briggs, "Cochlear's unique electrode portfolio now and in the future," *Cochlear Implants International*, vol. 15, no. 1, pp. S59–S61, 2014.

[10] T. S. Rau, O. Majdani, A. Hussong, T. Lenarz, and M. Leinung, "Determination of the curling behavior of a preformed cochlear implant electrode array," *International Journal of Computer Assisted Radiology and Surgery*, vol. 6, no. 3, pp. 421–433, 2011.

[11] J. Pile, M. Y. Cheung, J. Zhang, and N. Simaan, "Algorithms and design considerations for robot assisted insertion of perimodiolar electrode arrays," in *Proceedings of the IEEE International Conference on Robotics and Automation (ICRA '11)*, pp. 2898–2904, IEEE, Shanghai, China, May 2011.

[12] W. P. Liu, M. Azizian, J. Sorger et al., "Cadaveric feasibility study of da Vinci Si-assisted cochlear implant with augmented visual navigation for otologic surgery," *JAMA Otolaryngology—Head & Neck Surgery*, vol. 140, no. 3, pp. 208–214, 2014.

[13] O. Majdani, T. S. Rau, S. Baron et al., "A robot-guided minimally invasive approach for cochlear implant surgery: preliminary results of a temporal bone study," *International Journal of Computer Assisted Radiology and Surgery*, vol. 4, no. 5, pp. 475–486, 2009.

[14] S. Baron, H. Eilers, B. Munske et al., "Percutaneous inner-ear access via an image-guided industrial robot system," *Proceedings of the Institution of Mechanical Engineers Part H: Journal of Engineering in Medicine*, vol. 224, no. 5, pp. 633–649, 2010.

[15] L. B. Kratchman, G. S. Blachon, T. J. Withrow, R. Balachandran, R. F. Labadie, and R. J. Webster, "Design of a bone-attached parallel robot for percutaneous cochlear implantation," *IEEE Transactions on Biomedical Engineering*, vol. 58, no. 10, pp. 2904–2910, 2011.

[16] B. Bell, C. Stieger, N. Gerber et al., "A self-developed and constructed robot for minimally invasive cochlear implantation," *Acta Oto-Laryngologica*, vol. 132, no. 4, pp. 355–360, 2012.

[17] B. Bell, N. Gerber, T. Williamson et al., "In vitro accuracy evaluation of image-guided robot system for direct cochlear access," *Otology and Neurotology*, vol. 34, no. 7, pp. 1284–1290, 2013.

[18] J.-P. Kobler, J. Kotlarski, J. Öltjen, S. Baron, and T. Ortmaier, "Design and analysis of a head-mounted parallel kinematic device for skull surgery," *International Journal of Computer Assisted Radiology and Surgery*, vol. 7, no. 1, pp. 137–149, 2012.

[19] A. Hussong, T. S. Rau, T. Ortmaier, B. Heimann, T. Lenarz, and O. Majdani, "An automated insertion tool for cochlear implants: another step towards atraumatic cochlear implant surgery," *International Journal of Computer Assisted Radiology and Surgery*, vol. 5, no. 2, pp. 163–171, 2010.

[20] O. Majdani, D. Schurzig, A. Hussong et al., "Force measurement of insertion of cochlear implant electrode arrays in vitro:comparison of surgeon to automated insertion tool," *Acta Oto-Laryngologica*, vol. 130, no. 1, pp. 31–36, 2010.

[21] J.-P. Kobler, D. Beckmann, T. S. Rau, O. Majdani, and T. Ortmaier, "An automated insertion tool for cochlear implants with integrated force sensing capability," *International Journal of Computer Assisted Radiology and Surgery*, vol. 9, no. 3, pp. 481–494, 2014.

[22] D. Schurzig, R. F. Labadie, A. Hussong, T. S. Rau, and R. J. Webster III, "A force sensing automated insertion tool for cochlear electrode implantation," in *Proceedings of the IEEE International Conference on Robotics and Automation (ICRA '10)*, pp. 3674–3679, IEEE, May 2010.

[23] D. Schurzig, R. F. Labadie, A. Hussong, T. S. Rau, and R. J. Webster III, "Design of a tool integrating force sensing with automated insertion in cochlear implantation," *IEEE/ASME Transactions on Mechatronics*, vol. 17, no. 2, pp. 381–389, 2012.

[24] J. Zhang, W. Wei, J. Ding, J. T. Roland, S. Manolidis, and N. Simaan, "Inroads toward robot-assisted cochlear implant surgery using steerable electrode arrays," *Otology & Neurotology*, vol. 31, no. 8, pp. 1199–1206, 2010.

[25] J. Zhang and N. Simaan, "Design of underactuated steerable electrode arrays for optimal insertions," *Journal of Mechanisms and Robotics*, vol. 5, no. 1, Article ID 011008, 2013.

[26] R. F. Labadie, J. Mitchell, R. Balachandran, and J. M. Fitzpatrick, "Customized, rapid-production microstereotactic table for surgical targeting: description of concept and in vitro validation," *International Journal of Computer Assisted Radiology and Surgery*, vol. 4, no. 3, pp. 273–280, 2009.

[27] R. F. Labadie, R. Balachandran, J. E. Mitchell et al., "Clinical validation study of percutaneous cochlear access using patient customized micro-stereotactic frames," *Otology and Neurotology*, vol. 31, no. 1, pp. 94–99, 2010.

[28] T. R. McRackan, R. Balachandran, G. S. Blachon et al., "Validation of minimally invasive, image-guided cochlear implantation using Advanced Bionics, Cochlear, and Medel electrodes in a cadaver model," *International Journal of Computer Assisted Radiology and Surgery*, vol. 8, no. 6, pp. 989–995, 2013.

[29] B. Arcand, S. Shyamsunder, and C. Friedrich, "A fluid actuator for thin-film electrodes," *Journal of Medical Devices*, vol. 1, no. 1, pp. 70–78, 2007.

[30] L. Zentner, "Mathematical synthesis of compliant mechanism as cochlear implants," in *Proceedings of the 1st Workshop on Microactuators and Micromechanisms (MAMM '10)*, Aachen, Germany, May 2010.

[31] O. Majdani, T. Lenarz, N. Pawsey, F. Risi, G. Sedlmayr, and T. Rau, "First results with a prototype of a new cochlear implant electrode featuring shape memory effect," *Biomedizinische Technik*, vol. 58, pp. 1–2, 2013.

[32] K. S. Min, S. B. Jun, Y. S. Lim, S.-I. Park, and S. J. Kim, "Modiolus-hugging intracochlear electrode array with shape memory alloy," *Computational and Mathematical Methods in Medicine*, vol. 2013, Article ID 250915, 9 pages, 2013.

[33] B. Chen, H. N. Kha, and G. M. Clark, "Development of a steerable cochlear implant electrode array," in *3rd Kuala Lumpur International Conference on Biomedical Engineering 2006*, vol. 15 of *IFMBE Proceedings*, pp. 607–610, Springer, Berlin, Germany, 2007.

[34] O. Majdani, "Elektrodenentwicklung für Cochlea-Implantate zum Erhalt des restlichen Hörvermögens (GentleCI)," in *Proceedings of the MikroSystemTechnik*, pp. 12–15, 2009.

[35] J. F. Patrick, P. A. Busby, and P. J. Gibson, "The development of the Nucleus Freedom Cochlear implant system," *Trends in Amplification*, vol. 10, no. 4, pp. 175–200, 2006.

[36] B. Escudé, C. James, O. Deguine, N. Cochard, E. Eter, and B. Fraysse, "The size of the cochlea and predictions of insertion depth angles for cochlear implant electrodes," *Audiology and Neurotology*, vol. 11, supplement 1, pp. 27–33, 2006.

[37] S. H. Bartling, R. Gupta, A. Torkos et al., "Flat-panel volume computed tomography for cochlear implant electrode array examination in isolated temporal bone specimens," *Otology and Neurotology*, vol. 27, no. 4, pp. 491–498, 2006.

[38] S. Obenauer, C. Dullin, and M. Heuser, "Flat panel detector-based volumetric computed tomography (fpVCT): performance evaluation of volumetric methods by using different phantoms in comparison to 64-multislice computed tomography," *Investigative Radiology*, vol. 42, no. 5, pp. 291–296, 2007.

[39] T. S. Rau, A. Hussong, M. Leinung, T. Lenarz, and O. Majdani, "Automated insertion of preformed cochlear implant electrodes: evaluation of curling behaviour and insertion forces on an artificial cochlear model," *International Journal of Computer Assisted Radiology and Surgery*, vol. 5, no. 2, pp. 173–181, 2010.

[40] A. A. Eshraghi, N. W. Yang, and T. J. Balkany, "Comparative study of cochlear damage with three perimodiolar electrode designs," *Laryngoscope*, vol. 113, no. 3, pp. 415–419, 2003.

[41] T. S. Rau, M. Kluge, L. Prielozny, J.-P. Kobler, T. Lenarz, and O. Majdani, "Auf dem Weg zur klinischen Anwendung: Eine Weiterentwicklung des automatisierten Insertionstools für Cochlea-Implantate," in *Tagungsband der 12. Jahrestagung der Dt. Gesell. für Computer- und Roboterassistierte Chirurgie e.V. (CURAC)*, W. Freysinger, Ed., pp. 41–45, 2013.

14

The Relationship of the Facial Nerve to the Condylar Process: A Cadaveric Study with Implications for Open Reduction Internal Fixation

H. P. Barham,[1] P. Collister,[2] V. D. Eusterman,[2] and A. M. Terella[2]

[1]*Department of Otolaryngology-Head and Neck Surgery, Louisiana State University Health Sciences Center, 533 Bolivar Street, Suite 566, New Orleans, LA 70112, USA*

[2]*Department of Otolaryngology-Head and Neck Surgery, University of Colorado, Aurora, CO, USA*

Correspondence should be addressed to H. P. Barham; hpbarham@hotmail.com

Academic Editor: Jeffrey P. Pearson

Introduction. The mandibular condyle is the most common site of mandibular fracture. Surgical treatment of condylar fractures by open reduction and internal fixation (ORIF) demands direct visualization of the fracture. This project aimed to investigate the anatomic relationship of the tragus to the facial nerve and condylar process. *Materials and Methods.* Twelve fresh hemicadavers heads were used. An extended retromandibular/preauricular approach was utilized, with the incision being based parallel to the posterior edge of the ramus. Measurements were obtained from the tragus to the facial nerve and condylar process. *Results.* The temporozygomatic division of the facial nerve was encountered during each approach, crossing the mandible at the condylar neck. The mean tissue depth separating the facial nerve from the condylar neck was 5.5 mm (range: 3.5 mm–7 mm, SD 1.2 mm). The upper division of the facial nerve crossed the posterior border of the condylar process on average 2.31 cm (SD 0.10 cm) anterior to the tragus. *Conclusions.* This study suggests that the temporozygomatic division of the facial nerve will be encountered in most approaches to the condylar process. As visualization of the relationship of the facial nerve to condyle is often limited, recognition that, on average, 5.5 mm of tissue separates condylar process from nerve should help reduce the incidence of facial nerve injury during this procedure.

1. Introduction

The condylar process has been reported as most common site of mandibular fractures, accounting for 29% of all mandibular fractures [1]. Surgical treatment of condylar fractures by open reduction and internal fixation (ORIF) demands that internal fixation and anatomic reduction be completed under direct visualization of the fracture. One challenge of open surgery for condylar process fractures is navigating the anatomic complexity of the adjacent vital structures, specifically the facial nerve.

Several authors have described the location of the facial nerve in the preauricular area. Despite this, one of the most common complications of open reduction and internal fixation of subcondylar fractures remains facial nerve paresis and paralysis [2–4].

It is our feeling that the novice surgeon can benefit from a system of reference to enable the prediction of critical anatomic structures. This system must be based on anatomical landmarks that are (1) easily identifiable, (2) fixed in position during the procedure, and (3) independent of patient position [2].

This project aimed to describe pertinent anatomic relationships of the facial nerve in the preauricular region and relate these findings to ORIF procedures of the subcondylar region. Specifically, we describe the anatomic relationship of the nerve to subcondylar mandible and to easily palpable topographic landmarks, such as the tragus. We feel that these

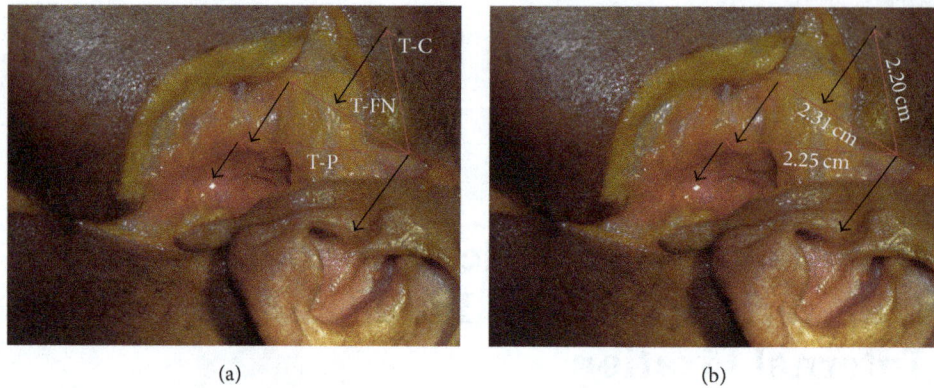

(a)   (b)

FIGURE 1: Illustrated in photo are the relationships of the temporozygomatic (upper) division of the facial nerve (FN) to the tragus (T), lateral pole of condyle (C), and pes anserinus (P).

relationships are especially germane to the less experienced surgeon performing ORIF for condylar process fractures.

2. Materials and Methods

Twelve hemicadavers heads were used. An extended preauricular/retromandibular approach was utilized to provide broad exposure of the facial nerve and subcondylar region. The incision was based parallel to the posterior edge of the ramus. Once parotid tissue was encountered, blunt dissection was carried out to the facial nerve branches.

Because of the ease of palpation and fixed location during ORIF of the subcondylar region, the posterior apex of the tragus and the lateral pole of the condyle were used as reference points for measurements.

Measurements were made as follows (Figure 1(a)):

(1) Depth of tissue separating facial nerve from the underlying condylar neck.

(2) Tragus (posterior apex) to the condyle (lateral pole).

(3) Tragus (posterior apex) to the point where the facial nerve crossed the posterior border of the condylar neck.

(4) Tragus (posterior apex) to the pes anserinus.

All dissections were performed by one of two authors (H. P. Barham or A. M. Terella). Measurements were made by one of the authors and verified independently by the other.

3. Results

The temporozygomatic (upper) division of the facial nerve was encountered during each of our dissections to the subcondylar region. This division of the facial nerve consistently emerged from posterior and medial to the condylar neck and traveled in an oblique plane. In all cases, this division crossed the mandible at the condylar neck. The mean depth from facial nerve to underlying condylar neck was 5.5 mm (standard deviation: 1.2 mm).

The mean distance from tragus (posterior apex) to condyle (lateral pole) was 2.20 cm (standard deviation: 0.04 cm),

TABLE 1: Reported rate of facial nerve injury.

Researcher	Approach	Sample size	Rate of facial nerve injury
Pereira et al. [2]	Preauricular	21	30%
Hammer et al. [3]	Preauricular	31	3.2%
MacArthur et al. [4]	Preauricular	13	15.4%
Meyer et al. [5]	High submandibular	64	0%

from tragus (posterior apex) to the point where the facial nerve crossed the posterior border of the condylar neck it was 2.31 cm (standard deviation: 0.10 cm), and from the tragus to pes anserinus it was 2.25 cm (standard deviation: 0.10 cm) (Figure 1(b)).

4. Discussion

An open approach to the treatment of condylar fractures has become increasingly common, and several surgical incisions including preauricular, rhytidectomy, retromandibular, submandibular, and postauricular incision have been described. A potential and devastating complication of ORIF in this region is facial paralysis or palsy. The reported incidence of facial nerve palsy varies widely, with a reported incidence of 0% utilizing a high submandibular approach to as high as 30% with a retromandibular approach [2–5] (Table 1). Our findings support those of authors prior in suggesting that the temporozygomatic division of the facial nerve has an intimate anatomic relationship to the condylar process. We attempt to expand on this work by highlighting the depth of tissue separating the nerve from the underlying condylar process. When approaching the condylar region from a retromandibular approach or preauricular approach, visualization of the facial nerve-condyle relationship is limited, and moderately strong retraction is frequently required to obtain an adequate visual field and working space for osteosynthesis.

Although the temporozygomatic (upper) division of the facial nerve should not be encountered during the submandibular or high submandibular approaches, the nerve is retracted laterally and easily stretched when attempting to achieve an ample working space and optical field. On average, only 5.5 mm of tissue separates the condylar process from the nerve. The surgeon must appreciate that blind and aggressive lateral or superior retraction of overlying soft tissue in this region can easily result in stretch injury and neuropraxis. Understanding this close relationship should help reduce the incidence of facial nerve injury during ORIF of the condylar region.

Additionally, on average, the pes anserinus of the facial nerve was located approximately 2.25 cm anterior-inferior to the tragus, while the facial nerve crossed the posterior border of the mandible on average 2.31 cm anterior-inferior to the tragus. The measurements and relationship of the facial nerve from this study should allow for nerve position to be estimated using the tragus and palpated posterior border of the mandible.

It is our opinion that the use of a palpable landmark is of greatest utility to the novice surgeon, less experienced in this region. Techniques and measurements to predict nerve location are only estimates and cannot replace the need for precise anatomic understanding and cautious dissection in the condylar region. Further, they must be interpreted understanding the inherent, well documented anatomic variation of the facial nerve.

Several studies have demonstrated efficacy of techniques for locating the facial nerve, with the work of de Ru et al. being the most complete and showing the single best anatomic landmark for locating the facial nerve trunk to be the tympanomastoid fissure (TMF), usually within 3 mm of this landmark [6]. These findings were confirmed by Pather and Osman. However, Pather and Osman noted that the TMF was not an ideal landmark because it often lay behind the sturdy tendon of the sternocleidomastoid muscle, thus requiring a complex dissection [7]. These techniques are excellent in localizing the nerve during dissection but do not help provide a preoperative estimate of nerve location in the condylar region.

Limitations to this study include those that are common to any cadaveric anatomic study. Tissues operated upon following a traumatic insult may undergo distortion due to edema or disruption of soft tissues. Presumably, a swelling process would increase distances between structures if uniformly distributed, so it may not significantly change the surgeon's operative strategy. Further, it is acknowledged that even careful anatomic dissection could lead to distortion of tissue in our specimens, thus affecting measurements. Lastly, our limited sample size enabled calculation of standard deviations, but not an evaluation of anatomic variation.

5. Conclusions

The temporozygomatic (upper) division of the facial nerve has an intimate relationship to the condylar process. It is critical to understanding both the course of the nerve and the depth of tissue separating it from the condylar neck. Soft tissue retraction to optimize the optical field can easily stretch the nerve resulting in neuropraxis. Understanding this close relationship should help reduce the incidence of facial nerve injury during ORIF of the condylar region.

Further the novice surgeon, less experienced in the subcondylar region, can benefit from estimates of facial nerve location using easily palpable topographic landmarks. We suggest that the tragus and lateral pole of the condyle can serve this function.

Ethical Approval

This study is IRB exempt.

Conflict of Interests

The authors declare that there is no conflict of interests regarding the publication of this paper.

References

[1] R. A. Olson, R. J. Fonseca, D. L. Zeitler, and D. B. Osbon, "Fractures of the mandible: a review of 580 cases," *Journal of Oral and Maxillofacial Surgery*, vol. 40, no. 1, pp. 23–28, 1982.

[2] J. A. Pereira, A. Meri, J. M. Potau, A. Prats-Galino, J. J. Sancho, and A. Sitges-Serra, "A simple method for safe identification of the facial nerve using palpable landmarks," *Archives of Surgery*, vol. 139, no. 7, pp. 745–748, 2004.

[3] B. Hammer, P. Schier, and J. Prein, "Osteosynthesis of condylar neck fractures: a review of 30 patients," *British Journal of Oral and Maxillofacial Surgery*, vol. 35, no. 4, pp. 288–291, 1997.

[4] C. J. MacArthur, P. J. Donald, J. Knowles, and H. C. Moore, "Open reduction-fixation of mandibular subcondylar fractures. A review," *Archives of Otolaryngology—Head and Neck Surgery*, vol. 119, no. 4, pp. 403–406, 1993.

[5] C. Meyer, S. Zink, B. Chatelain, and A. Wilk, "Clinical experience with osteosynthesis of subcondylar fractures of the mandible using TCP plates," *Journal of Cranio-Maxillofacial Surgery*, vol. 36, no. 5, pp. 260–268, 2008.

[6] J. A. de Ru, P. P. G. van Benthem, R. L. A. W. Bleys, H. Lubsen, and G.-J. Hordijk, "Landmarks for parotid gland surgery," *The Journal of Laryngology and Otology*, vol. 115, no. 2, pp. 122–125, 2001.

[7] N. Pather and M. Osman, "Landmarks of the facial nerve: implications for parotidectomy," *Surgical and Radiologic Anatomy*, vol. 28, no. 2, pp. 170–175, 2006.

What Are the Trends in Tonsillectomy Techniques in Wales? A Prospective Observational Study of 19,195 Tonsillectomies over a 10-Year Period

Hussein Walijee, Ali Al-Hussaini, Andrew Harris, and David Owens

Department of Otorhinolaryngology, Head and Neck Surgery, University Hospital of Wales, Cardiff CF14 4XW, UK

Correspondence should be addressed to Ali Al-Hussaini; alialhussaini@doctors.org.uk

Academic Editor: Peter S. Roland

There are a multitude of techniques to undertake tonsillectomy, with hot techniques such as diathermy and coblation being associated with a higher risk of secondary haemorrhage. The UK National Prospective Tonsillectomy Audit (2004) advocated cold steel dissection and ties to be the gold standard. This prospective observational study investigates the trends in tonsillectomy techniques across Wales in the last decade to establish if surgeons have adhered to this national guidance. Data relating to tonsillectomy were extracted over a 10-year period from 1 January 2003 to 31 December 2012 from the Wales Surgical Instrument Surveillance Programme database. A total of 19,195 patients were included. Time-series analysis using linear regression showed there was an increase in the number of bipolar diathermy tonsillectomies by 84% (Pearson's $r = 0.762$, $p = 0.010$) and coblation tonsillectomies by 120% ($r = 0.825$, $p = 0.003$). In contrast, there was a fall in the number of cold steel dissection tonsillectomies with ties by 60% ($r = -0.939$, $p < 0.001$). This observational study suggests that the use of bipolar and coblation techniques for tonsillectomy has increased. This deviation from national guidance may be due to these techniques being faster with less intraoperative bleeding. Further study for the underlying reasons for the increase in these techniques is warranted.

1. Introduction

Tonsillectomy is one of the oldest [1] and commonest [2, 3] surgical procedures performed by otorhinolaryngologists worldwide. The main indications for this procedure comprise recurrent tonsillitis and upper airway obstruction including obstructive sleep apnoea. Over time various techniques have been developed and employed in an attempt to reduce haemorrhage rates and improve postoperative morbidity, in particular postoperative pain.

Tonsillectomy can be performed in many different ways depending on the preference and experience of the surgeon. Generally, it may be divided into two stages: excision of the tonsil followed by control of bleeding. However, newer techniques combine these stages so that they are undertaken simultaneously. Cold dissection tonsillectomy involves cutting the pharyngeal mucosa with scissors followed by blunt dissection of the tonsil from the lateral pharyngeal wall, employing no form of heat or cautery. Haemostasis can then be achieved by ligatures or sutures [4].

Diathermy tonsillectomy is a technique that utilises electric current to cut tissue and coagulate blood vessels. Thus, the tonsil is excised and haemostasis is secured simultaneously. This has been advocated to reduce operative time [5]. Coblation is a technique that involves passing radiofrequency energy through a conductive medium such as isotonic sodium chloride creating a plasma field. This results in energetic charge carrying ions that have sufficient energy to break organic molecular bonds, providing simultaneous dissection and coagulation [6] at a temperature of 60–70°C. This is in contrast to monopolar cautery, which generates temperatures of up to 400–600°C. The lower operating temperatures are thought to reduce thermal damage to adjacent tissues and therefore cause less pain postoperatively and improve healing [7].

Although tonsillectomy is a worthwhile surgical intervention when indicated [8], it is not without its complications. The most serious risk associated with the procedure is postoperative haemorrhage, and a multitude of reports have discussed its relationship to operative technique [9, 10].

Different techniques have attracted controversy around their complication rates, in particular the incidence of haemorrhage. This controversy perseveres due to the difficulty in reliably proving or disproving a small difference in the rate of a relatively uncommon complication [11].

Notably, the UK National Prospective Tonsillectomy Audit [9] included 33,921 patients that underwent tonsillectomy between July 2003 and September 2004. This study found an overall haemorrhage rate around three times higher with "hot" surgical techniques for both dissection and haemostasis (diathermy or coblation) than with cold steel tonsillectomy without any use of diathermy. When cold steel was used for dissection and bipolar diathermy only for haemostasis the relative risk of postoperative haemorrhage was around 1.5. The study, however, reported no strong statistical evidence for variations in the risk of return to theatre among most techniques. The authors concluded by recommending that bipolar diathermy and coblation methods should be used with appropriate caution and only after proper training. This is in accordance with several large cohort studies published in the last decade, which also demonstrate an increased risk for the occurrence and/or severity of posttonsillectomy haemorrhage when hot instruments are utilised [12, 13].

Cold steel dissection with cold haemostasis is considered the gold standard technique [14]. However, there is an increasing pressure to reduce costs, operating time, hospital stay, and postoperative morbidity. This prospective observational study aims to investigate the trends in tonsillectomy techniques utilised across Wales in the last decade to explore if otorhinolaryngologists have adhered to or deviated from national guidance favouring cold steel dissection and cold haemostasis above hot tonsillectomy techniques.

2. Materials and Methods

Data were obtained from the Surgical Instrument Surveillance Programme (SISP) database [15] and the Patient Episode Database for Wales (PEDW) [16]. The SISP was established in 2003 to monitor the use of single-use instruments in all tonsil and adenoid surgery in Wales across 18 hospitals. Single-use instruments were introduced in Wales following fear of Creutzfeldt-Jakob prion transmission via reusable instruments. The SISP was designed to monitor the primary outcomes of instrument failure and postoperative haemorrhage. The data is anonymised and coded, and for this reason ethical approval was not required for the reuse of anonymous and open access population data.

Data relating to tonsillectomy were extracted using the Office of Population, Censuses and Surveys Classification of Surgical Operations and Procedures 4th revision (OPCS-4) [17] identifier code F34. Data were extracted over a 10-year period from 1st January 2003 to 31st December 2012 from the SISP database. Hospital stay data for tonsillectomy were extracted from the PEDW for the period between 2003 and 2012. Patients who had a tonsillectomy for recurrent infection and airway obstruction were included in the study. Patients undergoing an adenoidectomy alone, tonsillectomy as part of diagnosis or treatment of cancer, or tonsillectomy as part

of palatal surgery and incomplete datasets were excluded. There were no recorded cases of tonsillotomy/intracapsular tonsillectomy.

The respective number of patients was expressed as a percentage of the total number of tonsillectomies performed using each technique every individual year. Time-series analysis with a linear regression model was used to detect a change in the percentage of tonsillectomies performed using the technique in question. Pearson correlation analysis and the independent sample t-test were used to determine significance. Data were analysed in Microsoft Excel 2013 and IBM SPSS Statistics 20. A p value of <0.05 was considered statistically significant.

3. Results and Discussion

A total of 25,592 patients were identified from the SISP database as having undergone a tonsillectomy between 1st January 2003 and 31st December 2012; 6,397 patients were excluded from the study. Amongst those excluded, 5,676 patients had actually undergone an adenoidectomy as the only procedure, a tonsillar biopsy, and tonsillectomy for known cancer, uvulopalatoplasty, or poorly documented indication; the remaining 721 patients were excluded for the lack of documentation of the technique employed during the procedure. A total of 19,195 patients who underwent a tonsillectomy for recurrent tonsillitis (91%), peritonsillar abscess (5%), and upper airway obstruction (4%) were included in this study. Overall, gender variation within the cohort showed a significant female predominance with a gender ratio of 1.87 : 1 ($p < 0.001$). The median age of patients included in this study was 16 years (range: 2–74 years).

Time-series analysis using a linear regression model demonstrated that, between 2003 and 2012, there was a significant increase in the number of coblation tonsillectomies by 120% (Pearson's $r = 0.825$, $p = 0.003$) from an initial 8.3% in 2003 to 18.3% of all tonsillectomies in 2012. Furthermore, there was a significant increase in the use of bipolar diathermy by 84% ($r = 0.762$, $p = 0.010$). In contrast, time-series analysis demonstrated a significant fall in the number of cold steel tonsillectomies with ties by 60% ($r = -0.939$, $p < 0.001$) from an initial 45% in 2003 to 18% of all tonsillectomies in 2012. Cold steel dissection with the use of both diathermy and ties for haemostasis was the most prevalent technique in 2012, followed by bipolar diathermy. Additionally, there was a significant decrease in the use of laser, ultrasonic, and monopolar diathermy tonsillectomy techniques. Table 1 summarises the trends of tonsillectomy techniques utilised between 2003 and 2012 in Wales. Figure 1 depicts the trends in the techniques of coblation, bipolar diathermy dissection and haemostasis, cold steel dissection with ties, and cold steel dissection with haemostasis with ties and bipolar diathermy, in Wales between 2003 and 2012.

Time-series analysis using a linear regression model was also undertaken to examine the trends, if any, in tonsillectomy techniques utilised by otolaryngology consultants and specialist registrars (trainees) within the ten-year study period. With respect to the use of coblation, there was no significant change of its frequency of use by consultants but

TABLE 1: Trends in tonsillectomy techniques utilised in Wales between 2003 and 2012.

Tonsillectomy technique	% change	Pearson's correlation (r)	p value
Coblation	+120	0.825	0.003
Cold steel + ties	−60	−0.939	<0.001
Cold steel + both (diathermy haemostasis + ties)	+35	0.706	0.022
Bipolar diathermy (dissection & haemostasis)	+84	0.762	0.010
Laser	−115	−0.748	0.013
Ultrasonic	−133	−0.786	0.007
Monopolar diathermy	−103	−0.659	0.038

TABLE 2: Trends in tonsillectomy techniques utilised by consultants in Wales between 2003 and 2012.

Tonsillectomy technique	% change	Pearson's correlation (r)	p value
Coblation	+20	0.327	0.356
Cold steel + ties	−59	−0.958	<0.001
Cold steel + both (diathermy haemostasis + ties)	+22	0.704	0.023
Bipolar diathermy	+180	0.886	0.001

TABLE 3: Trends in tonsillectomy techniques utilised by specialist registrars in Wales between 2003 and 2012.

Tonsillectomy technique	% change	Pearson's correlation (r)	p value
Coblation	+2621	0.846	0.002
Cold steel + ties	−52	−0.817	0.004
Cold steel + both (diathermy haemostasis + ties)	+12	0.414	0.234
Bipolar diathermy	+252	0.665	0.036

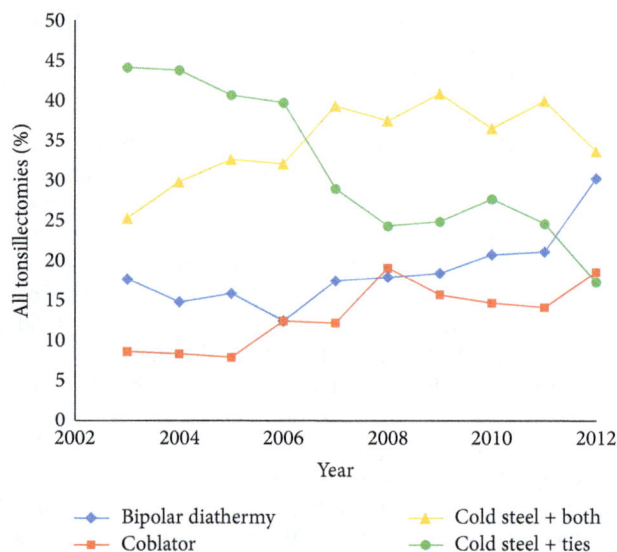

FIGURE 1: Time-series analysis of tonsillectomy techniques utilised in Wales between 2003 and 2012.

a significant increase of its use by specialist registrars (r = 0.846, p = 0.002). Although there was a large increase in the use of coblation by specialist registrars within the study period, this reflected virtually no use of this technique by this group in 2003 and it comprising fewer than 10% of all tonsillectomies performed by specialist registrars in 2012.

Time-series analysis also elicited that the use of traditional cold steel dissection and ties method had significantly decreased for both consultants (r = −0.958, p < 0.001) and specialist registrars (r = −0.817, p = 0.004) within the study period. In contrast, the use of bipolar diathermy (for dissection and haemostasis) had significantly increased for both consultants (r = 0.886, p = 0.001) and specialist registrars (r = 0.665, p = 0.036). Tables 2 and 3 summarise the trends of tonsillectomy techniques utilised between 2003 and 2012 in Wales for consultants and specialist registrars, respectively. Figures 2 and 3 depict the trends in tonsillectomy techniques utilised by consultants and specialist trainees, respectively, in Wales between 2003 and 2012.

Tonsil surgery has evolved greatly. Interestingly, its earliest report in the first century AD was by Aulus Cornelius Celsus, who first described removing the tonsil using a finger and washing the wound with vinegar or juice of comfrey [18]. "Hot" techniques for tonsillectomy first came into existence when Remington-Hobbs, in 1968, described the use of diathermy for tonsil dissection and haemostasis in a report of more than 5000 cases [19]. Coblation was later introduced in 2001, and a plethora of other techniques such as the harmonic scalpel, argon beam coagulator, and laser ablation have also been developed, each with their own risks and benefits.

The choice of technique to employ is inherently based on a number of factors, including risk of intraoperative blood loss, posttonsillectomy infection and haemorrhage, operating time, surgeons experience and preference, severity of postoperative pain, and early return to normal activities. A reduction

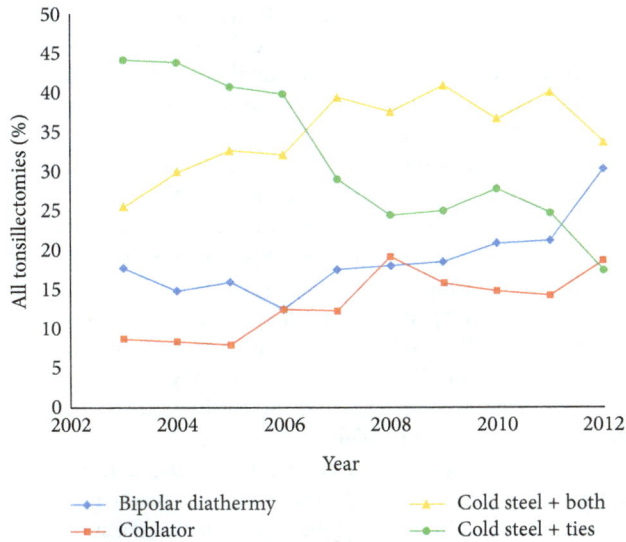

FIGURE 2: Time-series analysis of tonsillectomy techniques utilised by consultants in Wales between 2003 and 2012.

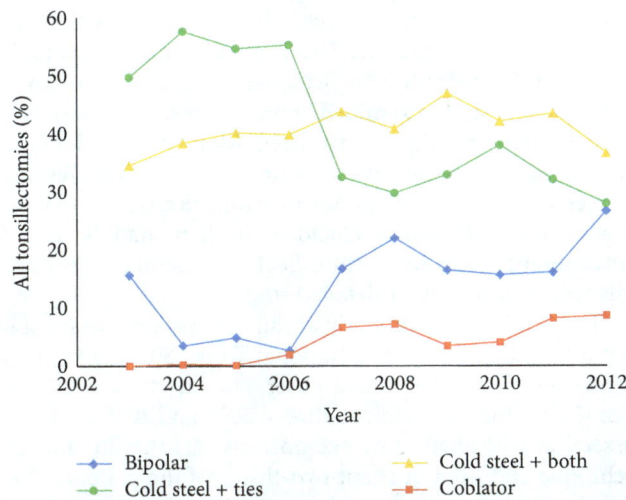

FIGURE 3: Time-series analysis of tonsillectomy techniques utilised by specialist trainees in Wales between 2003 and 2012.

in these parameters is thought to improve patient recovery time and satisfaction as well as bearing obvious social and economic implications [7].

The UK National Prospective Tonsillectomy Audit (NPTA) [9] included 33,921 patients. It reported varying primary (within the first 24 hours) haemorrhage rates from 0.4% (bipolar diathermy) to 1.1% (monopolar diathermy). Secondary (beyond 24 hours postoperatively) haemorrhage rates ranged from 1% (cold steel and ties) to 5.5% (monopolar diathermy). There was, however, no strong statistical evidence for differences in return to theatre (RTT) rates between most techniques. Only coblation had an elevated risk that was statistically significant with an adjusted odds ratio of 2.84 (95% CI 1.56–5.17) when compared to cold steel and ties. This is in contrast to findings from a recent study by Söderman et al. [20], which included 15,734 patients.

They reported an early haemorrhage rate of 3% for cold steel dissection and ties and a comparable 3.9% for coblation tonsillectomy. Late bleeding rates were 3.3% and 9.9% for cold steel with ties and coblation, respectively. Söderman et al. found the adjusted odds ratio for secondary RTT for patients undergoing coblation tonsillectomy was 2.20 (95% CI 0.93–5.19). The authors concluded that the risk for RTT was higher for all hot techniques except for coblation. Tomkinson et al. [21] found that methods utilising heat resulted in a significantly greater adjusted odds of secondary RTT as compared with cold steel dissection. This value ranged from 2.7 times greater for cold steel dissection that used diathermy and ties for haemostasis to a 7.0-fold increased likelihood of secondary RTT associated with coblation.

The NPTA recommended that hot techniques should be used with caution especially when used as a dissection tool and that trainee surgeons should become competent at cold steel dissection and cold haemostasis prior to embarking on other techniques in tonsillectomy. Being an observational study, the results of the NPTA are susceptible to bias. Inclusion within the study was incomplete, and this is apparent on comparison with Hospital Episode Statistics data. Lowe et al. [22] suggest one cause for this discrepancy as being the need for informed consent. The incomplete inclusion may have underestimated the differences in haemorrhage rates. Secondly, the results of the NPTA may be skewed by the modified definition of primary and secondary haemorrhage. A haemorrhage occurring after the first 24 hours postoperatively but during the initial stay is included in the NPTA's definition of primary haemorrhage but would be considered a secondary haemorrhage in other studies. This would result in minor bleeds not requiring intervention, unlikely to be recorded in the NPTA database. The difference in definition of postoperative haemorrhage also makes direct comparison of haemorrhage rates between the NPTA and other studies difficult.

Despite the national recommendations from the controversial, yet informative, NPTA, our prospective observational study of over 19,000 tonsillectomies within a national cohort elicits a sustained increase in the use of bipolar diathermy and coblation techniques for tonsillectomy with a simultaneous fall in the utilisation of the gold standard cold steel dissection and ties. The underlying reasons for the observation of increased use of hot tonsillectomy techniques ascertained by the present study may include shorter procedural time and less intraoperative blood loss [23] as such techniques allow virtually simultaneous dissection and haemostasis. This is a particularly important consideration in young children where minimising blood loss is paramount. The NPTA suggests another reason for the preference of bipolar dissection technique amongst trainee surgeons is that the technique is quicker to learn and requires less dexterity than cold steel dissection with the ligation of vessels [9].

The postulation of less intraoperative blood loss with hot tonsillectomy techniques is supported by evidence from a clinical trial undertaken by Kousha et al. [24], which demonstrated significantly less intraoperative blood loss and shorter operative duration with bipolar diathermy tonsillectomy compared to cold steel dissection with ties. In another prospective study, Pang [25] also made the observation of significantly shorter operating time and lower intraoperative blood loss using the bipolar diathermy technique compared to cold steel dissection and ties. Similarly, in a randomized controlled trial, Di Rienzo Businco and Coen Tirelli [26] ascertained that coblation tonsillectomy resulted in less intraoperative blood loss than cold steel dissection and ties.

Conversely, Hilton [11] argues that the perceived saving of operating time between diathermy dissection and cold steel with ties is no more than a few minutes, thereby unlikely to alter the potential throughput of cases on a standard operating list. A Cochrane review [23] addressed the issue of intraoperative haemorrhage, identifying a mean difference of about 21 mL per patient when comparing cold dissection with diathermy dissection (less bleeding). This figure is only 2% of the circulating blood volume of an average 2-year-old child, and most tonsillectomies are done on older children and adults.

Nevertheless, it may be argued that hot tonsillectomy techniques confer benefits in terms of reduced postoperative pain and earlier return to normal diet and hence the increase in their uptake. In a prospective randomized controlled trial (RCT) of 92 adults undergoing tonsillectomy for recurrent tonsillitis allocated to either coblation or cold steel dissection, Philpott et al. demonstrated there was no significant difference between the two groups in terms of postoperative pain and notably found the cold steel dissection group returned earlier to normal eating [7]. Conversely, in a prospective RCT of 19 adult patients undergoing a coblation tonsillectomy on one side and cold steel dissection on the other, postoperative pain levels in coblation tonsillectomy were significantly lower for the first 3 days following which the difference failed to show statistical significance [27]. Similarly, a prospective randomised double blinded trial including 79 paediatric patients aged between 4 and 16 years found no significant difference for pain scores, at the various time points measured in either the coblation or cold steel dissection group except for the 6th day in favour of the coblation technique [28]. In this study, the coblation group also required less analgesia in the first 12 hours postoperatively. In similarity, a prospective single blinded controlled trial including 34 patients found postoperative pain scores significantly less at 6 hours after operation in the coblation tonsillectomy group as compared to cold steel tonsillectomy. However, there were no differences in the pain scores on days 1, 2, and 3 postoperatively [29].

A retrospective audit of coblation tonsillectomies performed by a single surgeon over a 10-year period in Australia reported a 3.4% readmission rate with secondary haemorrhage and 1.3% RTT rate (0.4% primary haemorrhage and 0.9% secondary haemorrhage). The secondary haemorrhage rate and RTT are comparable to the NPTA; however, the primary RTT is vastly improved at 0.4% compared to 1.1% as seen in the NPTA. The authors conclude that coblation can be a safe method for tonsillectomy with low complication rates when performed by an experienced surgeon [30]. Moreover, in a meta-analysis of 24 prospective randomised controlled studies by Mösges et al. [31] comprising data of 796 patients who had undergone coblation tonsillectomy, the overall haemorrhage rate was 4.1% with a 95% confidence interval from 2.8 to 5.5%. This highlights that coblation is relatively safe and effective with bleeding rates that are comparable to other techniques. That noted, a Cochrane review reported inadequate evidence due to poor quality trials to determine whether coblation tonsillectomy is better or worse than other tonsillectomy techniques [32].

As is true for other surgical techniques, adequate training is required for surgeons new to coblation. Carney et al. [33] studied 2062 tonsillectomies and concluded the presence of a "learning curve" in that surgeon experience was statistically significant and accounted for 60% of the variability in primary bleeding rate and 8% of the variability in secondary bleeding rate. The NPTA recommended training prior to embarking on "hot" techniques and it may be a possibility that data presented in the current study reflects that very situation is occurring in Wales.

The present study is of course not without limitations. Being an observational study, the results of the current study are susceptible to bias; firstly, the study excluded a substantial number of patients with incomplete records. This could have undermined the differences in operative techniques used if the excluded patients underwent a technique to minimise various risks such as postoperative pain or intraoperative blood loss. Ultimately the technique employed is the surgeons' choice and may be based on patient or treatment characteristics as well as a personal preference. Moreover, although this study examined trends in how relatively new tonsillectomy techniques have been adopted using longitudinal data, it does not examine how these techniques and devices affect patient outcomes after tonsillectomy, and most importantly it does not elucidate if there had been any concomitant trends in posttonsillectomy haemorrhage rates. This will require further detailed study.

The findings of this study are in some ways comparable to published data from the National Tonsil Surgery Register in Sweden. In a prospective observational study analysing some 15,734 tonsillectomies between 2009 and 2013, cold steel dissection with diathermy haemostasis was the dominating technique and used in about two-thirds of the patients [20]. Bipolar diathermy was used in 15.7%, and coblation was the third most frequent technique (9.1%). Cold steel with cold haemostasis was only used in 7.4% during the study period. Interestingly, this study ascertained early and late postoperative haemorrhage rates for these techniques and demonstrated unambiguously that cold steel dissection and cold haemostasis should be considered the gold standard technique for tonsillectomy in terms of having the lowest risk of late postoperative haemorrhage, in spite of falling trends in its use.

4. Conclusions

Despite data from several studies reporting an increase in the likelihood of secondary haemorrhage with hot tonsillectomy techniques, there remains an increasing trend of hot tonsillectomy techniques being utilised in Wales. Inevitably, the decision of which technique to use is based on surgeon and patient factors and may be best decided on a case by case basis. However, as with all aspects of modern surgery, this decision should be evidence-based. The evidence remains insufficient but currently does not support the increased use of hot tonsillectomy techniques seen in this large cohort of patients. This trend and the underlying reasons for it should be examined further and reflected upon.

Conflict of Interests

The authors declare that there is no conflict of interests regarding the publication of this paper.

Acknowledgments

The authors would like to acknowledge ENT Wales and the Single-Use Instrument Surveillance Programme and Health Solution Wales for their help and support with the collection of data for this study.

References

[1] R. T. Younis and R. H. Lazar, "History and current practice of tonsillectomy," *Laryngoscope*, vol. 112, no. 8, part 2, supplement 100, pp. 3–5, 2002.

[2] J. A. Koempel, "On the origin of tonsillectomy and the dissection method," *The Laryngoscope*, vol. 112, no. 9, pp. 1583–1586, 2002.

[3] N. Charaklias, C. Mamais, and B. N. Kumar, "The art of tonsillectomy: the UK experience for the past 100 years," *Otolaryngology—Head and Neck Surgery*, vol. 144, no. 6, pp. 851–854, 2011.

[4] J. C. Ballantynem and D. F. N. Harrison, Eds., *Rob & Smith's Operative Surgery: Nose and Throat*, Butterworths, London, UK, 4th edition, 1986.

[5] A. Roy, C. De La Rosa, and Y. A. Vecchio, "Bleeding following tonsillectomy. A study of electrocoagulation and ligation techniques," *Archives of Otolaryngology*, vol. 102, no. 1, pp. 9–10, 1976.

[6] R. H. Temple and M. S. Timms, "Paediatric coblation tonsillectomy," *International Journal of Pediatric Otorhinolaryngology*, vol. 61, no. 3, pp. 195–198, 2001.

[7] C. M. Philpott, D. C. Wild, D. Mehta, M. Daniel, and A. R. Banerjee, "A double-blinded randomized controlled trial of coblation versus conventional dissection tonsillectomy on postoperative symptoms," *Clinical Otolaryngology*, vol. 30, no. 2, pp. 143–148, 2005.

[8] R. Fox, M. Temple, D. Owens, A. Short, and A. Tomkinson, "Does tonsillectomy lead to improved outcomes over and above the effect of time? A longitudinal study," *Journal of Laryngology and Otology*, vol. 122, no. 11, pp. 1197–1200, 2008.

[9] British Association of Otorhinolaryngologists—Head and Neck Surgeons Comparative Audit Group and the Clinical Effectiveness Unit. The Royal College of Surgeons of England, *National Prospective Tonsillectomy Audit Final Report*, The Royal College of Surgeons of England, London, UK, 2005.

[10] J. P. Windfuhr and Y.-S. Chen, "Incidence of post-tonsillectomy hemorrhage in children and adults: a study of 4,848 patients," *Ear, Nose & Throat Journal*, vol. 81, no. 9, pp. 626–634, 2002.

[11] M. Hilton, "Tonsillectomy technique—tradition versus technology," *The Lancet*, vol. 364, no. 9435, pp. 642–643, 2004.

[12] S. Sarny, G. Ossimitz, W. Habermann, and H. Stammberger, "Hemorrhage following tonsil surgery: a multicenter prospective study," *The Laryngoscope*, vol. 121, no. 12, pp. 2553–2560, 2011.

[13] S. O'Leary and J. Vorrath, "Postoperative bleeding after diathermy and dissection tonsillectomy," *The Laryngoscope*, vol. 115, no. 4, pp. 591–594, 2005.

[14] H. Blanchford and D. Lowe, "Cold versus hot tonsillectomy: state of the art and recommendations," *ORL*, vol. 75, no. 3, pp. 136–141, 2013.

[15] The Surgical Instrument Surveillance Programme Working Group, "Surgical instrument surveillance programme," All Wales Annual Tonsillectomy Surveillance Report, National Public Health Service for Wales, 2006.

[16] Patient Episode Database for Wales, "*Annual PEDW Data Tables*," http://www.infoandstats.wales.nhs.uk/page.cfm?orgid=869&pid=41010&subjectlist=Main%2bOperation%2b%284%2bcharacter%2bdetail%29&patientcoverlist=0&period=0&keyword=&action=Search.

[17] Office of Population Censuses and Surveys, *Tabular List of the Classification of Surgical Operations and Procedures*, Office of Population Censuses and Surveys, 4th edition, 1990.

[18] N. G. McGuire, "A method of guillotine tonsillectomy with an historical review," *The Journal of Laryngology and Otology*, vol. 81, no. 2, pp. 187–195, 1967.

[19] C. Remington-Hobbs, "Diathermy in dissection tonsillectomy and retrograde dissection adenoidectomy," *The Journal of Laryngology and Otology*, vol. 82, no. 11, pp. 953–962, 1968.

[20] A.-C. H. Söderman, E. Odhagen, E. Ericsson et al., "Posttonsillectomy haemorrhage rates are related to technique for dissection and for haemostasis. An analysis of 15734 patients in the National Tonsil Surgery Register in Sweden," *Clinical Otolaryngology*, vol. 40, no. 3, pp. 248–254, 2015.

[21] A. Tomkinson, W. Harrison, D. Owens, S. Harris, V. McClure, and M. Temple, "Risk factors for postoperative hemorrhage following tonsillectomy," *Laryngoscope*, vol. 121, no. 2, pp. 279–288, 2011.

[22] D. Lowe, J. van der Meulen, D. Cromwell et al., "Key messages from the national prospective tonsillectomy audit," *The Laryngoscope*, vol. 117, no. 4, pp. 717–724, 2007.

[23] D. K. Pinder, H. Wilson, and M. P. Hilton, "Dissection versus diathermy for tonsillectomy," *Cochrane Database of Systematic Reviews*, vol. 16, no. 3, Article ID CD002211, 2011.

[24] A. Kousha, R. Banan, N. Fotoohi, and R. Banan, "Cold dissection versus bipolar electrocautery tonsillectomy," *Journal of Research in Medical Sciences*, vol. 12, no. 3, pp. 117–120, 2007.

[25] Y. T. Pang, "Paediatric tonsillectomy: bipolar electrodissection and dissection/snare compared," *The Journal of Laryngology and Otology*, vol. 109, no. 8, pp. 733–736, 1995.

[26] L. Di Rienzo Businco and G. Coen Tirelli, "Paediatric tonsillectomy: radiofrequency-based plasma dissection compared to cold dissection with sutures," *Acta Otorhinolaryngologica Italica*, vol. 28, no. 2, pp. 67–72, 2008.

[27] N. Polites, S. Joniau, D. Wabnitz et al., "Postoperative pain following coblation tonsillectomy: randomized clinical trial," *ANZ Journal of Surgery*, vol. 76, no. 4, pp. 226–229, 2006.

[28] D. Parker, L. Howe, V. Unsworth, and R. Hilliam, "A randomised controlled trial to compare postoperative pain in children undergoing tonsillectomy using cold steel dissection with bipolar haemostasis versus coblation technique," *Clinical Otolaryngology*, vol. 34, no. 3, pp. 225–231, 2009.

[29] Z. Izny Hafiz, S. Rosdan, and M. D. Mohd Khairi, "Coblation tonsillectomy versus dissection tonsillectomy: a comparison of intraoperative time, intraoperative blood loss and postoperative pain," *The Medical Journal of Malaysia*, vol. 69, no. 2, pp. 74–78, 2014.

[30] M. A. Rogers, C. Frauenfelder, C. Woods, C. Wee, and A. S. Carney, "Bleeding following coblation tonsillectomy: a 10-year, single-surgeon audit and modified grading system," *The Journal of Laryngology and Otology*, vol. 129, supplement 1, pp. S32–S37, 2015.

[31] R. Mösges, M. Hellmich, S. Allekotte, K. Albrecht, and M. Böhm, "Hemorrhage rate after coblation tonsillectomy: a meta-analysis of published trials," *European Archives of Oto-Rhino-Laryngology*, vol. 268, no. 6, pp. 807–816, 2011.

[32] M. J. Burton and C. Doree, "Coblation versus other surgical techniques for tonsillectomy," *The Cochrane Database of Systematic Reviews*, vol. 18, no. 3, Article ID CD004619, 2007.

[33] A. S. Carney, P. K. Harris, P. L. MacFarlane, S. Nasser, and A. Esterman, "The coblation tonsillectomy learning curve," *Otolaryngology—Head and Neck Surgery*, vol. 138, no. 2, pp. 149–152, 2008.

Importance of "Process Evaluation" in Audiological Rehabilitation: Examples from Studies on Hearing Impairment

Vinaya Manchaiah,[1,2] Berth Danermark,[3] Jerker Rönnberg,[2] and Thomas Lunner[2,4]

[1] Department of Vision and Hearing Sciences, Anglia Ruskin University, Cambridge CB1 1PT, UK
[2] Linnaeus Centre HEAD, The Swedish Institute for Disability Research, Department of Behavioral Science and Learning, Linköping University, 58183 Linköping, Sweden
[3] The Swedish Institute for Disability Research, Örebro University, 702 81 Örebro, Sweden
[4] Eriksholm Research Centre, Oticon A/S, 20 Rørtangvej, 3070 Snekkersten, Denmark

Correspondence should be addressed to Vinaya Manchaiah; vinaya.manchaiah@anglia.ac.uk

Academic Editor: Leonard P. Rybak

The main focus of this paper is to discuss the importance of "evaluating the process of change" (i.e., process evaluation) in people with disability by studying their lived experiences. Detailed discussion is made about "why and how to investigate the process of change in people with disability?" and some specific examples are provided from studies on patient journey of persons with hearing impairment (PHI) and their communication partners (CPs). In addition, methodological aspects in process evaluation are discussed in relation to various metatheoretical perspectives. The discussion has been supplemented with relevant literature. The healthcare practice and disability research in general are dominated by the use of outcome measures. Even though the values of outcome measures are not questioned, there seems to be a little focus on understanding the process of change over time in relation to health and disability. We suggest that the process evaluation has an additional temporal dimension and has applications in both clinical practice and research in relation to health and disability.

1. Introduction

Disability and impairment have been defined in a number of ways, with either narrow or wider criteria. In general, wider criteria or definitions have been used when studying disability from social sciences perspective. Disability has also been studied, understood, and described by using various models both in practice and in research [1, 2], and some such models include biomedical, social, and biopsychosocial models [3–6]. In addition, disability has also been studied from perspectives such as systems theory [7, 8], intersectionality, and juridification [9].

Furthermore, various metatheoretical perspectives (i.e., philosophical standpoint) have been applied to disability research, for example, external realism (naïve realism), antirealism, and critical realism [10]. These metatheoretical perspectives can be complementary but some can be contradictory. Some of the perspectives are less inclusive (e.g., naïve

realist and antirealist) and others are of inclusive nature (e.g., critical realism) in studying and understanding disability. In addition, the experiences of people with disability and how it may change over time can also be studied (i.e., process evaluation).

In general, the healthcare practice and work with disability management are dominated by the use of "outcome measures." In a recent study focused on developing ICF core sets for hearing loss, it was found that there are over 100 different outcome measures in the literature related to adults with hearing impairment [11]. It was also highlighted that there are very few longitudinal studies in relation to adults with hearing impairment. Whilst the values of outcome measures are not at question, there seems to be a little focus on understanding the process of change over time in relation to health and disability. A recent study by Laplante-Lévesque et al. provides an example of study with a focus on process of change over time in adults with hearing impairment seeking help for the first time [12]. In addition, in recent years few researchers have highlighted the need for process evaluation in relation to evaluating health interventions [13, 14].

This paper aims at discussing the importance of "evaluating the process of change" (i.e., process evaluation) in understanding disability by studying their lived experiences. The paper written in two folds, in Section 2, we start with distinguishing between "outcome measurement" and "process evaluation," and we discuss the importance of process evaluation and provide some examples from our research on hearing impairment and make discussion about why and how to investigate the process of change in a person with disability. It is important to note that whilst the discussions are generally made about disability the empirical examples are provided from studies on hearing impairment. You can refer to a paper by Manchaiah and Stephens for detailed information about terminologies and definitions about hearing impairment [15]. In Section 3, discussions are made to highlight the methodological aspects in process evaluation (i.e., how different theoretical positioning may influence the "process evaluation") by relating it to ideas from various metatheoretical perspectives. Overall, the emphasis in Section 2 is method and the emphasis in Section 3 is to relate method to metatheory.

2. Outcome Measurement versus Process Evaluation

It is quite common to study and evaluate change when it comes to health and also health interventions. Outcome measures are tools used in assessing the change over time. However, in healthcare practice they are mainly used as baseline measurement during the initial consultation of the patient and after the intervention. The change in the outcome measures is usually assumed to be due to treatment and/or interventions. This is the typical design used in research trials with classical OXO model (one-group-pre-post) as proposed by Campbell and Stanley [16]. Outcome measures can have various purposes, for example, (a) to measure rehabilitative outcomes of an individual person with disability; (b) to access the effectiveness of the service provided by a particular clinical unit or agency; (c) to access the effectiveness of new technologies and treatment methods; and (d) to assess the effectiveness of rehabilitation services on quality of life [17]. In addition, outcome measures have also been used in formulating intervention strategies [18]. Whilst the outcome measures can be used longitudinally to measure change over time, they are mainly used just before and after the treatment. Furthermore, there is "almost no research on the rate of change in outcome measures throughout the episodes of treatment or how much treatment is required to produce a valued outcome" [19].

In recent years, there is more emphasis to measuring health outcomes in terms of function. For example, World Health Organisation-International Classification of Functioning, Disability and Health (WHO-ICF) is based on the biopsychosocial model which assumes an interplay of factors at different levels (e.g., biological, psychological, and social) and advocates understanding disability in terms of

impairment, ability, activity limitations, and participation restrictions [20]. In practice, the impairment is usually measured using clinical evaluations (i.e., objective measures) and disability (i.e., activity limitations and participation restrictions) is measured using self-reported outcome measures (i.e., subjective measures).

The term "process evaluation" in this paper has been used in the context of understanding and monitoring the change longitudinally (e.g., several days to several years). This aspect relates mainly to how the experiences of people with disability or a particular health condition change over time. For example, studies on "patient journey" have become popular in recent years which evaluate main phases they go through during their disease and treatment regime. There are examples of such studies in relation to hearing impairment [21–24].

2.1. Importance of Process Evaluation. Whilst the uses of outcome measures are most common, it can be argued that both outcome measurement and process evaluation are important. Some inspiration for process evaluation can be drawn from the area of marketing and business studies. For example, the concept of "product life cycle" refers to the stages through which product or its category bypasses, which may include stages such as introduction to the market, growth, maturity, and decline [25, 26]. This model provides important information about the product in the temporal dimension. However, it is important to note that length of each cycle in each product varies greatly. Despite the shortcomings that it may be difficult to identify where the product is in its life cycle and almost impossible to know with certainty when a product moves from one stage to another stage, the model is still very popular in the area of marketing and business management in formulating strategy.

To better understand the difference between process evaluation and outcome measurement, let us consider a simple scenario where a person is travelling from place A to place B. His main goal in this context is to reach B. In this example, if you use only outcome measurements we can capture whether or not a person reached place B. It can include more variables, for example, within a given time limit and using a particular route, and so forth. However, it does not capture the experience through this journey and how they changed over time. More importantly, what sort of factors may have positively or negatively influenced the journey? Even though most people may consider reaching to place B as a success, some may decide not to undertake that journey again because of the difficult experiences they had through this journey or the opposite. This example may suggest that the process evaluation may to some extent highlight various factors that may not be understood through outcome measures. We can apply this way of thinking to a particular health condition and disability.

Furthermore, it is important to note that there are benefits and shortcomings of both outcome measurement and process evaluation. A discussion paper by Mant compares process and outcome measures as performance indicators in healthcare and suggested that health care is one determinant of health and there could be other factors (e.g., nutrition, environment, lifestyle, etc.), which may influence the health outcomes [27]. The differences in outcomes (which are measured using outcome measures and can reflect wide range of aspects) may be due to various reasons such as types of cases on which the treatment was administered, how the data was collected, chance, and quality of care given. However, process evaluation could have some advantages as they are more sensitive to difference in quality of care and may act as a direct measure of quality. Mant also argued that the outcome measures are of use only where outcome indicator has the power to detect variation in healthcare leading to changes in health outcome (and such changes are sufficiently common so that it will produce enough power in outcome measures) [27]. For this reason, if these conditions are not met then other approaches such as process measurement and risk management of individual incidents could be more effective rather than looking at statistical variation of data from larger samples. Even though the perspectives expressed in this paper are based on looking at healthcare practice as a whole and to discuss the strengths and weakness of outcome measures and process measures as performance indicator for healthcare, the findings and recommendations have some use to each individual.

2.2. Outcome Measurement.

The outcome measures gives information about a specific aspect (e.g., depression, anxiety, level of hearing disability, etc.) depending on the measures we are using and also the extent to which the person is affected at that point of time. The Hearing Handicap Questionnaire (HHQ), which is used to measure the psychosocial aspects of hearing disability, is a good example of an outcome measure [28, 29]. Changes in outcome measures can be used to evaluate the degree of success of an intervention. For example, with HHQ lower perceived hearing disability after audiological management (e.g., hearing aids) suggests the benefits of the management approach used.

2.3. Process Evaluation.

The process evaluation refers to studying the experiences of person with disability in the form of a timeline to understand the main phases/stages they go through during the disease and the treatment. Studies on patient journey represent good examples of process evaluation [21–24]. Even though studies on patient's journey uncover important information about the process of change in a person with disability and factors influencing them, they may not capture the intensity by which the person is affected at one point of time. Although there is some amount of theme identification in this, time is an additional dimension in this approach. In addition, it can be argued that the use of outcome measures at multiple intervals may act as process evaluation (i.e., continuous monitoring of outcomes using outcome measures). However, devising such a measurement tool to capture both outcome and process could be challenging.

Overall, it is important to note that even though the approaches discussed above provide similar information, they give different perspectives in understanding the same condition. It can be argued that the combination of such

approaches may give better understanding of a person with disability than any other approach alone. It is also important to establish a link between such combined approaches in order to better understand what information they are providing. This discussion may highlight the fact that process evaluation has some use in disability research and may also have some clinical value.

2.4. Process Evaluation: Examples from Studies on Hearing Impairment.

It appears in the recent years that studying the lived experiences of persons with disability is becoming popular. Moreover, there is an "*increase in the instances that voices of disabled people are being heard or considered in all stages of research about their lives*" [1, 30]. Studies on patient journey represent one way of capturing the lived experiences of people with disability. In addition, such studies also explore the process of change by considering various experiences a person may have during the initial onset of the disease and realising that they have the condition, acceptance and help-seeking, assessment, rehabilitation, and continued experience living with a particular disability. Reported experiences can be analysed to identify relevant themes and be represented in the way the themes reflect the data. Such an approach is often used in disability research while attempting to understand the lived experiences of a person. A recent international study on perspectives of adults with hearing impairment towards help-seeking and rehabilitation is a good example of such an approach [31]. In a clinical setting this is done informally through case history.

The Ida Institute initially developed the possible patient journey of person with hearing impairment (PHI) and their communication partners (CPs) by considering the professionals' perspective [32, 33]. Our studies further developed these models by considering perspectives of PHIs and their CPs [21–24]. These models are indicated in Figure 1 which demonstrates the main phases the PHI and their CPs go through from the initial onset of the disease, diagnosis, treatment, and then continuing to live with the hearing impairment. It is important to note that the various stages in the model are not drawn to any scale and the progression from one phase to other may vary from person to person quite considerably (i.e., several days to several years). Even though the above model demonstrates the process of change from the perspective of PHI and their CPs, it does not measure the intensity at which they are affected at any one stage/point. For this reason, outcome measures would be helpful in measuring the intensity at which the person is affected at any point of time.

Studies on patient journey of PHI and CPs look at hearing disability from a different dimension (i.e., temporal) and have given some new insights. Moreover, studies on patient journey can also highlight some of the barriers to help-seeking process which may not be identified through structured outcome measurements. For example, in our recent study on sudden-onset hearing loss patient journey patients reported that the medical professionals did not always give them the correct information about the condition and expected prognosis which raises some general, ethical, and legal issues [23, 34].

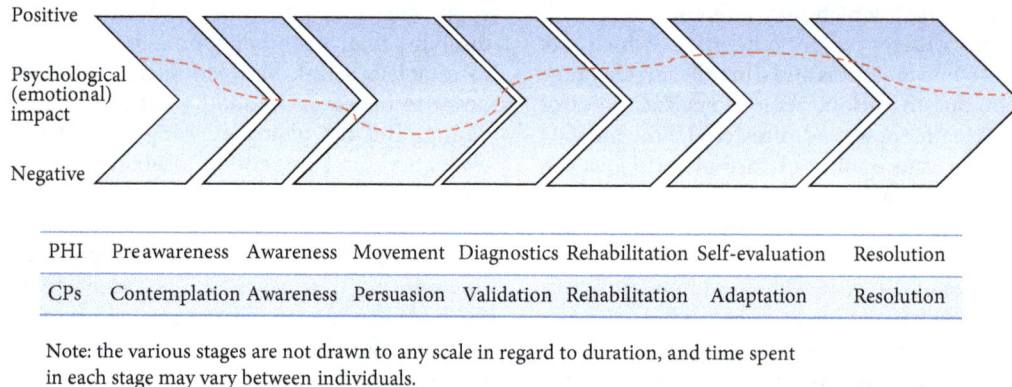

Note: the various stages are not drawn to any scale in regard to duration, and time spent in each stage may vary between individuals.

FIGURE 1: Models of persons with hearing impairment (PHI) and their communication partner's (CPs) journey through hearing impairment.

The phases represented in these patient journey studies related to hearing impairment seem to correlate well with the stages of change proposed in "transtheoretical model of change" (also known as stages of change theory) which was proposed in relation to health behaviour change [35, 36]. This theory suggested that health behaviour change involves six main stages, which include precontemplation, contemplation, preparation, action, maintenance, and termination. This model is cyclic or spiral model rather than linear which accounts for relapse and a restart. Such a model could be helpful while understanding the process of change through a disease and its treatment. The WHO has recently produced a document about "engaging in process of change," which highlights some facts and methods used to engage in the process of change [37].

2.5. How to Best Evaluate the Process of Change in a Person with Disability? Process evaluation can be studied and understood from perspectives of person with disability, their significant others (e.g., spouse, children, relatives, friends), and clinicians and in the wider context of society. However, it is important to note that priorities from each of these perspectives could be different. For example, (a) for people with disability and their significant others, their activity, participation, and quality of life could be key factors; (b) for clinicians, cure of impairment, reducing disability, and to some extent quick fix to the problems reported could be important; and (c) for society, less dependency of people with disability on society and a larger contribution from them could be important. Even though it is difficult and to some extent impossible to answer which of these perspectives are more important, considering the emphasis on "shared decision making" in recent years, the combined approach could be helpful. Moreover, the process of change can also be evaluated from different analytical levels, which may include biological, psychological, psychosocial, and socioeconomic.

In our research on patient journey of PHI and their CPs, we have focused on individual level by studying the reports of the PHI, their CPs, and clinicians [21–24]. Moreover, these studies had relatively small sample sizes and employed research designs, which were based on reported experiences and may have been influenced by various aspects including

perceptions and memory of the individuals. However, considering that the journey of PHI and their CPs may take several years, longitudinal designs may be more appropriate. In addition, evaluating such models in a large population is necessary.

3. Metatheoretical Approaches and Their Implications to Process Evaluation

As discussed in the earlier section disability and impairment have been studied and understood using various metatheoretical perspectives. In this section we will consider three perspectives and discuss their advantages and limitations. Detailed information about the metatheoretical perspectives in relation to the assessment of audiological rehabilitation can be found in the paper by Danermark [10].

Metatheory refers to a formal system that describes the structure of some other system (i.e., a theory about theory). Metatheory belongs to the philosophical specialty of epistemology (i.e., knowledge production) and also to assumptions about reality (ontological issues). The metatheoretical approaches are the key aspects, which determine our views on reality, to what extent it is possible to gain in-depth knowledge about reality, and also how we choose to study a particular phenomenon and/or problem. There are various metatheoretical approaches which can be grouped in some main categories: naïve realism (or empiricism), antirealism (e.g., social constructionism), critical realism, neo-Kantianism, and hermeneutics [10, 38–40].

It is important to note that all these perspectives have benefits and shortcomings and some of them are more inclusive when it comes to disability research than others. Moreover, they have some key assumptions. For example, (a) naïve realism is the most common approach which assumes that reality can be studied and understood by collecting empirical evidence in an objective nature and our senses help us in understanding reality (i.e., our senses provide us with direct knowledge of the external world); (b) antirealism (e.g., social constructionism) is that reality is socially constructed and there is no reality independent of our perception (or there is no objective truth and we can only understand the reality by personal accounts of people experiences which could differ) [41, 42]; and (c) critical realism is that reality exists at different analytical levels (i.e., stratified) and there is reality independent of our knowledge about it (or we can get closer to reality by understanding different levels of analytical truth and its interaction, but we may never get the complete truth). Moreover, critical realists make a distinction between empirical (i.e., our experience of what actually happens); actual (i.e., all the things that happen independently whether they are observable or not); and real (i.e., reality consists of mechanisms with generative powers).

Even though any of these three metatheoretical approaches can be used in studying hearing impairment from each of the methods discussed above (i.e., outcome measurement, process evaluation, and identifying themes from narratives), some approaches have been used for a certain dimension more often than others. For example, outcome measurements, which provide numerical quantification, have been an approach from a naïve realist perspective; and identifying themes from narratives has been the choice for antirealists.

Critical realism has a great advantage in process evaluation but also in the other two dimensions when compared with naïve realism and antirealism. This is because the "process evaluation" involves similar aspects which could be studied using outcome measures or identifying themes through reported experiences; however, this requires recontextualization and redescription of data from different theoretical perspective. For example, in patient journey studies the stages of change theory have been used to study the process of change through PHI and their CPs journey through hearing loss.

Moreover, one of the important steps in research from critical realist perspective is "abduction inference" which refers to "interpret and recontextualise individual phenomenon within a conceptual framework or a set of ideas, to be able to understand something in a new way by observing and interpreting this something in a new conceptual framework" [43]. There are no fixed criteria from which the abduction inference is done. However, this involves recontextualization and redescription of data, creativity, and imagination. It is important to note that most researchers follow such a process even though they may not be aware of the term abduction inference. This is an important concept in the process evaluation (i.e., studying process of change). This is because the experiences reported in the PHI and their CP journey studies can be found in the previous literature, for example, in a recent international study on perspectives of adults with hearing impairment towards help-seeking and rehabilitation [31]. However, the patient journey studies involved new theoretical framework (i.e., stages of change theory), which evaluates the experiences of hearing impairment and how they change over time.

Critical realism is also a fruitful perspective when it comes to outcome measures, because this perspective clearly demonstrates the boundaries for drawing conclusions based on quantitative analysis in order to avoid conclusions about causality that is beyond the capacity of the conducted research. It highlights the importance to not only include the "surface" in terms of observed empirical events but also

include analysis of underlying structures and mechanisms [43]. Furthermore it also stresses the importance to take the contexts into consideration (i.e., mechanisms + context = outcome). In short it aims for answering the question "*for whom, works what in which context?.*" However, ultimately the aspiration is to make the results generalisable.

4. Discussion

Disability is a complex phenomenon, which needs to be studied and managed with a holistic perspective. Moreover, disability experienced by an individual due to a specific condition (e.g., hearing impairment) may be diverse in its nature. Kerr and Cowie suggested that "*impact of acquired deafness cannot be understood simply by measuring its intensity and documenting the objective limitations that it imposes*" [44]. For this reason, it is important to clarify and understand why acquired hearing disability affects people the way it does [45]. However, this may require a multidimensional approach and it appears that studying "lived experiences" could be important.

Söder argued that there are various tensions in disability research (e.g., theory and political action, impairment versus disability, and theoretical and empirical research) [9]. Such tensions could arise from the metatheoretical approaches we take. For example, naïve realists believe that our sense provides us with the direct knowledge of the external world. According to this perspective empirical observations are central to research and objective assessment is the key aspect of gaining knowledge. Naïve realism approach to process evaluation requires quantification. This way of precisely quantifying which stage the PHI might be at one point could be done by designing structured questionnaires to capture different phases of the journey.

However, according to antirealists no objective statements about reality are possible due to the distinction first formulated by the German philosopher Emanuel Kant, things-in-themselves versus things-for-us (German: *Dinge-an-sich versus Dinge-für-uns*), and hence negotiation is important to come to agreement of what is working and what is not working in, for example, audiological rehabilitation. A quotation "*there are no facts, only interpretations*" is a good example of this way of thinking [46]. This statement illustrates that everything is subject for negotiations and there is no right or wrong based on objective facts. If we take antirealists (e.g., social constructionists) view it may not be possible to come up with any model, which can be empirically generalised to large group of population as it is against their underplaying assumption towards reality.

From a critical realist perspective to process evaluation, it is important to have theories about how mechanisms are working in different contexts and how they produce the outcomes. Specifically, when such a concept is applied to patient journey studies, it is important to consider forming theories on how patient journey may be influenced by various biological, social, cultural, and economical aspects. Such an approach is challenging and requires interdisciplinary work. Moreover, critical realism as a metatheoretical choice may have advantages to process evaluation, as the concepts such as "abduction inference" are central to research from critical realist perspective.

Overall, it is important to note that disability and impairment have been be studied and understood from various models and perspectives and there are significant differences in how it is understood based on the metatheoretical perspectives we take. The discussion made in this paper and also our studies on patient journey highlight the importance of process evaluation based on critical realism and suggest that such an approach could make an important contribution to better understand disability. We suggest that the process evaluation has an additional temporal dimension and has applications in both clinical practice and research. Furthermore, whether to choose the metatheoretical approaches based on the aim (e.g., outcome measurement or process evaluation) or vice versa (i.e., metatheoretical positioning guiding the choice of method) may create a dilemma for researchers. However, it is most important that the researchers are aware of the benefits and shortcomings of the choices made and also that such aspects should be discussed while reporting the research findings.

Conflict of Interests

The authors declare that there is no conflict of interests regarding the publication of this paper.

Acknowledgments

The inspiration for this paper came from "*Philosophy of Science*" course at the Swedish Institute of Disability Research (SIDR), Sweden. The authors also like to acknowledge late Professor Dafydd Stephens who provided useful insights in developing these concepts.

References

[1] M. Oliver, "Theories of disability in health practice and research," *British Medical Journal*, vol. 317, no. 7170, pp. 1446–1449, 1998.

[2] E. DePoy and S. F. Gilson, *Studying Disability: Multiple Theories and Responses*, Sage Publications, California, Calif, USA, 2011.

[3] N. B. Anderson, "Levels of analysis in health science: a framework for integrating sociobehavioral and biomedical research," in *Annals of the New York Academy of Sciences*, S. McCann and J. M. Lipton, Eds., vol. 840, pp. 563–576, Academy of Sciences, New York, NY, USA, 1998.

[4] J. F. Smart, "Challenging the biomedical model of disability," in *Advances in Medical Psychotherapy and Psychodiagnosisr*, vol. 12, pp. 41–44, American Board of Medical Psychotherapists, 2006.

[5] J. Suls and A. Rothman, "Evolution of the biopsychosocial model: prospects and challenges for health psychology," *Health Psychology*, vol. 23, no. 2, pp. 119–125, 2004.

[6] S. Thomas, "How is disability understood? An examination of sociological approaches," *Disability and Society*, vol. 19, no. 6, pp. 569–583, 2004.

[7] U. Bronfenbrenner, *The Ecology of Human Development: Experiments by Nature and Design*, Harvard University Press, Cambridge, Mass, USA, 1979.

[8] N. Luhmann, *Introduction to Systems Theory*, Polity Press, Cambridge, UK, 2012.

[9] S. M. Tensions, "Tensions, perspectives and themes in disability studies," *Scandinavian Journal of Disability Research*, vol. 11, no. 2, pp. 67–81, 2009.

[10] B. Danermark, "Different approaches in the assessment of audiological rehabilitation: a meta-theoretical perspective," *International Journal of Audiology*, vol. 42, no. 1, pp. S112–S117, 2003.

[11] S. Granberg, "ICF Core Sets for Hearing Loss Preparatory studies," in *Proceedings of the ICF Consensus Conference 2012*, Eriksholm, Denmark, 2012.

[12] A. Laplante-Lévesque, L. Hickson, and L. Worrall, "Stages of change in adults with acquired hearing impairment seeking help for the first time: application of the transtheoretical model in audiologic rehabilitation," *Ear and Hearing*, vol. 34, no. 4, pp. 447–457, 2013.

[13] A. Oakley, V. Strange, C. Bonell, E. Allen, and J. Stephenson, "Process evaluation in randomised controlled trials of complex interventions," *British Medical Journal*, vol. 332, no. 7538, pp. 413–416, 2006.

[14] A. Grant, S. Treweek, T. Dreischulte, R. Foy, and B. Guthrie, "Process evaluations for cluster-randomised trials of complex interventions: a proposed framework for design and reporting," *Trials*, vol. 14, no. 1, article 15, 2013.

[15] V. K. C. Manchaiah and D. Stephens, "Perspectives on defining "hearing loss" and its consequences," *Hearing, Balance and Communication*, vol. 11, no. 1, pp. 6–16, 2013.

[16] D. Campbell and J. Stanley, *Experimental and Quasi-Experimental Evaluations in Social Research*, Rand McNally, Chicago, Ill, USA, 1963.

[17] R. Cox, M. Hyde, S. Gatehouse et al., "Optimal outcome measures, research priorities, and international cooperation," *Ear and Hearing*, vol. 21, no. 4, pp. S106–S115, 2000.

[18] D. Stephens, G. Jones, and I. Gianopoulos, "The use of outcome measures to formulate intervention strategies," *Ear and Hearing*, vol. 21, no. 4 supplement, pp. 15S–23S, 2000.

[19] K. Grimmer-Somers, S. Milanese, and S. Kumar, "Managing the quality of allied health services in Australia: is it a case of "more we learn the less we know?"," *Journal of Healthcare Leadership*, vol. 4, pp. 71–81, 2012.

[20] World Health Organisation, *International Classification of Functioning, Disability and Health*, World Health Organisation, Geneva, Switzerland, 2001.

[21] V. K. C. Manchaiah, D. Stephens, and R. Meredith, "The patient journey of adults with hearing impairment: the patients' views," *Clinical Otolaryngology*, vol. 36, no. 3, pp. 227–234, 2011.

[22] V. K. C. Manchaiah and D. Stephens, "The patient journey: living with acquired hearing impairment," *Journal of the Academy of Rehabilitative Audiology*, vol. 44, pp. 29–40, 2011.

[23] V. K. C. Manchaiah and D. Stephens, "The "patient journey" of adults with sudden-onset acquired hearing impairment: a pilot study," *The Journal of Laryngology and Otology*, vol. 126, no. 5, pp. 475–481, 2012.

[24] V. K. C. Manchaiah, D. Stephens, and T. Lunner, "Communication partners journey through their partners hearing impairment," *International Journal of Otolaryngology*, vol. 2013, Article ID 707910, 11 pages, 2013.

[25] P. S. Segerstrom, T. C. A. Anant, and E. Dinopoulos, "A schumpeterian model of the product life cycle," *American Economic Review*, vol. 80, no. 5, pp. 1077–1091, 1990.

[26] S. Klepper, "Entry, exit, growth, and innovation over the product life cycle," *The American Economic Review*, vol. 86, no. 3, pp. 562–583, 1996.

[27] J. Mant, "Process versus outcome indicators in the assessment of quality of health care," *International Journal for Quality in Health Care*, vol. 13, no. 6, pp. 475–480, 2001.

[28] S. Gatehouse and W. Noble, "The speech, spatial and qualities of hearing scale (SSQ)," *International Journal of Audiology*, vol. 43, no. 2, pp. 85–99, 2004.

[29] W. Noble, R. Tyler, C. Dunn, and N. Bhullar, "Hearing handicap ratings among different profiles of adult cochlear implant users," *Ear and Hearing*, vol. 29, no. 1, pp. 112–120, 2008.

[30] C. Barnes and D. Mercer, *Doing Disability Research*, Disability Press, Leeds, UK, 1997.

[31] A. Laplante-Lévesque, L. V. Knudsen, J. E. Preminger et al., "Hearing help-seeking and rehabilitation: perspectives of adults with hearing impairment," *International Journal of Audiology*, vol. 51, no. 2, pp. 93–102, 2012.

[32] Ida Institute, "A possible patient journey," Ida Institute, Denmark, 2009, http://idainstitute.com/tool_room/self_development/patient_journey/.

[33] Ida Institute, *Communication Partner Journey*, Ida Institute, Nærum, Denmark, 2010, http://idainstitute.com/fileadmin/user_upload/Tools%20for%20Website%202011/Partner%20Journey%20-%20Ida%20Institute%20Tool.pdf.

[34] V. K. C. Manchaiah, D. Stephens, and T. Lunner, "Information about the prognosis given to sudden sensorineural hearing loss patients: implications to "patient journey" process," *Audiological Medicine*, vol. 10, no. 3, pp. 109–113, 2012.

[35] J. O. Prochaska and C. C. di Clemente, "Transtheoretical therapy: toward a more integrative model of change," *Psychotherapy*, vol. 19, no. 3, pp. 161–173, 1982.

[36] J. O. Prochaska and W. F. Velicer, "The transtheoretical model of health behavior change," *American Journal of Health Promotion*, vol. 12, no. 1, pp. 38–48, 1997.

[37] World Health Organization, *Engage in the Process of Change; Facts and Methods*, WHO Regional Office for Europe, Copenhagen, Denmark, 2012.

[38] B. Danermark, "Interdisciplinary research and critical realism: the example of disability research," *International Journal of Critical Realism*, vol. 1, pp. 56–64, 2002.

[39] R. Bhaskar, *A Realist Theory of Science*, Verso, London, UK, 2008.

[40] R. Bhaskar and B. Danermark, "Interdisciplinarity and disability research—a critical realist perspective," *Scandinavian Journal of Disability Research*, vol. 4, pp. 278–297, 2006.

[41] A. F. Chalmers, *What Is This Thing Called Science?* University of Queensland Press, Queensland, Australia, 3rd edition, 1999.

[42] I. Hacking, *Social Construction of What?* Harvard University Press, 2008.

[43] B. Danermark, M. Ekström, L. Jakobsen, and J. C. Karlsson, *Explaining Society: Critical Realism in the Social Sciences*, Taylor & Francis, 2002.

[44] P. C. Kerr and R. I. D. Cowie, "Acquired deafness: a multidimensional experience," *British Journal of Audiology*, vol. 31, no. 3, pp. 177–188, 1997.

[45] D. Stephens and R. Hétu, "Impairment, disability and handicap in audiology: towards a consensus," *Audiology*, vol. 30, no. 4, pp. 185–200, 1991.

[46] *Stanford Encyclopedia of Philosophy*, Friedrich Nietzsche, Stanford, Calif, USA, 2011, http://plato.stanford.edu/entries/nietzsche/.

17

Branchial Anomalies: Diagnosis and Management

Sampath Chandra Prasad,[1] Arun Azeez,[2] Nikhil Dinaker Thada,[1] Pallavi Rao,[3] Andrea Bacciu,[4] and Kishore Chandra Prasad[1]

[1] Department of Otolaryngology, Head and Neck Surgery, Srinivas Institute of Medical Sciences and Research,
   5-7-712/3 ASRP Street, Dongerkery, Kodialbail, Mangalore, Karnataka 575001, India
[2] Department of Otolaryngology, Head and Neck Surgery, Kasturba Medical College, Mangalore, Karnataka, India
[3] Department of Radiodiagnosis, Kasturba Medical College, Mangalore, Karnataka, India
[4] Department of Clinical and Experimental Medicine, Otolaryngology Unit, University Hospital of Parma, Parma, Italy

Correspondence should be addressed to Sampath Chandra Prasad; sampathcp@yahoo.co.in

Academic Editor: Leonard P. Rybak

Objective. To find out the incidence of involvement of individual arches, anatomical types of lesions, the age and sex incidence, the site and side of predilection, the common clinical features, the common investigations, treatment, and complications of the different anomalies. *Setting.* Academic Department of Otolaryngology, Head and Neck Surgery. *Design.* A 10 year retrospective study. *Participants.* 30 patients with clinically proven branchial anomalies including patients with bilateral disease totaling 34 lesions. *Main Outcome Measures.* The demographical data, clinical features, type of branchial anomalies, and the management details were recorded and analyzed. *Results and Observations.* The mean age of presentation was 18.67 years. Male to female sex ratio was 1.27 : 1 with a male preponderance. Of the 34 lesions, maximum incidence was of second arch anomalies (50%) followed by first arch. We had two cases each of third and fourth arch anomalies. Only 1 (3.3%) patients of the 30 presented with lesion at birth. The most common pathological type of lesions was fistula (58.82%) followed by cyst. 41.18% of the lesions occurred on the right side. All the patients underwent surgical excision. None of our patients had involvement of facial nerve in first branchial anomaly. All patients had tracts going superficial to the facial nerve. *Conclusion.* Confirming the extent of the tract is mandatory before any surgery as these lesions pass in relation to some of the most vital structures of the neck. Surgery should always be the treatment option. injection of dye, microscopic removal and inclusion of surrounding tissue while excising the tract leads to a decreased incidence of recurrence.

1. Introduction

Branchial fistulas and cysts, involving soft tissues of neck, are uncommon anomalies of embryonic development that are commonly encountered by otolaryngologists. In fact, approximately 17% of all pediatric cervical masses are due to branchial anomalies. Although branchial cleft cysts are benign, superinfection, mass effect, and surgical complications account for its morbidity. Branchial apparatus, seen in the early embryonic life, has a vital role to play in the development of head and neck structures. "Branchia" is the Greek word for gill, and the same word represents these anomalies owing to their resemblance to gills of certain species as fish. Six paired branchial arches, which appear

in the fourth week of embryonic life, give rise to many structures of the head and neck. Each branchial arch consists of core of mesenchyme covered externally by ectoderm and internally by endoderm. The fifth arch disappears and the sixth arch is rudimentary. Many anomalies of the head and neck region have been attributed to the aberrant development of these structures. Depending on the anatomic location, branchial anomalies are classified into first, second, third, and fourth anomalies. The course of a particular branchial anomaly is caudal to the structures derived from the corresponding arch and dorsal to the structures that develop from the following arch. Branchial anomalies are further typed into cysts, sinuses, and fistulas. Cysts are considered to be entrapped remnants of branchial cleft or

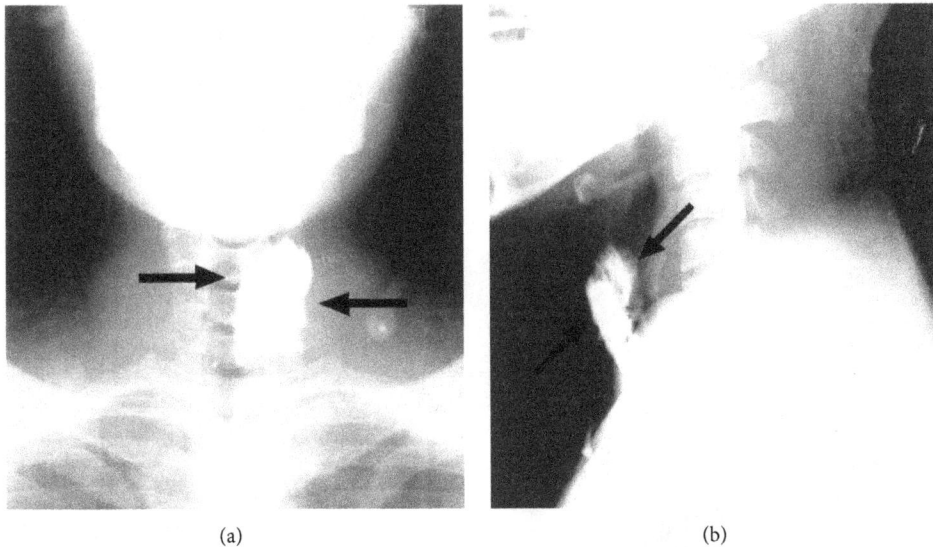

FIGURE 1: Contrast X-ray showing 4th branchial anomaly.

sinuses; sinuses are remnants of cleft or pouches; and fistulae result from persistence of both pouch and cleft [1]. Different anomalies of the head and neck area have been attributed to the maldevelopment of branchial apparatus. The importance of knowing the development of branchial apparatus and their anomalies is in applying the knowledge during surgery, as vital structures like facial nerve and parotid are in intimate relation with many of these anomalies. We performed a ten-year retrospective study to analyze the pathophysiology, clinical features, and management of branchial anomalies.

2. Materials and Methods

Ours is a retrospective study of 30 cases of branchial anomalies, which presented to the Department of Otolaryngology, Head and Neck Surgery, Kasturba Medical College, over a period of 10 years from 2000 to 2010. This study was cleared by the Manipal University Ethics Committee for Research and Publication. Age, sex, and duration of symptoms were noted from the case records. Family history and previous history of infection and/or surgery were noted. The side and site of the lesion and the site of opening of sinuses and fistula were noted. All the patients underwent routine blood examination. Patients with sinus and fistulas underwent sino-/fistulogram, by injecting contrast material urografin into the tract (Figure 1). The cystic lesions were investigated with ultrasound and CT scan. All patients were operated upon. In cases of acute infection, patients were put on intravenous antibiotics and in cases of abscess incision and drainage were done. Such patients were taken up for surgical excision of tract four weeks later. During surgery, a conscious attempt was made to remove some fascia and tissues adjacent to the branchial tracts along their path to avoid leaving behind ramifications that might lead to recurrences. The excised specimens were subjected to histopathological examination. Surgeries were performed under general anesthesia.

2.1. Excision of Collaural Fistula. This fistulous communication between the external auditory canal and the neck in the upper part of anterior border of sternocleidomastoid (SCM) muscle was identified by injecting methylene blue dye into the neck opening which was seen coming of an opening in the external auditory canal. A parotidectomy incision was given and facial nerve identified after superficial parotidectomy. The tract was then dissected from the surrounding tissue and followed till its opening in the external auditory canal (Figure 2). The tract was excised off its attachment to the external auditory canal and wound closed in layers.

2.2. Excision of Branchial Cyst. Skin incision was given over the cyst. Subplatysmal layer was elevated. SCM muscle was retracted away from the field taking care not to injure the greater auricular nerve. The cyst was carefully separated from the surrounding structures without damaging the wall. After complete excision, the wound was closed in layers.

2.3. Excision of Branchial Fistula. The tracts were identified by injecting methylene blue. Elliptical skin incision was made over the skin opening and the dissection proceeded in the direction of the tract. Step-ladder incision was used for the complete excision of the tract. This second incision was given at the level of the hyoid and the whole tract was brought out through this incision. It was then followed to its opening into the pharynx. During their course towards the oropharynx, the second branchial fistulae, were seen passing between the carotid bifurcations, where they were in close relation to the hypoglossal nerve. The third branchial fistulae were seen piercing the thyrohyoid membrane to open into the pyriform fossa (Figure 3). The tracts were followed to the pharynx and were excised; the pharyngeal defects were sutured. The suture lines were reinforced by a second layer of suture in the pharyngeal musculature. Wounds were closed in layers after placing a drain. The fourth branchial fistulae were seen

TABLE 1: Incidence of individual anomalies.

Branchial arch involved	Cyst		Fistula		Total	
	No.	%	No.	%	No.	%
1st branchial arch ($n = 13$) (38.24%)						
Work I	6	17.65%			6	17.65%
Work II			7	20.59%	7	20.59%
2nd branchial arch ($n = 17$) (50%)						
Branchial cyst	8	23.53%			8	23.53%
Branchial fistula			9	26.47%	9	26.47%
3rd branchial arch ($n = 2$) (5.88%)	—	—	2	5.88%	2	5.88%
4th branchial arch ($n = 2$) (5.88%)	—		2	5.88%	2	5.88%
Total ($n = 34$)	14	41.18%	20	58.82%	34	100%

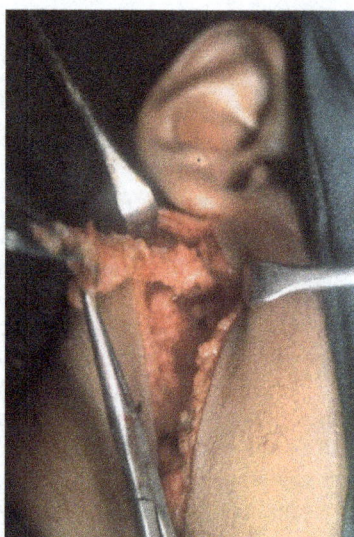

FIGURE 2: Collaural fistula.

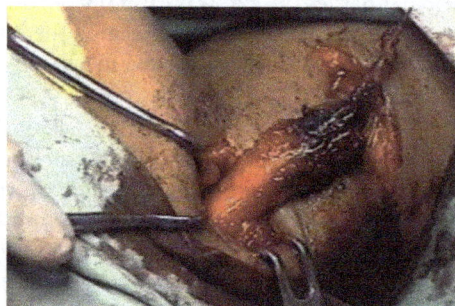

FIGURE 3: Excision of third branchial fistula.

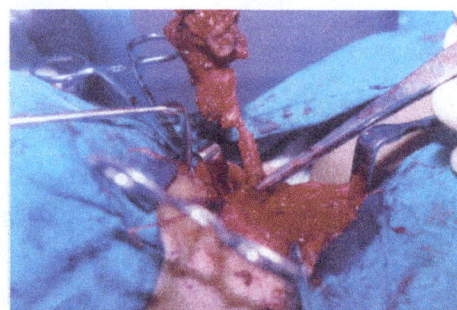

FIGURE 4: Excision of fourth branchial anomaly.

opening into the lower part of neck near the SCM muscle. The tract then passed inferiorly into the mediastinum, looping around the arch of aorta in the left and subclavian artery in the right and back in to the neck, ascending posterior to the carotid. Then it passed between the thyroid and cricoid cartilages opening into the pyriform fossa. The tract was followed from its neck opening into the mediastinum using blunt finger dissection. The intramediastinal part of the fistulae was left behind with their ends ligated and the rest of the tract was dissected out from the superior mediastinum up to the pyriform fossa (Figure 4).

3. Results and Observations

Thirty patients with 34 branchial anomalies were studied retrospectively over a period of 10 years from 2000 to 2010 in the Department of Otolaryngology, Head and Neck Surgery, Kasturba Medical College, Mangalore.

3.1. Type of Anomalies (Table 1). There was maximum incidence of second branchial anomalies with 17(50%) cases. Among the first branchial anomalies, seven (20.59%) cases belonged to Work II, while six (17.65%) cases belonged to Work I (according to the Work classification). Second branchial arch anomalies were seen in 17 cases (50%). Of these, branchial cyst constituted eight (26.53%) cases while branchial fistula constituted nine (26.47%) cases. Third branchial arch anomaly was seen in two (5.88%) patients. Fourth branchial arch anomaly was seen in two (5.88%) patients (Figure 5).

Among the anatomical types of the lesion, we had a maximum incidence of fistula seen in 20 (58.82%) cases, followed by cyst in 14 (41.12%) cases.

TABLE 2: Age and sex incidence.

Age in years	1st arch				2nd arch		3rd arch		4th arch	
	Work I		Work II							
	No.	%	No.	%	No.	%	No.	%	No.	%
0–5										
M	—	—	—	—	—	—	—	—	—	—
F	—	—	—	—	1	2.96%	—	—	—	—
6–10										
M	—	—	1	2.94%	2	5.88%	—	—	—	—
F	—	—	3	8.82%	2	5.88%	—	—	—	—
11–20										
M	2	5.88%	—	—	4	11.76%	—	—	1	2.94%
F	1	2.94%	2	5.88%	3	8.82%	—	—	—	—
21–40										
M	2	5.88%			3	8.82%	1	2.94%	1	2.94%
F	1	2.94%	—	—	2	5.88%	—	—	—	—
≥41										
M	—	—	—	—	—	—	1	2.94%	—	—
F	—	—	—	—	—	—	—	—	—	—
Total ($n = 34$)										
M	4	11.76%	2	5.88%	9	26.47%	2	2.94%	2	2.94%
F	2	5.88%	5	14.70%	8	23.53%	—	—	—	—

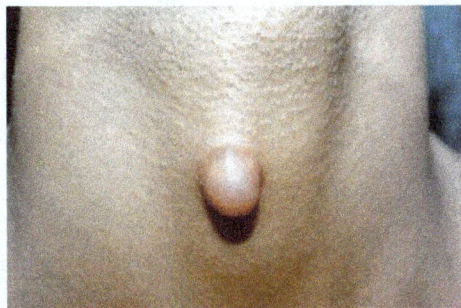

FIGURE 5: Fourth branchial anomaly.

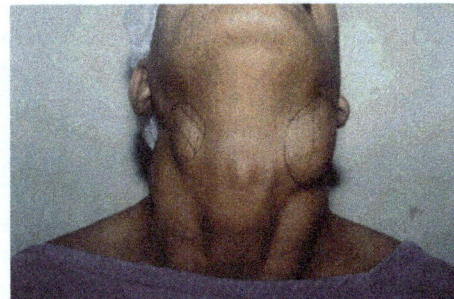

FIGURE 6: Bilateral branchial cyst.

3.2. Age and Sex Incidence (Table 2). The youngest patient in our study was one and a half years and the oldest one 48 years. The mean age of presentation was 18.67 years with a standard deviation of 11.06. Only 1 (3.3%) patient of the 30 presented with lesion at birth. The remaining 29 patients (96.7%) had a late onset of the disease. The mean age of onset among this late onset group was 15.97 years.

Among the first branchial anomalies, the maximum incidence of the lesion was seen in the 11–20 age group with 5 (14.70%) cases followed by 4 (11.76%) cases in the 6–10 and 21–40 age groups. In the second arch anomalies, we had four (11.76%) cases in the 6–10 age group and seven (20.59%) cases in the 11–20 and five (14.70%) in 20–40 age groups. Considering all the anomalies together, 55.88% were males and 44.12% were females with a male to female ratio of 1.27 : 1. In the first branchial anomalies, the incidence in males was 17.65% and 20.59% in females. Among the second arch anomalies 26.47% were males, while 23.53% were females. Third and fourth anomalies were seen only in males.

3.3. Side Incidence. The overall incidence of the anomalies was more on the right side (57.08%) while 42.92% of the lesions occurred on the left side. In the first arch anomalies, 8 (23.53%) cases were present on the right and 5 (14.71%) cases on the left. In the second arch anomalies 11 (32.35%) cases occurred on the right side and six (17.65%) cases on the left including one patient with bilateral branchial cysts (Figure 6). The third anomalies occurred on the right side and the fourth anomalies on the left side.

3.4. Clinical Features (Table 3). In all anomalies put together, the most common clinical feature was a swelling seen in 21 (61.76) and fistula opening in 18 (52.94%) cases. Discharge from the lesion was presented by 41.58% of the patients. 26.47% of the patients had pain at the site of the lesion.

TABLE 3: Clinical features.

Clinical features	1st arch No.	1st arch %	2nd arch No.	2nd arch %	3rd arch No.	3rd arch %	4th arch No.	4th arch %	Total No.	Total %
Swelling										
Neck	3	8.82%	9	26.47%	1	2.94%	1	2.94%	14	41.18%
Postauricular	7	20.59%	—	—	—	—	—	—	7	20.59%
Sinus										
Neck	8	23.53%	8	23.53%	1	2.94%	1	2.94%	18	52.94%
Pain	5	14.71%	3	8.82%	—	—	1	2.94%	9	26.47%
Fever	2	5.88%	3	8.82%	—	—	—	—	5	14.71%
Discharge	5	14.71%	7	20.59%	1	2.94%	1	2.94%	14	41.18%

Among the first arch anomaly patients, swelling in the neck and postauricular region was the most common presenting feature (29.41%). Pain and discharge were seen in 14.71%. The most common presenting feature of second branchial arch anomaly was neck swelling, seen in 26.47%, while 23.53% presented with opening in the neck. 20.59% had discharge from the lesion. Pain and fever were present in 8.82% of patients each. The third arch anomaly patient had swelling and opening in the neck along with discharge. The fourth arch anomaly patient had swelling and opening in the neck along with discharge and pain.

Fourteen patients had history of previous infection for which they had taken treatment. Five patients with second branchial arch anomalies had previous history of infection. The third and fourth arch anomaly patients also had history of previous infection.

3.5. Investigations. Sinogram/fistulogram was performed in all the cases. Ultrasound and CT scans were each done in 13.84% of patients. CT scan and ultrasound were done in all cases of third and fourth arch anomalies and nine cases of second arch anomaly. FNAC was done in five cases of branchial cysts.

3.6. Treatment (Table 4). Acute infection was treated by a course of antibiotics in 18 (60%) cases and incision and drainage in one case (before proceeding to the excision of the lesion). All the patients underwent surgical excision of the lesion. 73.33% of the cases were managed by single incision, while 23.33% required stepladder incision.

3.7. Complications (Table 5). Wound infection developed in 14.71% of the cases. Majority of this occurred in first branchial arch anomalies (11.76%). Wound gaping, which required secondary suturing, was seen in 8.82%. The recurrence rate in our series was 1.2%.

4. Discussion

Though described first in the early nineteenth century, the origin and classification of different branchial anomalies are highly controversial even today. The earliest description of branchial apparatus has been attributed to Von Baer in 1827. Rathke in 1828 had described the development of

pharyngeal arches in the human fetus. Acherson in 1832 first recognized branchial fistula and gave branchial cyst its name. Virchow first described the branchial cleft anomalies in 1865. Cervicoaural or collaural fistula was first described by Sir James Paget in 1878. Second branchial anomalies are considered to be the commonest with figures up to 95% being reported [2]. The remainder of branchial anomalies is derived from first branchial remnants (1–8%) with third and fourth branchial anomalies being quite rare [1]. There is still a controversy regarding the origin of branchial anomalies. Several theories proposed for the development of branchial anomalies include branchial apparatus theory, cervical sinus theory, thymopharyngeal theory, and inclusion theory. Of these, the widely accepted theory is that branchial anomalies result from incomplete involution of the branchial apparatus [1].

4.1. Age, Sex, and Side Incidence. According to Ford et al., [3] most of the branchial anomalies arise from the second branchial cleft (92.45%). Remaining is derived from first arch remnants (4.72%) and third (1.87%) and fourth arch anomalies (0.94%) are quite rare. Bajaj et al. [4] also reported higher incidence of second branchial anomalies (78%) in their series of 80 patients. Choi and Zalzal [1] who reported a higher incidence of first branchial arch anomalies (25%) in their series still had the maximum incidence of second branchial arch anomalies (40%). In our series, we had the maximum incidence of second arch anomalies (50%) followed by first arch anomalies (38.24%). Third and fourth arch anomalies accounted 5.88% each. Cysts, sinuses, and fistulae are the three anatomical types of branchial anomalies. Choi and Zalzal [1] reported a maximum incidence of sinuses, followed by fistula. In our series cysts were the most common lesion followed by sinuses.

Though a congenital lesion, branchial anomaly usually presents late in life. The age of onset of these anomalies has been seen to vary according to the type of the lesion. Choi and Zalzal [1] have noted that mean age of presentation of cyst (18.35 years) was late compared to that of fistulae (6.28 years) and sinuses (7.82 years). This finding was confirmed in our study. In our group, it was found that fistulas (1.14 years) had an early age of onset followed by that of sinuses (4.21 years). Cysts (7.51 years) were found to have a late onset compared to the other two lesions. Ford et al. [3] have pointed out that

TABLE 4: Treatment.

	1st arch		2nd arch		3rd arch		4th arch		Total	
	No.	%	No.	%	No.	%	No.	%	No.	%
Antibiotics	12	40%	4	13.33%	1	3.33%	1	3.33%	18	60%
I and D	1	3.33%	—	—	—	—	—		1	3.33%
Excision										
(i) Single incision	13	43.33%	7	23.33%	1	3.33%	1	3.33%	22	73.33%
(ii) Stepladder incision	—	—	7	23.33%	—	—	—		7	23.33%

TABLE 5: Complications.

	1st arch		2nd arch		3rd arch		4th arch		Total	
	No.	%	No.	%	No.	%	No.	%	No.	%
Wound infection	4	11.76%	1	2.94%	—	—	—	—	5	14.71%
Wound gaping	2	5.88%	1	2.94%	—	—	—	—	3	8.82%
Neurological deficit	—	—	1	2.94%	—	—	—	—	1	2.94%
Dermatitis	1	2.94%	—	—	—	—	—	—	1	2.94%
Total (34)	7	20.59%	3	8.82%	—	—	—	—	10	29.41%

the branchial anomalies occur more on the right side. They had 60% incidence on the right side and 40% on the left side. In the present study, we have a similar picture with right side incidence of 55.38% and left side incidence of 44.62%.

4.2. Clinical Features. In the study by Choi and Zalzal [1], the most common presenting features were discharge from the openings, cervical mass, and repeated infection. In our study, the most common clinical feature was a swelling seen in 21 (61.76). Discharge from the lesion was presented by 41.58% of the patients. 26.47% of the patients had pain at the site of the lesion.

4.3. Investigations. The diagnosis of branchial anomalies may be straightforward. However atypical lesions can be misdiagnosed. An initial correct diagnosis is crucial because experience shows that recurrence rates after surgical excision of branchial anomalies are 14% and 22% with previous infection and surgery, respectively, whereas the recurrence rate for primary lesion is 3% [5]. Although physical examination and history are the most important elements in the diagnosis, radio-diagnostic studies can add valuable information to the evaluation of a congenital neck mass. A CT scan is an accurate and noninvasive diagnostic tool, which can confirm the diagnosis or suggest an alternative diagnosis, define both the location and extent of a neck lesion, and delineate infectious process or possible malignant degeneration [6]. CT scan is useful in evaluating first branchial anomaly and the position of facial nerve. CT scan is reported to be more useful than MRI in evaluating branchial anomalies [1]. In case of sinus or fistula, sinogram or Conray contrast study can delineate the course of branchial anomaly. In the series by Choi and Zalzal [1], CT scan was performed on 15.38% of patients, sonogram/contrast study was performed on 7.69% of patients, and ultrasound/MRI was done on 1.92% of patients.

In our series, intraoperative methylene blue injection was performed in all cases; CT scan was done in 10.77% of cases. Ultrasound was done in 10.77% of cases. None of the patients underwent MRI.

4.4. Treatment. Surgery is definitive mode of treatment because there is lack of spontaneous regression, a high rate of recurrent infection, the possibility of other diagnoses, and rare malignant degeneration. Acute inflammation is treated medically unless incision and drainage or aspiration of an abscess is required. Three to four weeks should pass after an acute infection before a definitive surgical exploration is undertaken. In our series 60% of patients took medical treatment and 3.33% underwent drainage of abscess before definitive surgical excision of the lesion. Surgical excision of lesion was done in all patients.

4.5. Complications. In the series by Ford et al. [3], there was a postoperative recurrence rate of 3%. In our series recurrence rate was 1.2%. It is our observation that while methylene blue dye enhances visualization of the larger and more proximal (in relation to the punctum) part of the tracts and ramifications, it does not demarcate the most peripheral ramifications and hence a conscious attempt must be made to follow the tracts till the end. Using magnification loops or the microscope at the time of dissection may enhance prospects of complete removal. While it may be impossible to guarantee a complete removal, injection of dye and microscopic removal may be vital in preventing recurrences. We believe that this along with the practice of excision of the tract along with surrounding tissue has led to a low recurrence rate seen in our series. In our series, postoperative wound infection was the most common postoperative complication seen in 14.71% patients. This relatively high incidence can be attributed to the fact that a high percentage of the patients in this series were from a low socioeconomic stratum. 8.82% had wound gaping requiring secondary suturing. Though facial nerve paralysis/weakness has been reported in patients undergoing superficial parotidectomy for first branchial cleft anomalies, none of our patients had involvement of facial nerve.

5. Individual Branchial Anomalies

5.1. First Branchial Cleft Anomalies. First branchial cleft anomalies are thought to develop as a result of incomplete obliteration of the cleft between the mandibular process of the first arch and the second arch. A sinus will have an opening in the upper neck or in the floor of the external auditory canal, and a fistula will have an opening in both of these sites. The first branchial cleft anomalies have been classified as Type I or Type II by work [6].

Type I is considered to be a duplication of cartilaginous external auditory canal. A cystic mass in the postauricular area extends medially and anteriorly along the external auditory canal. It usually passes lateral to the facial nerve and ends at the bony meatus. No external opening is present except after infection. Type II is considered to be a duplication of the cartilaginous external auditory canal and pinna. A sinus passes from an external opening high in the neck along the anterior border of SCM muscle, superficial or deep to the facial nerve and closely related to parotid gland. It can either end blindly at the floor of the cartilaginous external auditory canal or open in to the external auditory canal, which is called the collaural fistula. In both types entrapment of desquamating squamous epithelium will result in the production of a cholesteatoma process resulting in erosion of bony external meatus, tympanic annulus, and hypotympanum [7].

In the series by Belenky and Medina [8] 66.66% of patients belonged to Work I and 33.33% to Work II. In the study by Nofsinger et al. [9] 27.27% had Work I and 72.73% had Work II lesions. In our study, Work I constituted 17.65% and Work II constituted 20.59%. In the study by Triglia et al. [10] on the first branchial cleft anomalies, 30.77% were male and 69.23% female. In the study by Belenky and Medina [8] the incidence in male was 22.22% and in female was 77.77%. In our study, 17.65% were male and 20.59% were female. All these studies show a higher incidencev of first branchial cleft among female. The symptoms and signs related to these anomalies in this series are similar to those described by various authors. In general, both types of anomalies may present as a progressively enlarging or recurrent mass or as a draining sinus. The diagnosis is usually made after infection has taken place. Incision and drainage of an abscess are frequently needed before definitive surgical treatment can be performed. Histopathology of the Work I lesions in our study showed that 100% of cases lined by squamous epithelium and 20% had cartilage components in the subepithelial layer. In the study by Belenky and Medina [8] 16.7% of Work I had cartilage component in the subepithelium. Intraoperatively

the lesion was found superficial to the facial nerve in 100% of our cases. Belenky and Medina [8] reported that the lesion was superficial to facial nerve in 88.88% of cases. In the study by Triglia et al. [10] lesion was deep to facial nerve in 39% cases. In the series by Nofsinger et al. [9], the lesion was deep to the facial nerve in 55% of cases. We agree with Bajaj et al. [4, 11] that it is advisable to perform a superficial parotidectomy in cases of first cleft anomalies while identifying the tract in relation to the facial nerve.

5.2. Second Branchial Cleft/Pouch Anomalies. During embryonic development, the second arch grows caudally, enveloping the third, fourth, and sixth arches and fusing with skin caudal to these arches, forming a deep groove (cervical sinus). The edges of this grove then meet and fuse. The ectoderm within the fused tube then disappears. Persistence of the ectoderm gives rise to a branchial cyst. A branchial fistula results from the breakdown of the endoderm. A persistent fistula of the second branchial cleft and pouch usually has its external opening in the neck near mid or lower part of SCM muscle. As it ascends it pierces platysma. At the level of hyoid it curves medially and passes between the external and internal carotids in relation to the hypoglossal and glossopharyngeal nerves. It opens in to the oropharynx usually in the intratonsillar cleft of palatine tonsil. In series of 98 cases by Ford et al. [3] 78% presented by the age of five years and in vast majority there was history of intermittent discharge and infection of neck sinus since birth. In seven percent there was history of incision and drainage of an associated neck abscess. In his series 60% sinus opening was on the right side and 40% on left. In our series of 17 cases 70% presented at age above 11 years. Only one patient presented at birth. 64.7% occurred on the right side and 35.3% on the left.

Second arch anomalies may take several forms. There may be only a simple sinus opening that extends up the neck for a variable distance. Branchial fistulas commonly present with persistent mucoid discharge from an opening in the skin of the neck. But rare and unusual presentation have also been documented. They have been documented as to present as parapharyngeal mass located in the supratonsillar fossa and extending to the lateral nasopharynx [12]. Exceedingly rarely, a branchial cleft anomaly may be found to be malignant on presentation [13]. A complete branchial fistula with external and internal opening is rare. The completeness of a fistula is diagnosed by a dye test in which methylene blue is injected through the outer opening and appears in the throat. A negative preoperative outcome on the test might become positive under general anaesthesia because of muscle relaxation. Occasionally, the fistula tract may be blocked by secretion or granulation giving negative fistula test [14]. In many a case, saliva is seen dribbling from the neck opening, which itself proves the completeness of the tract (Figure 7). In the 62 pediatric second branchial cleft anomalies, Bajaj et al. [4] reported 50 of them to be unilateral and 12 to be bilateral.

Several surgical approaches have been described for the management of a branchial fistula. The stepladder approach

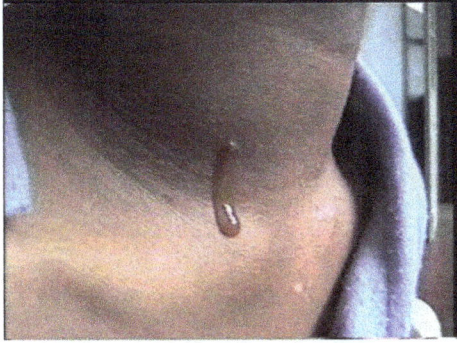

FIGURE 7: Saliva coming out of third branchial fistula.

[15] was described in 1933. The fistulous tract can be approached through a series of stepladder incision first encompassing the sinus opening and second overlying the carotid bifurcation. Subsequently the parapharyngeal portion of the fistula can be approached perorally after tonsillectomy. A wide cervicotomy incision (hockey stick) [16] can also be used which allows for adequate exposure of neck structure for accurate dissection. In all our cases, we traced the fistula up to the tonsillar area and excised the tract.

5.3. Third and Fourth Branchial Cleft/Pouch Anomalies. Third branchial anomalies are rare and constitute less than 1% of all such cases. Here the fistula opening is seen in the lower neck and it passes along the carotid sheath and then passes between the glossopharyngeal and hypoglossal nerve, piercing the thyrohyoid membrane to enter pharynx in the region of pyriform fossa. Anomalies of this type are very rare. Third pouch remnants are described as passing superior to superior laryngeal nerve and posterior to the common carotid artery. The tract emerges above the thyroid cartilage.

A persistent fistula of the fourth branchial cleft and pouch is theoretically possible but is very rare. Here the fistula opens in to the lower part of neck near the SCM muscle. The tract then passes inferiorly between superior and recurrent laryngeal nerve into the mediastinum, looping around the arch of aorta in the left and subclavian artery in the right and passes back in to the neck, ascending posterior to the carotid. Then it passes between the thyroid and cricoid cartilages and opens in to the pyriform fossa. According to Godin et al. [17], almost all the fourth arch anomalies reported occurred in the left side. In our series also, the fourth arch fistula occurred in the left side.

Third and fourth branchial remnants have been reported at any age. In neonates, these anomalies can be dangerous because of rapid enlargement leading to tracheal compression and respiratory distress. Noncommunicating or noninfected communicating cysts may present as cold thyroid nodules [18]. When infected, diagnosis and successful excision of a pyriform fossa sinus are very challenging and require meticulous approach. A history of recurrent upper respiratory tract infection, neck or thyroid pain and tenderness, and neck mass is common. Other presentations include cellulites,

hoarseness, odynophagia, thyroiditis, abscess, and stridor. A combination of ultrasound and CT with or without oral contrast will assist in the diagnosis.

We had two cases each of third and fourth branchial anomalies. All these patients came to us with after recurrences following surgeries done elsewhere. In cases of fourth cleft anomalies, CT with contrast through the neck opening demonstrated dye in the mediastinum. The third branchial anomalies showed a fistulous opening in the lower neck, which, on dissection, passed between the glossopharyngeal and hypoglossal nerve as classically described, piercing the thyrohyoid membrane to enter pharynx in the region of pyriform fossa. In the cases of fourth branchial anomalies, the intramediastinal part of the fistula was left behind with their ends ligated and the rest of the tract was dissected out from the superior mediastinum up to the pyriform fossa.

6. Highlights

(1) Our series confirms a higher incidence of first branchial cleft anomaly among females, the cause of which needs to be investigated.

(2) None of our patients had involvement of facial nerve. All patients had tracts going superficial to the facial nerve.

(3) All the fourth arch anomalies in our series occurred on the left side which is consistent with the literature.

(4) While it may be impossible to guarantee a complete removal, injection of dye and microscopic removal may be vital in preventing recurrences. We believe that this along with the practice of excision of the tract along with surrounding tissue has led to a low recurrence rate seen in our series.

7. Conclusion

Branchial apparatus plays an important role in the development of head and neck structures. Aberrant development of these structures can lead to formation of different anomalies. Most of these anomalies remain asymptomatic and might present later in life. Diagnosis is rather easy with a proper knowledge of the anatomy of the branchial anomalies. Confirming the extent of the tract is mandatory before any surgery as these lesions pass in relation to some of the most vital structures of the neck. Surgery must always be the treatment option for these lesions due to the fact that these lesions do not regress spontaneously and they have a high incidence of recurrent infection. Surgery also gives a chance to diagnose by means of histopathology, the rare occurence of branchogenic carcinoma.

Conflict of Interests

The authors declare that there is no conflict of interests regarding the publication of this paper.

References

[1] S. S. Choi and G. H. Zalzal, "Branchial anomalies: a review of 52 cases," *Laryngoscope*, vol. 105, no. 9, part 1, pp. 909–913, 1995.

[2] J. F. Kenealy, A. J. Torsiglieri Jr., and L. W. Tom, "Branchial cleft anomalies: a five-year retrospective review," *Transactions of the Pennsylvania Academy of Ophthalmology and Otolaryngology*, vol. 42, pp. 1022–1025, 1990.

[3] G. R. Ford, A. Balakrishnan, J. N. G. Evans, and C. M. Bailey, "Branchial cleft and pouch anomalies," *Journal of Laryngology and Otology*, vol. 106, no. 2, pp. 137–143, 1992.

[4] Y. Bajaj, S. Ifeacho, D. Tweedie et al., "Branchial anomalies in children," *International Journal of Pediatric Otorhinolaryngology*, vol. 75, no. 8, pp. 1020–1023, 2011.

[5] D. Reiter, "Third branchial cleft sinus: an unusual cause of neck abscess," *International Journal of Pediatric Otorhinolaryngology*, vol. 4, no. 2, pp. 181–186, 1982.

[6] F. Coppens, P. Peene, and S. F. Lemahieu, "Diagnosis and differential diagnosis of branchial cleft cysts by CT scan," *Journal Belge de Radiologie*, vol. 73, no. 3, pp. 189–196, 1990.

[7] S. A. Hickey, G. A. Scott, and P. Traub, "Defects of the first branchial cleft," *Journal of Laryngology and Otology*, vol. 108, no. 3, pp. 240–243, 1994.

[8] W. M. Belenky and J. E. Medina, "First branchial cleft anomalies," *Laryngoscope*, vol. 90, no. 1, pp. 28–39, 1980.

[9] Y. C. Nofsinger, L. W. C. Tom, D. LaRossa, R. F. Wetmore, and S. D. Handler, "Periauricular cysts and sinuses," *Laryngoscope*, vol. 107, no. 7, pp. 883–887, 1997.

[10] J. Triglia, R. Nicollas, V. Ducroz, P. J. Koltai, and E. Garabedian, "First branchial cleft anomalies: a study of 39 cases and a review of the literature," *Archives of Otolaryngology—Head and Neck Surgery*, vol. 124, no. 3, pp. 291–295, 1998.

[11] Y. Bajaj, D. Tweedie, S. Ifeacho, R. Hewitt, and B. E. J. Hartley, "Surgical technique for excision of first branchial cleft anomalies: how we do it," *Clinical Otolaryngology*, vol. 36, no. 4, pp. 371–374, 2011.

[12] F. A. Papay, C. Kalucis, I. Eliachar, and H. M. Tucker, "Nasopharyngeal presentation of second branchial cleft cyst," *Otolaryngology—Head and Neck Surgery*, vol. 110, no. 2, pp. 232–234, 1994.

[13] A. K. Ohri, R. Makins, C. E. T. Smith, and P. W. Leopold, "Primary branchial cleft carcinoma—a case report," *Journal of Laryngology and Otology*, vol. 111, no. 1, pp. 80–82, 1997.

[14] A. H. Ang, K. P. Pang, and L. K. Tan, "Complete branchial fistula: case report and review of the literature," *Annals of Otology, Rhinology and Laryngology*, vol. 110, no. 11, pp. 1077–1079, 2001.

[15] D. L. Mandell, "Head and neck anomalies related to the branchial apparatus," *Otolaryngologic Clinics of North America*, vol. 33, no. 6, pp. 1309–1332, 2000.

[16] F. C. Agaton-Bonilla and C. Gay-Escoda, "Diagnosis and treatment of branchial cleft cysts and fistulae. A retrospective study of 183 patients," *International Journal of Oral and Maxillofacial Surgery*, vol. 25, no. 6, pp. 449–452, 1996.

[17] M. S. Godin, D. B. Kearns, S. M. Pransky, A. B. Seid, and D. B. Wilson, "Fourth branchial pouch sinus: principles of diagnosis and management," *Laryngoscope*, vol. 100, no. 2, part 1, pp. 174–178, 1990.

[18] M. Liberman, S. Kay, S. Emil et al., "Ten years of experience with third and fourth branchial remnants," *Journal of Pediatric Surgery*, vol. 37, no. 5, pp. 685–690, 2002.

Mucin Gene Expression in Reflux Laryngeal Mucosa: Histological and *In Situ* Hybridization Observations

Mahmoud El-Sayed Ali,[1,2] **David M. Bulmer,**[2] **Peter W. Dettmar,**[3] **and Jeffrey P. Pearson**[2]

[1] *Department of Otolaryngology, Mansoura University Hospital, Mansoura University, Egypt*
[2] *Institute for Cell and Molecular Biosciences, Newcastle University, Faculty of Medical Sciences, Newcastle upon Tyne NE2 4HH, UK*
[3] *Castle Hill Hospital, Castle Road, Cottingham, East Yorkshire HU16 5JQ, UK*

Correspondence should be addressed to Mahmoud El-Sayed Ali; msamomar@yahoo.co.uk

Academic Editor: Charles Monroe Myer

Objectives/Hypothesis. To determine if laryngopharyngeal reflux alters mucin gene expression in laryngeal mucosa. *Methods. In situ* hybridization was employed to study the expression of the 8 well-characterised mucin genes MUC1-4, 5AC, 5B, 6, and 7 in reflux laryngeal mucosa from laryngeal ventricles, posterior commissures, and vocal folds compared to control/normal laryngeal mucosa. *Results.* MUC1-5 genes are expressed in normal and reflux laryngeal mucosa. MUC1, 3 and 4 are expressed in respiratory and squamous mucosa whereas MUC2 and 5AC are expressed in respiratory mucosa only. MUC3, 4 and 5AC are downregulated in reflux mucosa. MUC5AC expression is significantly reduced in the 3 mucosal sites and when mucosal type was taken into account, this remains significant in combined laryngeal and ventricular mucosa only. *Conclusions.* MUC3, 4 and 5AC expression is downregulated in laryngopharyngeal reflux. This may be due to laryngeal mucosal metaplasia and/or alteration of mucin gene expression in the preexisting mucosa. Altered mucin gene expression might predispose laryngeal mucosa to the damaging effect of reflux.

1. Introduction

Mucin gene expression is tissue specific in order to afford protection for the relevant mucosa. In certain conditions such as inflammation, metaplasia, and neoplasia, mucin gene expression patterns can be altered through changes in the nature of the mucosal tissue. An example is Barrett's oesophageal metaplasia when lower oesophageal mucosa changes from squamous to gastrointestinal mucosa containing mucus secreting cells [1]. This appears to result from repetitive insult to oesophageal mucosa by gastric refluxate leading to altered mucin expression from normal membrane-bound mucins and submucosal gland secretory mucins to the secretory gel-forming mucins similar to those found in the gastrointestinal tract. MUC2 expression found in Barrett's metaplasia is lost as the cells become dysplastic [2].

Laryngopharyngeal reflux (LPR) has become more commonly attributed as an etiology of many upper airway disorders for which there has previously been no known aetiology.

The anecdotal evidence as to the increased laryngeal mucus noted in reflux patients during laryngoscopy has not been fully elucidated. It is not known whether this increased mucus is laryngeal or tracheobronchial in origin and whether it is due to increased mucus expression or reduced mucus clearance. Although mucin expression in laryngeal cancers has been studied before [3–5], the effect of LPR on laryngeal mucin gene expression has been documented in only a few studies [6, 7]. Furthermore, mucin gene expression in different regions of the laryngeal mucosa has not been studied in detail.

2. Aim of Study

This study aims to investigate mucin gene expression in laryngeal mucosa of LPR patients in contrast to control/normal laryngeal mucosa. *In situ* hybridization was employed as it offers not only high specificity but also provides cellular

TABLE 1: Histological types of reflux mucosa from three laryngeal locations.

Mucosa	Respiratory only		Squamous only		Mixed	
	Control	LPR	Control	LPR	Control	LPR
Posterior commissure	0/3	0/27	1/3	18/27	2/3	9/27
Ventricles	3/3	17/22	0/3	0/3	0/3	5/22
Vocal folds	0/3	00	0/3	14/22	3/3	8/22
Total	3/9	17/71	1/9	40/71	5/9	14/71
	33%	24%	11%	56%	56%	20%

The quoted numbers indicate how many patients from whom laryngeal mucosal samples were taken.

expression details in histological sections. The study includes the first 8 mucin genes, MUC1-4, 5AC, 5B, 6 and 7, the best characterized mucin genes so far.

3. Methods

3.1. Control Laryngeal Mucosa. Clinically and histo-pathologically normal human laryngeal mucosa was obtained from 3 nonsmoker patients with no documented history of LPR. The first 2 patients had ischemic heart disease. The third patient had localised laryngeal cancer and mucosal samples were taken well away from the cancer. Mucosal samples were obtained from 3 anatomical locations: vocal folds, laryngeal ventricles and posterior commissure as these are the areas often involved in reflux laryngeal disorders.

3.2. Reflux Laryngeal Mucosa. Laryngeal mucosal samples from patients with LPR were donated by Professor Koufman, Wake Forest Medical School, NC, USA. All tissues were obtained in accordance with ethical guidelines, with informed consent obtained for each sample, and the study was approved by the institutional review board of Newcastle University. Mucosal samples were taken from the vocal folds, laryngeal ventricles and posterior commissure during microlaryngoscopic examination. Three samples were taken from a total of 27 LPR patients. Due to the small size of some of the laryngeal mucosal samples, the numbers of samples from the 3 anatomical sites were not equal.

3.3. In Situ Hybridization. The protocol followed a modified version of that of Aust et al. [8] using 48 bp Oligonucleotide probes with sequences complimentary to the most frequently occurring base-pair sequences within the tandem repeat domain of the mucin mRNA. This was to obtain signal amplification by hybridizing the largest number of probes with the tandem repeat regions in the same mRNA molecule. Positive control tissues were obtained from tissues known to strongly express the investigated mucin gene. Human breast tissue was used as a control for MUC1; human colon for MUC2, 3 and 4; human gastric mucosa for MUC5AC and 6; human bronchial mucosa for MUC5B, and human submandibular salivary gland for MUC7. Negative controls consisted of sections from normal human liver, as it does not express any of these mucin genes. Steps of the experiment

were detailed elsewhere [9]. Whenever possible, all mucin genes were tested on the available samples and duplicates were carried out as tissue allowed.

Sections were lightly counterstained in Harris' haematoxylin before immersing in Scott's modified tap water (bluing reagent) and mounted using gelatin and a coverslip. Light microscopy was performed on sections using Nikon Labophot microscope fitted with a trinocular mount and photographed using an Olympus Camedia C-3030 Zoom digital camera at magnification of 100X and 200X. Image clarity was enhanced by adjusting brightness, hue, and contrast with Adobe Photoshop software (Adobe Systems, Mountain view, CA). Histological details were also observed in each slide before looking for the hybridization signals. Positive signal were identified as an intense blue/black darkening in the cytoplasm of cells. *In situ* hybridization data was analysed by a chi square test comparing the two subsets of data and the significance level was considered at $P < 0.05$.

4. Results

4.1. Histological Observations. In control laryngeal mucosa, posterior commissures were covered by mixed (respiratory and squamous) mucosa in 2/3 of samples and in 1/3 the covering mucosa was squamous epithelium. Vocal cord mucosa was mixed (respiratory and squamous) in the 3 samples whereas ventricular mucosa was covered by respiratory epithelium only. Squamous metaplasia was noted in reflux laryngeal mucosa from the 3 locations. Reflux vocal cord and posterior commissure mucosa was predominantly covered by squamous mucosa in 2/3 of samples and the other 1/3 was covered by mixed epithelium. Mixed mucosa appeared in 23% of ventricular mucosal samples and the remaining 77% was still covered by respiratory epithelium (Table 1).

4.2. Mucin Gene Expression in Control Laryngeal Mucosa (Figure 1). Control laryngeal mucosa expressed MUC1-4 and 5AC depending on the type of mucosa. Thus, the secretory mucin genes MUC2 and 5AC were present only in respiratory mucosa of the ventricles and vocal folds and were absent in squamous mucosa of the posterior commissure and vocal cords. MUC1, 3 and 4 were expressed in both mucosal types. MUC4 was the most prevalent mucin gene expressed in 78% of samples (7/9 of samples) followed by MUC3 and 5AC (67% each). MUC1 and 2 were less prevalent (11% each)

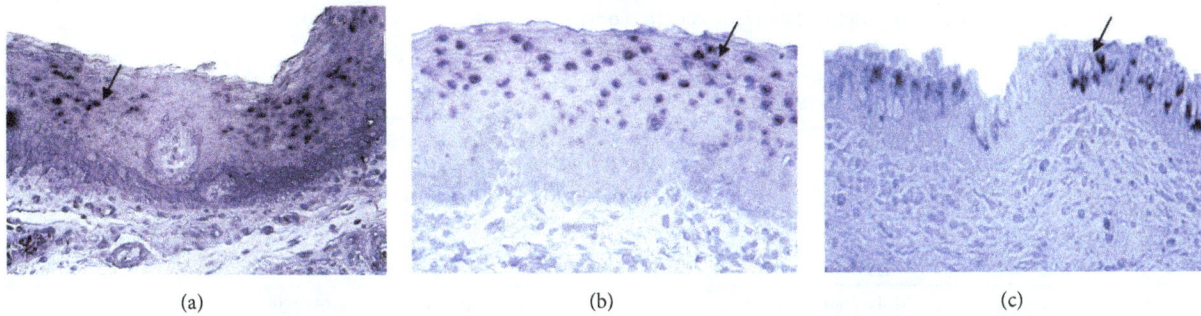

(a)   (b)   (c)

FIGURE 1: Mucin gene expression in normal laryngeal mucosa. *In situ* hybridization photographs of the expression of MUC3 and 4 in vocal cords mucosa ((a) and (b), resp.) and MUC5AC in laryngeal ventricles mucosa (c). Sections were lightly counterstained in Harris' hematoxylin and then immersed in Scott's modified tap water (bluing reagent). Arrows indicate areas of mucin gene expression. Magnification 200X.

TABLE 2: *In situ* hybridisation results of mucin gene expression in the control laryngeal mucosa from 3 control cases.

Mucosa	MUC1	MUC2	MUC3	MUC4	MUC5AC
Posterior commissure	0/3	0/3	2/3	2/3	2/3
Ventricles	1/3	1/3	2/3	3/3	3/3
Vocal folds	0/3	0/3	2/3	2/3	1/3
Total	1/9	1/9	6/9	7/9	6/9
%	11%	11%	67%	78%	67%

Samples were taken from 3 laryngeal mucosal samples from each control case and the total was taken for each area for each mucin gene.

(Table 2). MUC6 and 7 were not expressed in any of the control laryngeal samples. MUC5B results were not explored as the positive control for this mucin gene (human bronchial mucosa) consistently failed to show positive expression.

4.3. Mucin Gene Expression in Reflux Laryngeal Mucosa (Figure 2). MUC6 and 7 were not expressed in any of the tested (vocal folds, laryngeal ventricles and posterior commissure) samples. MUC3 and 4 were downregulated (52% in LPR mucosa versus 67% in control mucosa for MUC3 and 69% in LPR mucosa versus 78% in control mucosa for MUC4) whereas MUC1 and 2 were upregulated (21% in LPR mucosa versus 11% in control mucosa for MUC1 and 29% in LPR mucosa versus 11% in control mucosa for MUC2). The only mucin gene which showed significant expression change was MUC5AC which was down regulated in LPR samples from the 3 anatomical sites (16% in LPR mucosa versus 67% in control mucosa) ($P < 0.001$, chi square test) (Table 3).

4.4. Topographic Mucin Gene Expression in Reflux Laryngeal Mucosa. Mucin gene expression in individual areas of reflux laryngeal mucosa showed similar patterns as observed in control laryngeal mucosa as a whole.

4.4.1. Posterior Commissure. MUC1 and 2 were expressed in LPR posterior commissure mucosa whereas these 2 mucin genes were not expressed in control mucosa. This however

was not statistically significant. MUC4 was slightly up regulated. Although MUC3 and 5AC were down regulated, this was statistically significant only for MUC5AC ($P < 0.05$).

4.4.2. Laryngeal Ventricles (Figure 3). All the expressed mucin genes were down regulated in the mucosa of laryngeal ventricles to variable extents; however, the only mucin gene which showed significant downregulation was MUC5AC ($P < 0.001$). MUC4 was expressed in only 70% of reflux versus 100% expression in control ventricular mucosa.

4.4.3. Vocal Folds. MUC1 and 2 were expressed in LPR (32% and 14% for MUC1 and 2, resp.) whereas these 2 mucin genes were not expressed in the 3 control vocal cord mucosal samples. However, this was not statistically significant. The other 3 mucin genes MUC3, 4 and 5AC were downregulated although this was not statistically significant.

Secretory mucin expression was analysed taking into account the type of mucosa, that is, the expression of secretory mucin genes by respiratory mucosa only and expression of membrane-bound mucin genes in both mucosal types. This resulted in no difference of MUC2 expression in LPR versus control laryngeal mucosa. MUC5AC down regulation was still significant in respiratory mucosa of the combined laryngeal and ventricular mucosa ($P < 0.05$) while statistical significance was lost in respiratory mucosa of posterior commissure mucosa.

5. Discussion

Mucin gene expression in control and reflux laryngeal mucosa is similar to that in other parts of airway mucosa such as tracheal [10], bronchial [11] and nasal mucosa [8, 12]. Although MUC3 is considered as an intestinal mucin gene, it has been found to be expressed in airway mucosa [13, 14] and in nasal polyps [9]. Expression patterns were different among the different laryngeal mucosal sites. This could be accounted for by specific mucin gene expression related to a specific type of mucosa.

There is an overall upregulation of MUC1 and 2 and down regulation of MUC3 4 and 5AC mucin gene expression in

TABLE 3: Mucin gene expression in control versus reflux laryngeal mucosa.

Laryngeal mucosa	MUC1		MUC2		MUC3		MUC4		MUC5AC	
	Control	LPR	Control	LPR	Control	LPR	Control	LPR	Control	LPR
Posterior commissure	0/3	4/26	0/3	6/26	2/3	15/26	2/3	17/24	2/3	3/24
Ventricle	1/3	4/22	1/3	5/20	2/3	11/20	3/3	14/20	3/3	3/24
Vocal folds	0/3	7/22	0/3	3/22	2/3	9/21	2/3	14/21	1/3	5/21
Total/average	1/9	15/70	1/9	14/68	6/9	35/67	7/9	45/65	6/9	11/69
	11%	21%	11%	29%	67%	52%	78%	69%	67%	16%

Numbers of mucosal samples for each area of laryngeal mucosa expressing the mucin gene in question are divided by total numbers of samples studied and resultant % calculated. LPR: laryngopharyngeal reflux mucosa.

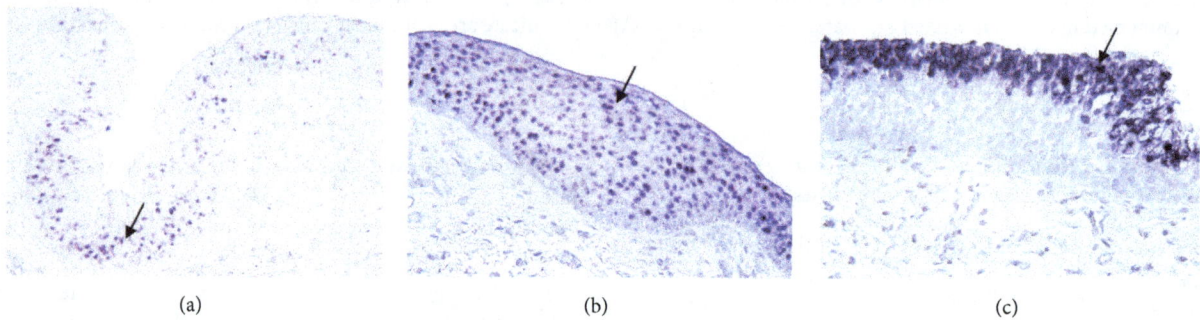

(a)   (b)   (c)

FIGURE 2: Mucin gene expression in laryngopharyngeal reflux mucosa. *In situ* hybridization photographs of the expression of MUC3 in laryngeal ventricle (a), MUC4 in posterior commissure (b), and MUC5AC in laryngeal ventricle (c). Sections were lightly counterstained in Harris' haematoxylin and then immersed in Scott's modified tap water (bluing reagent). Arrows indicate areas of mucin gene expression. Magnification 200X.

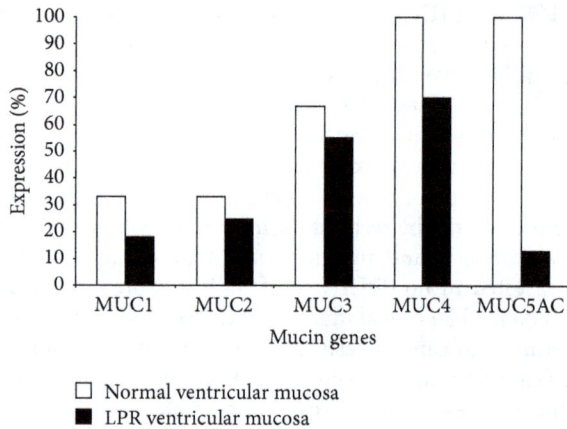

FIGURE 3: Mucin gene expression in ventricular mucosa of control and laryngopharyngeal reflux mucosa.

reflux laryngeal mucosa. Samuels et al. [7] employed RT-PCR to 2 normal and 3 LPR mucosal samples and reported down regulation of MUC2, 3 and 5AC in LPR compared to normal laryngeal mucosa. They found that exposure of normal hypopharyngeal mucosal cell to low pH *in vitro* up regulated these mucins whereas pepsin inhibited this up regulation. They postulated that depletion of mucosal secretions may contribute to the progression of reflux injury. Although the net effect of acid and pepsin was still one of up regulation

of MUC2 and 3 and completely abolished up regulation of MUC1 and 5AC in hypopharyngeal cell culture, Samuel et al. postulated that, after repeated exposure to gastric refluxate, pepsin could deregulate the protective stimulation of mucin gene expression and may ultimately lead to the overall down regulation of a subset of mucin genes.

MUC3 and 4, the two main mucin genes controlling the expression of membrane-bound mucins, are down regulated in reflux laryngeal mucosa. The contribution of membrane-bound mucins in laryngeal mucosal protection is unknown. However, the structure of membrane-bound mucins may provide antidesiccating and protective mechanism against passage of air, inhaled particles, vibratory stress (as a result of phonation) and other insults such as contact with noxious refluxed materials. Alteration of this protective mechanism may predispose the laryngeal mucosa to damage and metaplasia.

Secretory mucins MUC2 and 5AC would provide lubricating and protective barrier. MUC2 was expressed only in control ventricular mucosa and was absent in posterior commissure and vocal fold mucosa whereas MUC5AC was moderately expressed in the three locations to various extents. In LPR mucosa, low expression of MUC2 in vocal fold mucosa was associated with moderate expression of MUC5AC and moderate expression of MUC2 in posterior commissure and ventricular mucosa was associated with low expression of MUC5AC. This suggests that respiratory MUC2 and 5AC are not mutually inclusive or exclusive in pathological respiratory mucosa. This is similar to our previous results on sinus mucin expression where an inverse relationship was found between the expression of these two mucins [12]. Airway mucin expression could be contributing to a finite pool, so if for example MUC2 is up regulated, compensatory MUC5AC down regulation results.

MUC5AC was significantly down regulated in LPR mucosa from the ventricular and posterior commissure mucosa not in the vocal fold mucosa. However, when squamous mucosa was excluded from the calculation, the significant reduction of MUC5AC expression in the LPR posterior commissure mucosa was lost. This indicates that MUC5AC down regulation in the posterior commissure mucosa could be, at least in part, due to the replacement of respiratory epithelium by squamous epithelium which is unable to express MUC5AC.

MUC5AC down regulation in laryngeal ventricles was still significant in the respiratory mucosa after exclusion of squamous mucosa. A direct inhibitory effect of reflux on MUC5AC expression independent of squamous metaplasia could be responsible for MUC5AC down regulation in ventricular mucosa. It is to be noted also that respiratory mucosa of laryngeal ventricles demonstrated no total squamous metaplasia in any of the studied samples. The samples which showed squamous metaplasia had areas of respiratory mucosa (mixed mucosa). This was also noted in only 23% of samples in contrast to the posterior commissures and vocal folds where 67% and 64% of samples demonstrated squamous metaplasia and were covered by squamous epithelium only. The low incidence of squamous metaplasia in ventricular mucosa compared to posterior commissures and vocal fold mucosa could be related to the anatomy of the ventricular mucosa being sequestered between ventricular and vocal folds and thus being less likely to be exposed to reflux components. However, this does not agree with the significant down regulation of MUC5AC expression in reflux ventricular mucosa. An explanation for this could be that the exposure of ventricular mucosa to the reflux insult triggers MUC5AC down regulation as the main insult effect rather than altering the nature of the covering epithelium.

The appearance of squamous metaplasia in an initially respiratory mucosa would decrease the quantity of secretory mucins. It is a possible consequence that any protective effect imparted to the tissue by the expression of these mucins would decrease, so further increasing the susceptibility of the mucosal surface to damage by noxious agents such as reflux components. On the other hand, this squamous metaplasia may indicate another way of tissue defence by creating a multilayer of dead cells which could then incur stronger physical barrier against injurious effect of refluxate. It has been reported that ciliated bronchiolar epithelial cells undergo squamous metaplasia after bronchiolar injury with naphthalene and new squamous cells spread beneath injured epithelial cells maintaining the integrity of the epithelium [15].

Down regulation of membrane-bound mucins MUC3 and 4 would be solely due to direct effect of reflux on laryngeal mucosa as these mucin genes are expressed in respiratory and squamous mucosa. This is in contrast to down regulation of the secretory mucin MUC5AC which could be due to an indirect effect of reflux through squamous metaplasia of laryngeal mucosa in addition to the direct effect on respiratory mucosal mucin gene expression. The possible dual mechanisms of MUC5AC down regulation would explain the significant alteration of this mucin gene in reflux laryngeal mucosa compared to MUC3 and 4. It would also suggest a significant contribution of MUC5AC down regulation in the development of endoscopic laryngeal mucosal changes noted in reflux laryngitis.

Histological sections of laryngeal mucosa did not show submucosal glands. This suggests that MUC5B which is mainly expressed in submucosal gland of airway epithelium [16, 17] might not be a significant member of the laryngeal mucin genes family. This could imply that laryngeal mucosal defence depends mainly on the integrity of the surface mucosa and therefore a change in the nature of laryngeal mucosa could have a significant impact on its protective functions. Therefore, the lack of information about this mucin gene in the current study, due to technical difficulty, does not seem to significantly alter the drawn picture of normal and reflux laryngeal mucin gene expression.

5.1. Further Works/Studies Required. Further studies with larger numbers of samples are needed to clarify these observations to create a clearer picture of the impact of reflux on mucin gene expression in laryngeal mucosa. Comparative histological analysis of the spread of respiratory and squamous epithelia in normal versus reflux laryngeal mucosa is important to clarify the possible interplay of laryngeal mucosal changes and mucin gene expression in LPR.

5.2. Strength and Weakness of the Study. This study explores mucin gene expression in normal and reflux laryngeal mucosa with some interesting observations. The number of control/normal laryngeal mucosal samples is small. It is a clinical and ethical challenge to get normal laryngeal mucosa from healthy volunteers or patients with nonlaryngeal pathologies. Although clinically normal mucosa can be obtained from laryngectomy samples, subtle changes at the molecular levels may exist and could alter the normal mucin gene expression. Furthermore, laryngeal cancer patients are usually elderly smokers and these, among other factors, could alter mucin gene expression in control laryngeal mucosa.

6. Conclusion

LPR tends to downregulate mucin gene expression particularly MUC5AC, a secreted and gel-forming mucin. This change could be due to laryngeal mucosal metaplastic changes and/or alteration of mucin gene expression in the preexisting mucosa. The expression of mucin genes in laryngeal mucosa may offer some protection to laryngeal mucosa and alteration of the mucosal type or the gene expressed may predispose laryngeal mucosa to the damaging effects of reflux. Down regulation of MUC5AC could be involved in the development of reflux-related laryngeal mucosal changes noted in clinical settings.

Conflict of Interests

The authors declare that there is no conflict of interests regarding the publication of this paper.

Acknowledgments

The authors thank Dr. David Hopwood and Dr. Neil Kernhan of the Department of Molecular Pathology, Ninewells Hospital and Medical School, Dundee, for histological analysis of laryngeal mucosa.

References

[1] N. R. Barrett, "Chronic peptic ulcer of the oesophagus and 'oesophagitis'," *The British Journal of Surgery*, vol. 38, no. 150, pp. 175–182, 1950.

[2] C. N. Chinyama, R. E. K. Marshall, W. J. Owen et al., "Expression of MUC1 and MUC2 mucin gene products in Barrett's metaplasia, dysplasia and adenocarcinoma: an immunopathological study with clinical correlation," *Histopathology*, vol. 35, no. 6, pp. 517–524, 1999.

[3] M. V. Croce, "Detection and isolation of MUC1 mucin from larynx squamous cell carcinoma," *Pathology and Oncology Research*, vol. 6, no. 2, pp. 93–99, 2000.

[4] J.-P. Jeannon, V. Aston, F. W. Stafford, J. V. Soames, and J. A. Wilson, "Expression of MUC1 and MUC2 glycoproteins in laryngeal cancer," *Clinical Otolaryngology and Allied Sciences*, vol. 26, no. 2, pp. 109–112, 2001.

[5] V. Paleri, J. P. Pearson, D. Bulmer, J.-P. Jeannon, R. G. Wight, and J. A. Wilson, "Expression of mucin gene products in laryngeal squamous cancer," *Otolaryngology*, vol. 131, no. 1, pp. 84–88, 2004.

[6] D. Bulmer, P. E. Ross, S. E. Axford et al., "Cell biology of laryngeal epithelial defenses in health and disease: further studies," *Annals of Otology, Rhinology and Laryngology*, vol. 112, no. 6, pp. 481–491, 2003.

[7] T. L. Samuels, E. Handler, M. L. Syring et al., "Mucin gene expression in human laryngeal epithelia: effect of laryngopharyngeal reflux," *Annals of Otology, Rhinology and Laryngology*, vol. 117, no. 9, pp. 688–695, 2008.

[8] M. R. Aust, C. S. Madsen, A. Jennings, and J. L. Kasperbauer, "Mucin mRNA expression in normal and vasomotor inferior turbinâtes," *American Journal of Rhinology*, vol. 11, no. 4, pp. 293–302, 1997.

[9] M. S. Ali, J. A. Wilson, M. Bennett, and J. P. Pearson, "Mucin gene expression in nasal polyps," *Acta Oto-Laryngologica*, vol. 125, no. 6, pp. 618–624, 2005.

[10] C. J. Reid, S. Gould, and A. Harris, "Developmental expression of mucin genes in the human respiratory tract," *American Journal of Respiratory Cell and Molecular Biology*, vol. 17, no. 5, pp. 592–598, 1997.

[11] A. López-Ferrer, V. Curull, C. Barranco et al., "Mucins as differentiation markers in bronchial epithelium squamous cell carcinoma and adenocarcinoma display similar expression patterns," *American Journal of Respiratory Cell and Molecular Biology*, vol. 24, no. 1, pp. 22–29, 2001.

[12] M. S. Ali, D. A. Hutton, J. A. Wilson, and J. P. Pearson, "Major secretory mucin expression in chronic sinusitis," *Otolaryngology*, vol. 133, no. 3, pp. 423–428, 2005.

[13] A. Dohrman, T. Tsuda, E. Escudier et al., "Distribution of lysozyme and mucin (MUC2 and MUC3) mRNA in human bronchus," *Experimental Lung Research*, vol. 20, no. 4, pp. 367–380, 1994.

[14] S. H. Bernacki, A. L. Nelson, L. Abdullah et al., "Mucin gene expression during differentiation of human airway epithelia in vitro MUC4 and MUC5b are strongly induced," *American Journal of Respiratory Cell and Molecular Biology*, vol. 20, no. 4, pp. 595–604, 1999.

[15] K.-S. Park, J. M. Wells, A. M. Zorn et al., "Transdifferentiation of ciliated cells during repair of the respiratory epithelium," *American Journal of Respiratory Cell and Molecular Biology*, vol. 34, no. 2, pp. 151–157, 2006.

[16] P. Sharma, L. Dudus, P. A. Nielsen et al., "MUC5B and MUC7 are differentially expressed in mucous and serous cells of submucosal glands in human bronchial airways," *American Journal of Respiratory Cell and Molecular Biology*, vol. 19, no. 1, pp. 30–37, 1998.

[17] Y. Chen, Y. H. Z. Yu Hua Zhao, Y.-P. Di, and R. Wu, "Characterization of human mucin 5B gene expression in airway epithelium and the genomic clone of the amino-terminal and $5'$-flanking region," *American Journal of Respiratory Cell and Molecular Biology*, vol. 25, no. 5, pp. 542–553, 2001.

Chronic Maxillary Rhinosinusitis of Dental Origin: A Systematic Review of 674 Patient Cases

Jerome R. Lechien,[1,2] **Olivier Filleul,**[1] **Pedro Costa de Araujo,**[1] **Julien W. Hsieh,**[3] **Gilbert Chantrain,**[4] **and Sven Saussez**[1,4]

[1] *Laboratory of Anatomy and Cell Biology, Faculty of Medicine, UMONS Research Institute for Health Sciences and Technology, University of Mons (UMons), Avenue du Champ de Mars 6, B7000 Mons, Belgium*
[2] *Laboratory of Phonetics, Faculty of Psychology, Research Institute for Language Sciences and Technology, University of Mons (UMons), B7000 Mons, Belgium*
[3] *Laboratory of Neurogenetics and Behavior, Rockefeller University, 1230 York Avenue, New York City, NY 10065, USA*
[4] *Department of Otorhinolaryngology, Head, and Neck Surgery, CHU Saint-Pierre, Faculty of Medicine, Université Libre de Bruxelles (ULB), B1000 Brussels, Belgium*

Correspondence should be addressed to Sven Saussez; sven.saussez@hotmail.com

Academic Editor: Charles Monroe Myer

Objectives. The aim of this systematic review is to study the causes of odontogenic chronic maxillary rhinosinusitis (CMRS), the average age of the patients, the distribution by sex, and the teeth involved. *Materials and Methods*. We performed an EMBASE-, Cochrane-, and PubMed-based review of all of the described cases of odontogenic CMRS from January 1980 to January 2013. Issues of clinical relevance, such as the primary aetiology and the teeth involved, were evaluated for each case. *Results*. From the 190 identified publications, 23 were selected for a total of 674 patients following inclusion criteria. According to these data, the main cause of odontogenic CMRS is iatrogenic, accounting for 65.7% of the cases. Apical periodontal pathologies (apical granulomas, odontogenic cysts, and apical periodontitis) follow them and account for 25.1% of the cases. The most commonly involved teeth are the first and second molars. *Conclusion*. Odontogenic CMRS is a common disease that must be suspected whenever a patient undergoing dental treatment presents unilateral maxillary chronic rhinosinusitis.

1. Introduction

Chronic rhinosinusitis (CRS) is the most frequent pathology in USA, since it affects 33.7 million people each year [1], representing nearly 14% of the American population [2]. According to various reports, a dental origin is found in 5 to 40% of cases of chronic maxillary rhinosinusitis (CMRS) [1, 3, 4]. CMRS is defined by the presence of ongoing rhinosinusal symptoms for at least 12 weeks [5, 6]. Its incidence is consistently growing and it is more frequent among women [7]. The majority of CMRS patients are between 30 and 50 years old. From an anatomic perspective, maxillary sinus are air-filled cavities situated laterally to the nasal fossae and communicate with them through an ostium which is approximately 4 millimetres in diameter and vulnerable

to occlusion during mucosal inflammation [8]. The maxillary sinus anatomical relationships involve the dental roots inferiorly, explaining the easy extension of the infectious processes from some teeth to the maxillary sinus [3, 9]. The paranasal sinuses and the whole nasal fossae are covered with a ciliated pseudostratified epithelium. The essential role of this epithelium is the secretion of respiratory mucus and its movement to the nasopharynx, ensuring elimination of sinus secretions towards the nasal fossa. Normal mucociliary clearance requires an adequate permeability of the sinus ostium as well as good secretory and ciliary functions [10]. From a pathophysiological point of view, CMRS is due to a temporary and reversible mucociliary dyskinesia [11], which could be favoured by several factors: gastroesophageal reflux disease [12], atmospheric pollution [13], smoking [14], nasosinusal polyposis [15], arterial hypertension [15], dental infections, anatomic malformations such as septal deviations, concha bullosa, allergic reactions, and immune deficits [16–20]. Odontogenic CMRS occurs when the Schneiderian membrane is irritated or perforated, as a result of a dental infection, maxillary trauma, foreign body into the sinus, maxillary bone pathology, the placing of dental implants in the maxillary bone, supernumerary teeth, periapical granuloma, inflammatory keratocyst, or dental surgery like dental extractions or orthognathic osteotomies [3, 21]. Among the CMRS induced by foreign bodies, one might distinguish between exogenous or, less frequently, endogenous foreign bodies. The most frequent types of exogenous foreign bodies are endodontic material used in dental obturation [9]; these foreign bodies can trigger an inflammatory response and an alteration of the ciliary function [22, 23]. A CMRS caused by a dental infection can take two different routes to spread the infection. It can extend into the sinus through the pulp chamber of the tooth, causing an apical periodontitis. If the "tooth height" is altered due to a chronic infection and destruction of the tooth socket, we call it a marginal periodontitis.

Once the drainage is compromised by mucosal oedema, sinus infection may start involving various microorganisms. In bacteriological studies, it is well recognised that anaerobes can be isolated in up to two-thirds of patients who have CRS, mostly in the setting of a polymicrobial infection [24]. α-hemolytic *Streptococcus* spp., microaerophilic *Streptococcus* spp., and *Staphylococcus aureus* are predominant aerobes and the predominant anaerobes are *Peptostreptococcus* spp. and *Fusobacterium* spp. [3]. There is a difference between the bacteriology of odontogenic CMRS and that of other cases; however, in clinical practice, taking an uncontaminated bacteriological sample might turn out to be difficult. In addition, fungal superinfections are frequent and increased by immunodeficiency, diabetes mellitus, sinus radiotherapy and, excessive antibiotic and corticosteroid use [10, 17, 25]. Dental amalgams may sometimes contain minerals such as zinc oxide, sulphur, lead, titanium, barium, calcium salts, and bismuth that may accelerate fungal growth [17]. Microbiological findings often reveal *Aspergillus fumigatus* and, more rarely, *Aspergillus flavus*, which may be much more aggressive [17, 25, 26]. Different theories are put forward to explain those *aspergillus* superinfections. Following a French etiologic hypothesis, an *Aspergillus* infection would also be odontogenic, requiring an oroantral fistula to allow sinus contamination. Other hypotheses favour a mixed origin or strict aerogenic contamination via heavy spore inhalation over an extended period of time [22, 27]. CMRS is clinically characterised by a variable association of symptoms including anterior or posterior, unilateral or sometimes bilateral discharge (purulent, watery, or mucoid), sinus or dental pain, nasal obstruction, hypo- or anosmia facial headaches that intensify in the evening while bending, halitosis, and occasionally coughing [17]. Even if there is no significant difference between classic and odontogenic CMR, anterior discharge, sinus pain, nagging pain of the upper teeth of the damaged side that increases during occlusion and tooth mobilisation, and halitosis seem to be more frequent in

the latter [21, 25]. Percussion of the causal tooth may reveal an abnormal sensitivity, unless endodontic filling has been performed. Most cases are unilateral, although bilateral cases have been described as well [7]. The time interval between symptoms onset and the causal dental procedure may be highly variable: according to Mehra and Murad, 41% of patients developed CMRS in the following month, 18% between one and three months after the procedure, 30% from three months to one year, and 11% of patients after more than one year [8]. Computed tomography (CT) of the sinus is essential. Some authors also recommend the Valsalva test for diagnosing an oroantral communication [10]. Most of the literature concerning odontogenic CMRS consists of either prospective or retrospective reports, and the guidelines on how to deal with the disease are often based on expert opinions.

2. Materials and Methods

2.1. Aim. The aim of this review is to define the aetiologies of odontogenic CMRS and the teeth involved.

2.2. Literature Search and Data Extraction. The literature was reviewed independently by three different authors (Jerome R. Lechien, Pedro Costa de Araujo, and Julien W. Hsieh) to minimise inclusion biases. The authors were not blinded to the study author(s), their institutions, the journal, or the results of the studies. The search for articles was done through PubMED, Cochrane Library, and EMBASE (Figure 1). It included all articles written in English, French, and other languages and published between January 1980 and January 2013. We focused only on published papers. The keywords used were "odontogenic, chronic, maxillary sinusitis, dental, cyst, foreign body, iatrogenic, and periodontitis." The initial 190 references (including case reports, retrospective and prospective studies) were manually sorted to extract all descriptions of patients meeting the diagnostic criteria of chronic maxillary rhinosinusitis proposed by the European position paper on rhinosinusitis and nasal polyps 2012 [6]. Methodologic quality was assessed by the authors to determine the validity of each study. When important data were missing in some studies, the first author (Jerome R. Lechien) tried to contact the authors to obtain the additional information. In addition, references were obtained from citations within the retrieved articles. To avoid multiple inclusions of patients, we checked for the age, gender, author, and geographic area, whenever they were available. If a patient was described in more than one publication, we used only the data reported in the larger and more recent publication. Patient demographic data, age, gender, and the teeth involved in odontogenic cases were only recorded on the basis of individual data; if it was impossible to obtain these data from the authors, they were considered missing.

2.3. Inclusion and Exclusion Criteria. The diagnosis of CMRS was based on;

(1) the presence of ongoing rhinosinusal symptoms for at least 12 weeks secondary to a clearly identified dental

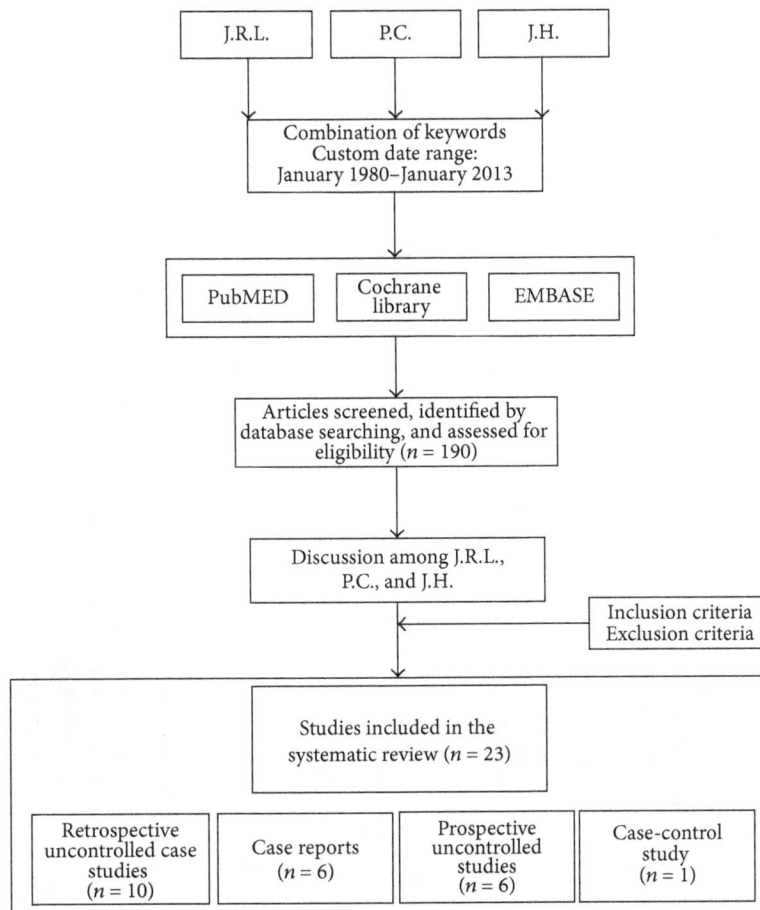

FIGURE 1: Flow chart shows the process of article selection for this study.

cause (including traumatic, iatrogenic, tumour, and dental infectious);

(2) the diagnosis of CMRS should be confirmed by computed tomography or by panoramic radiography.

Concerning periodontal infections, they were defined as clearly identified infections around the teeth that were concomitant of CMRS. Immunocompromised patients, cases of acute and subacute rhinosinusitis, and unclear causes of dental origin and cases where the type of rhinosinusitis is not clear were excluded.

3. Results

Our database search yielded 190 articles. From these, we selected 23 articles, including 6 isolated case reports, 10 retrospective uncontrolled case studies describing 389 patients, 6 prospective uncontrolled studies describing 192 patients, and one case-control study describing 91 patients [11, 15, 22, 23, 26–44]. The description of all articles and ventilation of cases is displayed in Table 1. Among the 23 papers, 18 were published in English, two in both English and Spanish, and three in French. Fifty-four percent of all patients were women, and average patient age at diagnosis was 45.6 years (ranging between 12 and 81 years). The different aetiologies

found in the literature search are summarized in Figure 2. Based on the 674 patients for whom it was displayed, iatrogenic causes were the most frequent, accounting for 65.7% of cases of described odontogenic maxillary rhinosinusitis. They included impacted tooth after dental care, artificial implants, dental amalgams in the sinus, and oroantral fistula. They were followed by apical periodontal pathologies, accounting for 25.1% of the cases. Apical periodontal pathologies include apical periodontitis (16.8%), apical granulomas (5.8%), and odontogenic cysts (2.5%). Unfortunately, the paucity of clinical descriptions limited the data of the involved teeth to only 236 cases. Nevertheless, as shown in Figure 3, the first and second molars were the most commonly affected teeth when reported, representing 35.6% and 22% of cases, respectively. They were followed by the third molar (17.4%) and the second premolar (14.4%).

4. Discussion

The aim of our study was to describe the aetiologies of odontogenic CMRS, the teeth involved, and age and sex distribution. To our knowledge, this paper is the first review studying the causes of CMRS. Further descriptions of CMRS causes were displayed in consecutive case series. In a case series of 70 patients with odontogenic CMRS, published by

TABLE 1: General characteristics of the studies. General table describing the studies characteristics (including category of evidence following the European position paper on rhinosinusitis and nasal polyps 2007 recommendations [6]) number of cases, middle age, sex, and the involved teeth. CA: category of evidence, NA: not available.

Authors	Year	Review	Language	Study design	CA	n tot	Aetiology	n	Middle age (ranged)	Sex F	Sex M	Tooth	n
Lindahl et al. [39]	1981	Acta Otolaryngol	English	Prospective case series	III	29	Marginal periodontitis	13	52	NA	NA	Canina	2
							Apical periodontitis	14	42			1st premolar	5
							Iatrogenia	2	40			2nd premolar	11
												1st molar	17
												2nd molar	10
Melen et al. [22]	1986	Acta Otolaryngol	English	Prospective case series	III	99	Iatrogenia	17	48	NA	NA	2nd Incisiva	1
							Marginal periodontitis	43				Canina	4
							Granuloma apical	39				1st premolar	11
												2nd premolar	23
												1st molar	56
												2nd molar	34
												3rd molar	9
Fligny et al. [27]	1991	Ann Oto-Laryng	French	Prospective case series	III	14	Iatrogenesis	14	42 (22–60)	NA	NA	NA	
Lin et al. [40]	1991	Ear Nose Throat J	English	Retrospective case series	III	16	Iatrogenesis	16	11–60	4	12	Canina	1
												1st premolar	5
												2nd molar	3
												3rd molar	2
Thevoz et al. [28]	2000	Schweiz Med Wochenschr	French	Retrospective case series	III	10	Iatrogenesis	10	48	NA	NA	NA	
Doud Galli et al. [29]	2001	Am J Rhinology	English	Retrospective case series	III	14	Iatrogenesis	14	(21–80)	10	4	NA	
Lopatin et al. [30]	2002	Laryngoscope	English	Retrospective case series	III	70	Iatrogenesis	60	(16–62)	NA	NA	3rd molar	26
							Odontogenic cyst	10					
Cedin et al. [31]	2005	Braz J Otorhinolaryngol	English	Retrospective case series	III	4	Iatrogenesis	4	NA	NA	NA	NA	
Nimigean et al. [32]	2006	B-ENT	English	Retrospective case series	III	125	Apical periodontitis	99	46 (12–81)	69	56	NA	
							Iatrogenesis	26					
Selmani and Ashammakhi [33]	2006	J craniofac surgery	English	Prospective case series	III	13	Iatrogenesis	13	45 (26–81)	8	5	NA	
Ugincius et al. [15]	2006	Stomatologjia	English	Retrospective case series	III	136	Iatrogenesis	136	NA	NA	NA	NA	
Macan et al. [41]	2006	Dentomaxillo-facial Radiology	English	Case Report	III	1	Iatrogenesis	1	61	1	0	NA	

TABLE 1: Continued.

Authors	Year	Review	Language	Study design	CA	n tot	Aetiology	n	Middle age (ranged)	Sex F	Sex M	Tooth	n
Srinivasa Prasad et al. [42]	2007	Indian J Dent Res	English	Case Report	III	1	Ectopic tooth	1	45	1	0	3rd molar	1
Mensi et al. [34]	2007	OOOOE	English	Case Control	IIB	91	Iatrogenesis	91	NA	NA	NA	NA	
Costa et al. [23]	2007	Oral and Maxillofacial Surgery	English	Prospective case series	III	17	Iatrogenesis Odontogenic cyst Peri-implantis	8 7 2	NA	NA	NA	NA	
Crespo del Hierro et al. [35]	2008	Acta Otorrinolaringol Esp	Spanish/English	Case Report	III	1	Odontoma	1	24	1	0	NA	
Rodrigues et al. [11]	2009	Med Oral Patol Oral Cir Bucal	English	Case Report	III	1	Iatrogenesis	1	62	0	1	NA	
Bodet Augustí et al. [36]	2009	Acta Otorrinolaringol Esp	Spanish/English	Retrospective case series	III	10	Iatrogenesis	10	NA	NA	NA	NA	
Andric et al. [37]	2010	OOOOE	English	Retrospective case series	III	14	Iatrogenesis	14	40	5	9	1st premolar 1st molar 2nd molar 3rd molar	1 6 5 2
Hajiioannou et al. [26]	2010	J Laryngol Otol	English	Prospective case series	III	4	Iatrogenesis	4	NA	NA	NA	NA	
Lechien et al. [38]	2011	Revue medicale de Bruxelles	French	Retrospective case series	III	2	Iatrogenesis	2	36	2	0	NA	
Mohan et al. [43]	2011	National Journal of Maxillofacial Surgery	English	Case report	III	1	Ectopic tooth	1	28	1	0	3rd molar	1
Khonsari et al. [44]	2011	Rev St Chir Maxillofac	English	Case report	III	1	Osteoma	1	52	1	0	NA	

Note: the incidence of oroantral communication is estimated at 0,58% of all premolar and molar extraction (ref); one can assume that the incidence of oroantral fistula is even smaller, keeping in mind that some oroantral communications were treated immediately after their creation or healed spontaneously. ref = Punwutikorn J, Waikakul A.

Aetiologies proportions

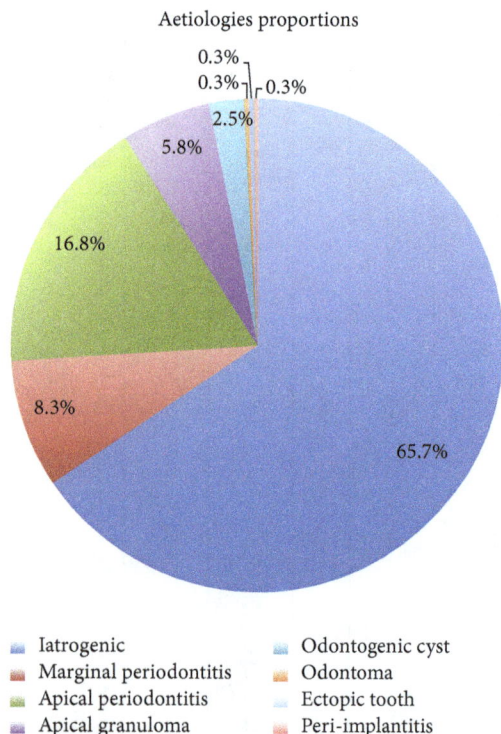

FIGURE 2: *Aetiology of odontogenic CMRS*. The main cause of odontogenic CMRS is iatrogenic and accounts for 65.7% of cases. Apical periodontal pathologies (including apical periodontitis, apical granulomas, and odontogenic cysts) and marginal periodontitis follow them and account for 25.1% and 8.3%, respectively. Peri-implantitis, ectopic tooth, and odontoma remain rare causes of odontogenic CMRS.

Lopatin et al., an exogenous foreign body from the teeth was found in 10 cases (14%), of which 7 dental amalgam fillings and 3 dental packings, and an endogenous foreign body (i.e. a tooth root) in 11 cases [30]. Thirty-nine patients (56%) also presented an oroantral fistula. Although rare, the foreign body was sometimes inserted in the sinus through trauma or accident [32]. In another case series of 125 patients suffering from odontogenic CMRS, the main aetiology was periapical chronic periodontitis (79% of patients), followed by complications of endodontic treatment (21% of cases) [32]. In addition, in two prospective studies of Melen et al. and Lindahl et al., most cases of CMRS were secondary to a dental infectious process such as marginal periodontitis and apical diseases [22, 39]. We compared the results of their studies with ours, specifically looking at aetiologies. Our results are consistent with the study of Lopatin et al., showing a majority of iatrogenic causes in comparison with infectious aetiologies. Our results in favor of the iatrogenic cause can be explained in part by the high proportion of studies reporting only a large number of iatrogenic etiology [15, 27, 29, 34, 37]. However, patient selection criteria were not described in most of the studies. Therefore, we were unable to control for selection bias, and our study may be subject to under- and overreporting bias. Finally, in a case series written by Krause et al., focusing on the foreign bodies found in any of

the sinus, 60% of all foreign bodies were found to be iatrogenic and 25% of industrial accidents [45]. The sinuses affected were mainly the maxillary (75%) and frontal sinus (18%), foreign bodies in ethmoidal or sphenoid sinus being rare. Several studies found in the literature are limited by different biases. So the size of the clinical series is often relatively small, which may allow for undetected infrequent variants, and the retrospective design of the studies included did not let us make incidence estimations. Putting these limitations aside, the larger size of the sample studied allows for a better description of the pathology than what could be made based on a single case series, something crucial for a frequently overlooked condition. Concerning the gender distribution, our data show that women (57%) were slightly more affected by odontogenic CMRS than men (43%). Most clinical series are also characterized by a ratio in favour of women [29, 32, 33]. Among the dental characteristics found in the literature, information about the teeth involved is rare. Indeed, apart from the study of Lopatin et al. who reported involvement of the third molar, only three publications accurately investigated the teeth involved. The prospective study from Melen et al. shows that the most commonly involved teeth are the first (40.6%) and second molars (24.6%) [22]. Even with a smaller sample, Andric et al. observed similar proportions in their retrospective analysis where first and second molars account for 42% and 35%, respectively [37]. Finally, Lindahl et al. reported a higher proportion of the first molar (38%), followed by the second premolar (24%) and second molar (22%) [39]. These results can easily be explained by the preferential anatomical relationships between the floor of the maxillary sinus and the various teeth concerned (premolars, first and second molars). These proportions are similar in our study. However, our work is limited by the retrospective nature of most reports, which may include selection bias in the overall description.

The diagnosis of unilateral chronic maxillary RS required systematic dental examination and sinus computed tomography (CT) [22]. CT, with reconstructions following the axial and coronal planes, classically reveals sinus filling or a chronic mucous swelling associated with a reaction to foreign body [46, 47]. Interestingly, secondary aspergillosis, which is often associated with dental foreign body and appeared as a luminal opacity, can be misinterpreted as calcified dental amalgam. Other types of sinus opacities include ectopic tooth fragments, calcified retention cysts, osteoma, condensing osteitis, calcified polyps, odontomas, osteosarcomas, cementomas, bone fibrous dysplasia, and metastases of carcinoma [10].

Odontogenic CMRS is managed by both a medical and surgical approach. The first step consists of addressing the dental pathology and the second is a functional endoscopic sinus surgery. Starting with the dental intervention allows for the elimination of the origin of the infection as well as the removal of any newly introduced foreign sinus material in the same sinus endoscopy. Usually, the stomatologist or dental practitioner repeats the endodontic treatment or proceeds to an extraction. Addressing the sinusal component with functional endoscopic sinus surgery allows for the removal of the foreign bodies with a curved aspiration or a curved forceps and opening the sinus cavities for a better drainage. Minimal

Involved teeth

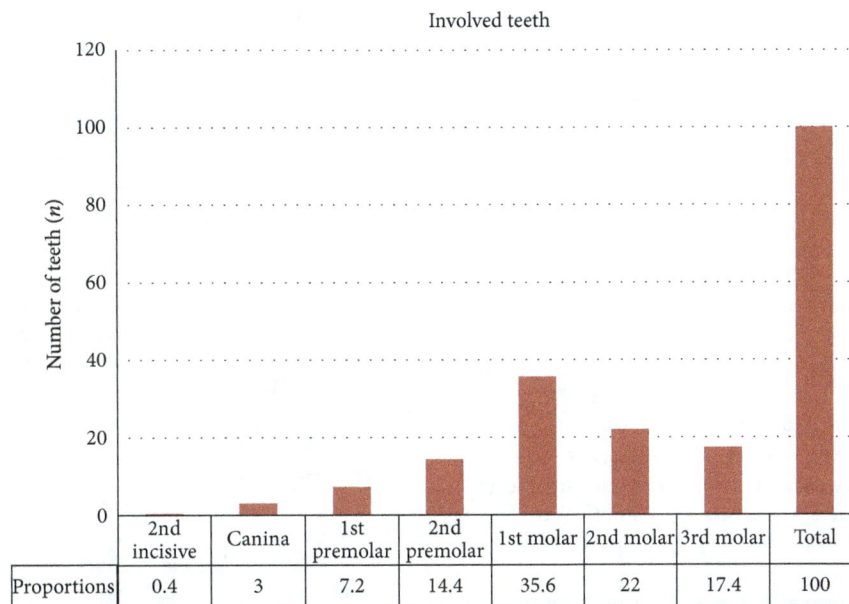

Proportions	2nd incisive	Canina	1st premolar	2nd premolar	1st molar	2nd molar	3rd molar	Total
	0.4	3	7.2	14.4	35.6	22	17.4	100

FIGURE 3: *Involved teeth.* The first and second molars were the most commonly affected teeth representing 35.6% and 22% of cases, respectively. They are followed by the third molar (17.4%), the second premolar (14.4%), and the first premolar (7.2%). The canina (3%) and the second incisiva (0.4%) remain rare and occasional.

invasive endoscopic sinus surgery [23] is safer [48], quicker [3], has less impact on the sinus mucus clearance, provokes less bleeding, and allows for a shorter hospitalisation time [49]. The endoscopic approach is also recommended to treat *Aspergillus* infections with the exception of invasive mycotic complications. Medical treatment is based on decongestants and antibiotics selected with bacterial cultures.

5. Conclusion

Odontogenic CMRS is a frequent ENT pathology. Our review summarized the current clinical knowledge about aetiologies, teeth involved, gender, and age of this clinical entity. This condition affects women slightly more than it affects men. Patients are relatively young, given the average age of 45 years. Iatrogenic cause is the most common aetiology, and thus medical and dental practitioners should keep it in mind whenever a patient presents unilateral RS after dental treatment. The first and second molars are the most affected teeth, and the diagnosis is based on a combination of nasal endoscopy and CT, which usually displays sinus filling and intraluminal opacity. Managing odontogenic CMRS requires collaboration between the ENT specialist, the dental practitioner, the stomatologist, and the radiologist. The treatment always starts with the dental treatment, and then the removal of the foreign body is achieved by endoscopic route. Even if a complete cure is achieved in most cases, clinical follow-up remains critical for this pathology.

Conflict of Interests

The authors declare that there is no conflict of interests regarding the publication of this paper.

Acknowledgments

S. Chhem and F. E. H. Sleiman (English M.D. students) are acknowledged for the collaboration in proofreading of the paper.

References

[1] B. F. Marple, J. A. Stankiewicz, F. M. Baroody et al., "Diagnosis and management of chronic rhinosinusitis in adults," *Postgraduate Medicine*, vol. 121, no. 6, pp. 121–139, 2009.

[2] L. Chee, S. M. Graham, D. G. Carothers, and Z. K. Ballas, "Immune dysfunction in refractory sinusitis in a tertiary care setting," *Laryngoscope*, vol. 111, no. 2, pp. 233–235, 2001.

[3] P. A. Clement and F. Gordts, "Epidemiology and prevalence of aspecific chronic sinusitis," *International Journal of Pediatric Otorhinolaryngology*, vol. 49, supplement 1, pp. S101–S103, 1999.

[4] I. Brook, "Sinusitis of odontogenic origin," *Otolaryngology—Head and Neck Surgery*, vol. 135, no. 3, pp. 349–355, 2006.

[5] P. Schleier, C. Bräuer, K. Küttner, A. Müller, and D. Schumann, "Video-assisted endoscopic sinus revision for treatment of chronic, unilateral odontogenic maxillary sinusitis," *Mund-, Kiefer- und Gesichtschirurgie*, vol. 7, no. 4, pp. 220–226, 2003.

[6] W. J. Fokkens, V. Lund, and J. Mullol, "EP3OS 2007: European position paper on rhinosinusitis and nasal polyps 2007. A summary for otorhinolaryngologists," *Rhinology*, vol. 50, no. 1, pp. 1–12, 2007.

[7] J. D. Osguthorpe and J. A. Hadley, "Rhinosinusitis: current concepts in evaluation and management," *Medical Clinics of North America*, vol. 83, no. 1, pp. 27–41, 1999.

[8] P. Mehra and H. Murad, "Maxillary sinus disease of odontogenic origin," *Otolaryngologic Clinics of North America*, vol. 37, no. 2, pp. 347–364, 2004.

[9] Y. Ariji, E. Ariji, K. Yoshiura, and S. Kanda, "Computed tomographic indices for maxillary sinus size in comparison

with the sinus volume," *Dentomaxillofacial Radiology*, vol. 25, no. 1, pp. 19–24, 1996.

[10] O. Arias-Irimia, C. Barona-Dorado, J. A. Santos-Marino, N. Martínez-Rodríguez, and J. M. Martínez-González, "Meta-analisis of the etiology of odontogenic maxillary sinusitis," *Medicina Oral, Patologia Oral y Cirugia Bucal*, vol. 15, no. 1, pp. e70–e73, 2010.

[11] M. T. Rodrigues, E. D. Munhoz, C. L. Cardoso, C. A. de Freitas, and J. H. Damante, "Chronic maxillary sinusitis associated with dental impression material," *Medicina Oral, Patologia Oral y Cirugia Bucal*, vol. 14, no. 4, pp. E163–E166, 2009.

[12] M. M. Al-Rawi, D. R. Edelstein, and R. A. Erlandson, "Changes in nasal epithelium in patients with severe chronic sinusitis: a clinicopathologic and electron microscopic study," *Laryngoscope*, vol. 108, no. 12, pp. 1816–1823, 1998.

[13] C. M. Tammemagi, R. M. Davis, M. S. Benninger, A. L. Holm, and R. Krajenta, "Secondhand smoke as a potential cause of chronic rhinosinusitis: a case-control study," *Archives of Otolaryngology—Head and Neck Surgery*, vol. 136, no. 4, pp. 327–334, 2010.

[14] L. Mfuna Endam, C. Cormier, Y. Bossé, A. Filali-Mouhim, and M. Desrosiers, "Association of IL1A, IL1B, and TNF gene polymorphisms with chronic rhinosinusitis with and without nasal polyposis: a replication study," *Archives of Otolaryngology—Head and Neck Surgery*, vol. 136, no. 2, pp. 187–192, 2010.

[15] P. Ugincius, R. Kubilius, A. Gervickas, and S. Vaitkus, "Chronic odontogenic maxillary sinusitis," *Stomatologija*, vol. 8, no. 2, pp. 44–48, 2006.

[16] S. J. Zinreich, D. E. Mattox, D. W. Kennedy, H. L. Chisholm, D. M. Diffley, and A. E. Rosenbaum, "Concha bullosa: CT evaluation," *Journal of Computer Assisted Tomography*, vol. 12, no. 5, pp. 778–784, 1988.

[17] R. Matjaz, P. Jernej, and K.-R. Mirela, "Sinus maxillaris mycetoma of odontogenic origin: case report," *Brazilian Dental Journal*, vol. 15, no. 3, pp. 248–250, 2004.

[18] L. J. Newman, T. A. E. Platts-Mills, C. D. Phillips, K. C. Hazen, and C. W. Gross, "Chronic sinusitis: Relationship of computed tomographic findings to allergy, asthma, and eosinophilia," *Journal of the American Medical Association*, vol. 271, no. 5, pp. 363–367, 1994.

[19] H. F. Krause, "Allergy and chronic rhinosinusitis," *Otolaryngology—Head and Neck Surgery*, vol. 128, no. 1, pp. 14–16, 2003.

[20] D. P. Kretzschmar and C. J. L. Kretzschmar, "Rhinosinusitis: Review from a dental perspective," *Oral Surgery, Oral Medicine, Oral Pathology, Oral Radiology, and Endodontics*, vol. 96, no. 2, pp. 128–135, 2003.

[21] C. Rudack, F. Sachse, and J. Alberty, "Chronic rhinosinusitis—need for further classification?" *Inflammation Research*, vol. 53, no. 3, pp. 111–117, 2004.

[22] I. Melen, L. Lindahl, L. Andreasson, and H. Rundcrantz, "Chronic maxillary sinusitis. Definition, diagnosis and relation to dental infections and nasal polyposis," *Acta Oto-Laryngologica*, vol. 101, no. 3-4, pp. 320–327, 1986.

[23] F. Costa, E. Emanuelli, M. Robiony, N. Zerman, F. Polini, and M. Politi, "Endoscopic surgical treatment of chronic maxillary sinusitis of dental origin," *Journal of Oral and Maxillofacial Surgery*, vol. 65, no. 2, pp. 223–228, 2007.

[24] I. Brook, "Microbiology of acute and chronic maxillary sinusitis associated with an odontogenic origin," *Laryngoscope*, vol. 115, no. 5, pp. 823–825, 2005.

[25] A. C. Pasqualotto, "Differences in pathogenicity and clinical syndromes due to Aspergillus fumigatus and Aspergillus flavus," *Medical Mycology*, vol. 47, supplement 1, pp. S261–S270, 2009.

[26] J. Hajiioannou, E. Koudounarakis, K. Alexopoulos, A. Kotsani, and D. E. Kyrmizakis, "Maxillary sinusitis of dental origin due to oroantral fistula, treated by endoscopic sinus surgery and primary fistula closure," *Journal of Laryngology and Otology*, vol. 124, no. 9, pp. 986–989, 2010.

[27] I. Fligny, G. Lamas, F. Rouhani, and J. Soudant, "Chronic maxillary sinusitis of dental origin and nasosinusal aspergillosis. How to manage intrasinusal foreign bodies?" *Annales d'Oto-Laryngologie et de Chirurgie Cervico-Faciale*, vol. 108, no. 8, pp. 465–468, 1991.

[28] F. Thevoz, A. Arza, and B. Jaques, "Dental foreign bodies sinusitis," *Schweizerische Medizinische Wochenschrift*, supplement 125, pp. 30S–34S, 2000.

[29] S. K. Doud Galli, R. A. Lebowitz, R. J. Giacchi, R. Glickman, and J. B. Jacobs, "Chronic sinusitis complicating sinus lift surgery," *The American Journal of Rhinology*, vol. 15, no. 3, pp. 181–186, 2001.

[30] A. S. Lopatin, S. P. Sysolyatin, P. G. Sysolyatin, and M. N. Melnikov, "Chronic maxillary sinusitis of dental origin: is external surgical approach mandatory?" *Laryngoscope*, vol. 112, no. 6, pp. 1056–1059, 2002.

[31] A. C. Cedin, F. A. De Paula Jr., E. R. Landim, F. L. P. Da Silva, L. F. De Oliveira, and A. C. Sotter, "Endoscopic treatment of the odontogenic cyst with intrasinusal extension," *Revista Brasileira de Otorrinolaringologia*, vol. 71, no. 3, pp. 392–395, 2005.

[32] V. R. Nimigean, V. Nimigean, N. Măru, D. Andressakis, D. G. Balatsouras, and V. Danielidis, "The maxillary sinus and its endodontic implications: clinical study and review," *B-ENT*, vol. 2, no. 4, pp. 167–175, 2006.

[33] Z. Selmani and N. Ashammakhi, "Surgical treatment of amalgam fillings causing iatrogenic sinusitis," *Journal of Craniofacial Surgery*, vol. 17, no. 2, pp. 363–365, 2006.

[34] M. Mensi, M. Piccioni, F. Marsili, P. Nicolai, P. L. Sapelli, and N. Latronico, "Risk of maxillary fungus ball in patients with endodontic treatment on maxillary teeth: a case-control study," *Oral Surgery, Oral Medicine, Oral Pathology, Oral Radiology and Endodontology*, vol. 103, no. 3, pp. 433–436, 2007.

[35] J. Crespo del Hierro, M. Ruiz González, M. Delgado Portela, E. García del Castillo, and J. Crespo Serrano, "Compound odontoma as a cause of chronic maxillary sinusitis," *Acta Otorrinolaringologica Espanola*, vol. 59, no. 7, pp. 359–361, 2008.

[36] E. Bodet Agustí, I. Viza Puiggrós, C. Romeu Figuerola, and V. Martinez Vecina, "Foreign bodies in maxillary sinus," *Acta Otorrinolaringologica Espanola*, vol. 60, no. 3, pp. 190–193, 2009.

[37] M. Andric, V. Saranovic, D. Drazic, B. Brkovic, and L. Todorovic, "Functional endoscopic sinus surgery as an adjunctive treatment for closure of oroantral fistulae: a retrospective analysis," *Oral Surgery, Oral Medicine, Oral Pathology, Oral Radiology and Endodontology*, vol. 109, no. 4, pp. 510–516, 2010.

[38] J. Lechien, V. Mahillon, E. Boutremans et al., "Chronic maxillary rhinosinusitis of dental origin: report of 2 cases," *Revue Medicale de Bruxelles*, vol. 32, no. 2, pp. 98–101, 2011.

[39] L. Lindahl, I. Melen, C. Ekedahl, and S. E. Holm, "Chronic maxillary sinusitis. Differential diagnosis and genesis," *Acta Oto-Laryngologica*, vol. 93, no. 1-2, pp. 147–150, 1981.

[40] P. T. Lin, R. Bukachevsky, and M. Blake, "Management of odontogenic sinusitis with persistent oro-antral fistula," *Ear, Nose and Throat Journal*, vol. 70, no. 8, pp. 488–490, 1991.

[41] D. Macan, T. Ćabov, P. Kobler, and Ž. Bumber, "Inflammatory reaction to foreign body (amalgam) in the maxillary sinus misdiagnosed as an ethmoid tumor," *Dentomaxillofacial Radiology*, vol. 35, no. 4, pp. 303–306, 2006.

[42] T. Srinivasa Prasad, G. Sujatha, T. M. Niazi, and P. Rajesh, "Dentigerous cyst associated with an ectopic third molar in the maxillary sinus: a rare entity," *Indian Journal of Dental Research*, vol. 18, no. 3, pp. 141–143, 2007.

[43] S. Mohan, H. Kankariya, B. Harjani et al., "Ectopic third molar in the maxillary sinus," *National Journal of Maxillofacial Surgery*, vol. 2, no. 2, pp. 222–224, 2011.

[44] R. H. Khonsari, P. Corre, P. Charpentier, and P. Huet, "Maxillary sinus osteoma associated with a mucocele," *Revue de Stomatologie et de Chirurgie Maxillo-Faciale*, vol. 112, no. 2, pp. 107–109, 2011.

[45] H. R. Krause, J. Rustemeyer, and R. R. Grunert, "Foreign body in paranasal sinuses," *Mund-, Kiefer- und Gesichtschirurgie*, vol. 6, no. 1, pp. 40–44, 2002.

[46] H. Lund, K. Gröndahl, and H. G. Gröndahl, "Cone beam computed tomography evaluations of marginal alveolar bone before and after orthodontic treatment combined with premolar extractions," *European Journal Oral Sciences*, vol. 120, no. 3, pp. 201–211, 2012.

[47] J. J. Cymerman, D. H. Cymerman, and R. S. O'Dwyer, "Evaluation of odontogenic maxillary sinusitis using cone-beam computed tomography: Three case reports," *Journal of Endodontics*, vol. 37, no. 10, pp. 1465–1469, 2011.

[48] X. Dufour, C. Kauffmann-Lacroix, F. Roblot et al., "Chronic invasive fungal rhinosinusitis: two new cases and review of the literature," *The American Journal of Rhinology*, vol. 18, no. 4, pp. 221–226, 2004.

[49] M. H. Dahniya, R. Makkar, E. Grexa et al., "Appearances of paranasal fungal sinusitis on computed tomography," *British Journal of Radiology*, vol. 71, pp. 340–344, 1998.

20

Changing Trends in the Management of Epistaxis

Henri Traboulsi, Elie Alam, and Usamah Hadi

Department of Otolaryngology-Head and Neck Surgery, American University of Beirut Medical Center, Phase I, 6th Floor, Room C-638, Bliss Street, P.O. Box 11-0236, Beirut, Lebanon

Correspondence should be addressed to Henri Traboulsi; henritrab@hotmail.com

Academic Editor: David W. Eisele

Epistaxis is a very common complaint seen by many types of physicians including otolaryngologists, family physicians, and others. Management of epistaxis is often challenging and requires many types of intervention. The following review describes the different types of past and current treatment modalities including cautery, nasal packing, maxillary artery ligation, anterior artery ligation, and sphenopalatine artery ligation. The paper also proposes an algorithm for managing such cases.

1. Introduction

Epistaxis is one of the commonest presenting symptoms to ENT physicians as well as to family and emergency physicians. It is thought to affect 10–12% of the population, of which 10% require medical attention [1]. Although most cases are self-limited, some do not resolve without intervention. New treatment options and approaches have developed in the past decade, especially with the advent of nasal endoscopy. The purpose of this paper is to review the different currently available treatment modalities for the management of epistaxis and to propose a comprehensive yet simple and modern algorithm for the treatment of epistaxis. The treatment options will be divided into medical, nonsurgical interventional, and surgical options and will be described along with their advantages, disadvantages, complications, and success/failures rates. The proposed algorithm will argue for an earlier role for surgical intervention with endoscopic ligation of the sphenopalatine artery (ESPAL) in view of recent literature regarding its efficacy, safety, and cost-effectiveness.

2. Medical Treatment

Topical decongestants are widely available, and their limited side effect profile makes them a convenient first-line therapy for the treatment of epistaxis. Chart reviews revealed that the use of topical oxymetazoline can be successful in treating posterior epistaxis in the emergency setting in up to 65–75%

of cases [2, 3]. They are, however, to be used with caution in hypertensive patients, especially when anxious patients with profuse epistaxis might have significantly elevated blood pressure in the acute setting. Another concern is the drug inability to reach its target areas when the nasal cavity is filled with blood.

Recently, a randomized control trial published by Zahed et al. compared the application of topical tranexamic acid (a drug used for patients with hereditary hemorrhagic telangiectasia) with the use of anterior packing for cases of anterior epistaxis presenting to the emergency department [4]. The study showed that the drug was more efficacious and resulted in more rapid discharge from the emergency department and higher satisfaction rates from patients. A more recent review, however, argued that there is insufficient evidence to date for the use of tranexamic acid in stable patients with spontaneous epistaxis [5].

3. Nonsurgical Interventions

3.1. Warm Water Irrigation. When nasal packing products came into the market, along with the advent of nasal endoscopy and endoscopic procedures, the technique of warm water irrigation fell out of favor [6]. But later, in 1999, a study by Stangerup et al. showed that warm water irrigation was more effective than nasal packing for the control of posterior epistaxis (55% success rate compared to 44%, resp.) [7]. A more recent article by Novoa and Schlegel-Wagner reports a success rate of 82% in cases of intractable posterior epistaxis with no complications [6]. The group utilize this technique as a first-line treatment for cases of posterior epistaxis. They describe the insertion of a modified bladder catheter that seals the choanae through which water at 50°C will be irrigated with the help of a caloric stimulator and will exit the catheter through a hole proximal to the inflated balloon. It is believed that the warm water causes edema of the nasal mucosa thereby compressing the bleeding vessels in addition to possibly stimulating the coagulation cascade [8].

3.2. Cautery via Anterior Rhinoscopy. Initial evaluation of a patient with epistaxis with anterior rhinoscopy might often reveal the source of the bleed if indeed this bleed is anterior.

Cautery options include chemical (with silver nitrate) and electric bipolar cautery. Since chemical cautery is less costly, easier to perform, and more readily available, it is more commonly used, especially by the non-ENT physician. The main risk of this procedure is septal perforation, which increases with bilateral cautery on opposing sides [9].

A recent chart review performed by Shargorodsky et al. reported that 77.1% of anterior epistaxis cases in their case review were treated with silver nitrate cautery with a 79% success rate on the first trial [10].

3.3. Nasal Packing. Nasal packing is often an effective and simple means of stopping nasal bleeds. The wide availability of packs, ease of use by nonspecialists, and low cost make this option a valid one as a first-line treatment.

However, nasal packing can be quite uncomfortable and may be responsible for a plethora of complications and adverse effects. Some of these can fortunately be mild and self-limited such as eustachian tube dysfunction, epiphora, and vasovagal reactions during insertion of the pack [11–17]. More importantly, nasal packing can also induce local infections of the nasal cavity and vestibule or can result in more extensive regional infections such as sinusitis and orbital cellulitis [18–21]. A nasal cavity giant pyogenic granuloma has also been described following nasal packs insertion [22]. Rarely, these infections can result in more severe and potentially lethal systemic responses such as toxic shock syndrome and infectious endocarditis [18]. The pressure effect caused by the presence of nasal packs can result in significant complications such as septal abscesses and perforations as well as necrosis of the inferior turbinates [23] and the nasal alae. Fracture of the lamina papyracea and perforation of the palate have also been described. The presence of the nasal packs has been also shown to disturb normal cardiopulmonary functions and can cause bradycardia and hypoxia [18]. Less commonly, nasal packs can be dislodged from the nasal cavity into the oropharynx resulting in a life-threatening upper airway obstruction [11, 12]. A case of cerebrospinal fluid leak was also reported following the application of a RapidRhino inflatable balloon pack [24]. These severe complications are fortunately rare, but the overall complication rate of nasal packing has been reported to be up to 69% [25].

The failure rate of nasal packing has been reported to be up to 52% [26], and the rate of rebleeding is increased to 70% in patients with bleeding disorders [27]. The traumatic insertion of nasal packs can also cause bleeding in areas different from the one responsible for the primary bleed [28]. These complications and high failure rates make the insertion of nasal packs an extremely unpleasant and often dangerous option for the control of epistaxis.

3.4. Embolizations. In an attempt to avoid complications during surgery, angiographic embolization for treating posterior epistaxis has first been described in 1974 [29]. The success of this procedure has been classically reported to be 71–95% [30]. In a recent study comprising 70 patients who underwent angiographic embolization of the sphenopalatine artery, 13% had recurring bleeds within 6 weeks of the procedure and another 14% at a later presentation [31].

The complications of this procedure have been extensively reported in the literature and include hemiplegia, ophthalmoplegia, facial paralysis/paresthesia, blindness, or other neurological deficits caused by accidental embolization of cerebral arteries [18, 32, 33]. These possible complications were shown to occur in up to 27% of cases [18, 20].

Interestingly, some authors advocate embolization of the internal maxillary artery instead of the sphenopalatine artery in children under the age of 10 [34]. Due to these relatively high failure rates and the introduction of the less risky and more successful endoscopic procedures, some advocate the use of angiographic embolization only when endoscopic procedures have failed or are contraindicated [21, 35, 36].

4. Surgical Intervention

4.1. Maxillary Artery Ligation. In 1965, Chandler and Serrins described the transantral ligation of the maxillary artery under local anesthesia [37]. This technique is classically performed through the Caldwell-Luc approach.

It has been associated with persistent pain in the upper teeth, infraorbital neuralgia, oroantral fistula, sinusitis, potential damage to sphenopalatine ganglion and vidian nerve, and, rarely, blindness [38]. Complications of this approach have been estimated to reach 28% [39].

Chandler and Serrins reported no failures in all 21 patients [37]. A more recent review of the failures of this technique was published in 1988 and reported 15 failures out of 100 patients who underwent the procedure [40]. The authors attributed these failures to the inability to properly locate the IMA and the inability to clip the branches of the internal maxillary artery to the pterygopalatine fossa.

Due to this somewhat invasive approach and potential complications, the transantral ligation of the maxillary artery technique has lost popularity, especially with the advent of the endoscopic procedures.

Ligation of the external carotid artery has also been described for refractory epistaxis; however, its failure was found to be quite high (45%) in a retrospective study conducted in 1992 [41].

4.2. Anterior Ethmoid Artery Ligation. The ligation of the anterior ethmoid artery has first been described through a Lynch incision in 1946 [42]. The advances in endoscopic procedures facilitated the development of the endoscopic ligation of this technique. In a recent study [43], a cadaveric dissection examined the feasibility of the procedure as well as the surgical anatomy of the anterior ethmoid artery, which was correctly identified in 98.5% of cases.

A study conducted in 2006 suggested the use of endoscopic anterior ethmoid artery ligation only when the artery is in a mesentery and is clearly visible (present in 20% of cases according to the study). Otherwise, the authors rather suggested an external approach [44].

The surgeon should be familiar with the anatomy of the anterior ethmoid artery and should recognize its intraorbital and ethmoid components in order to properly identify it intraoperatively and to avoid complications, such as bleeding and CSF leak [45, 46]. Interestingly, the anterior ethmoid artery has also been considered to be one of the landmarks for the cranial base [47]. Other reported complications include scarring, edema, facial ecchymosis, and damage to the medial canthal ligament [48].

4.3. Endoscopic Nasal Cautery. Cautery under endoscopic vision is another option for the control of epistaxis that may avoid the uncomfortable insertion of nasal packs in the case of an unidentified bleeder. While this can be performed in the operating room, a well-equipped clinic or emergency department can also be adequate settings for this procedure. While some authors report a very high success rate [49], others report a relatively significant risk of failure (17–33%) [21], which may be due to the fact that cauterizing the nasal mucosa may also damage an area that will bleed persistently.

Additionally, nasal cautery for epistaxis has been associated with palatal numbness [50] as well as thermal damage to neural structures, obstruction of the nasolacrimal duct, and trauma of the optic nerve, especially if the patient has previously undergone ethmoidectomy [18].

Cautery of the bleeding nasal mucosa seems to be simple and effective means of epistaxis control; however, the restricted availability of endoscopes and endoscopic surgeons in small centers limits the use of this technique.

4.4. Endoscopic Ligation of the Sphenopalatine Artery. The ESPAL was first described over 20 years ago [36]. Interrupting the blood flow in a sufficiently distal area provides an advantage over the previously described techniques by avoiding the possible revascularization from the internal maxillary artery [32].

Despite being a relatively simple procedure, the endoscopic surgeon should have a good knowledge of the technique and the anatomy of the sphenopalatine artery (SPA) as well as the possible anatomical variations in order to achieve a successful surgery. The SPA is an end branch of the internal maxillary artery and enters the nasal cavity through the sphenopalatine foramen at the posterior lateral nasal wall (Figure 1). It is anteriorly bounded by the crista ethmoidalis, an apparently flawless bony anatomical landmark during surgery [51, 52], which is often taken down to better expose the artery. When the latter or its branches are properly identified, they can be either cauterized or clipped. A study of 67 patients by Nouraei et al. concluded that diathermy is more efficacious than ligation and that not using diathermy

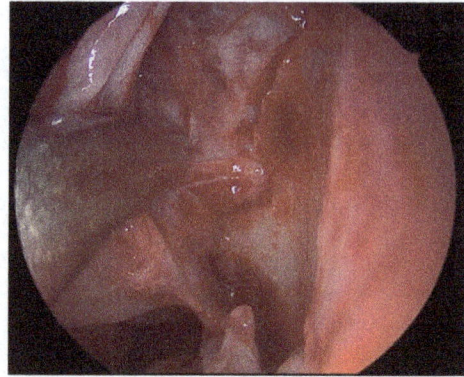

FIGURE 1: Endoscopic exposure of the left sphenopalatine artery.

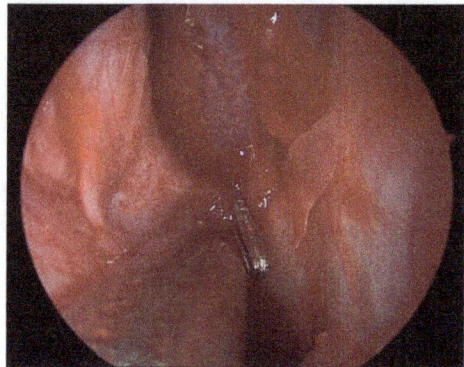

FIGURE 2: Endoscopic clipping of the left sphenopalatine artery.

was an independent risk factor for failure of the procedure [53].

The branching patterns of the SPA have been extensively studied. It may form two, three, or even four branches [54–56]. However, it appears that two branches are almost consistently present: the posterior lateral nasal artery and the nasal septal branch [54, 55]. Moreover, it seems that the location of the sphenopalatine foramen itself is also variable, for which a classification has been proposed by Wareing and Padgham [56].

If performed correctly in the hands of an experienced endoscopic surgeon, the success rate of this procedure approaches 95–100% [18, 21, 51, 57]. Other authors report a failure rate of 5–10% [39, 58] and early failures are attributed by some to the release of clips or to the failure of identification and clipping of all branches [39] (Figure 2).

The study by Nouraei et al., however, revealed a 90% efficacy rate at 5 years for SPA diathermy. It has also shown that the complication rate has not been associated with any predictive data, such as bilateral surgery, surgery for nasal polyps, or concomitant septoplasty.

A systematic review by Kumar et al. showed that ligation of the SPA and cautery were efficacious in 98% and 100%, respectively [57].

5. Discussion of the Proposed Algorithm

The traditional approach to manage patients with intractable epistaxis is to rely on surgery as a last-line treatment once

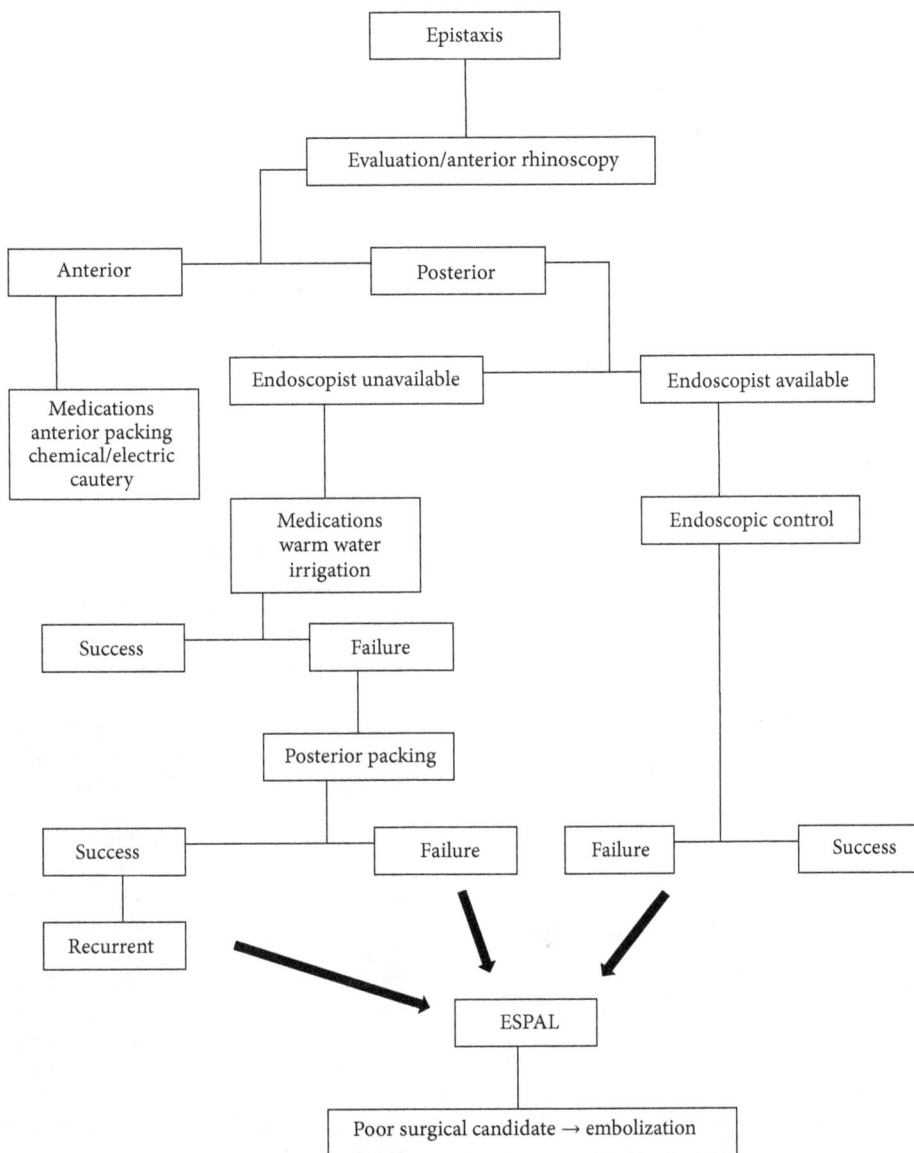

FIGURE 3: Algorithm for the management of epistaxis.

all conservative and nonsurgical treatments (such as nasal packing) have failed. The ease of use of ESPAL technique, its high success rate, and low complication rates have led some authors to propose revision of this management strategy and an earlier deployment of ESPAL. During the past decade, there has been interest in the literature in comparing the cost-effectiveness of ESPAL with other treatment strategies.

A prospective randomized trial by Moshaver et al. in 2004 compared treatment costs of ESPAL with conventional packing. Their reported calculated costs were $5,133 and $12,213, respectively [59].

Additionally, Dedhia et al. conducted a review study in 2013 to determine event probabilities while comparing current practice algorithms (initial nasal pack insertion for 3 days) and first-line ESPAL [60]. Taking into account costs of the respective procedures and the management of recurrences, the authors concluded that the traditional practice arm and first-line ESPAL cost approximately $6,450

and $8,246, respectively. Therefore, according to this study, ESPAL as a first-line treatment for epistaxis might actually be more cost-effective than traditional approaches that rely on prolonged insertion of nasal packs initially.

Similarly, a study conducted by Rudmik and Leung in 2014 compared the cost-effectiveness of ESPAL and emboliza-tion for intractable epistaxis, defined as failure of posterior nasal packing after 3 days [61]. Taking incremental cost-effectiveness ratio (ICER) as an outcome measure and a modeling-based economic evaluation using a decision tree analysis to incorporate postprocedural outcomes, the authors concluded that embolization was more costly compared to ESPAL ($22,324.70 and $12,484.14, resp.). The time horizon of the decision tree analysis was 2 weeks, and a multivariate sensitivity analysis confirmed that this economic conclusion was correct at a 74% certainty at least.

More recently, the same group published a modeling-based simulation of a 50-year-old male with intractable epistaxis [62]. The risk model took into account the probabilities of the complications of each intervention, in 6 laddered management algorithms, using posterior packing, embolization, and ESPAL, in different sequences. The severity of each complication was monetized. They found that all 6 laddered strategies would achieve 99% success rate after 2 interventions; however, ESPAL and embolization were more likely to succeed after a single procedure. Strategies starting with packing and ESPAL had the lower risk.

When combining the results of this risk analysis with data on cost-effectiveness, the authors advocated a laddered approach to intractable epistaxis starting with ESPAL first.

In addition to that, there are other advantages of ESPAL over embolization, which include a reduced risk of major complications (such as stroke and blindness), direct endoscopic visualization of the bleeding site, potential diagnosis of rare causes of bleeding such as neoplasms with the possibility of biopsy, an opportunity to perform a concurrent anterior ethmoid artery ligation if required, and a reported lower health care cost [63].

On the other hand, many patients only experience one episode of epistaxis which may never recur, while others have only mild anterior epistaxis that may only require minimal definitive intervention. It would be difficult to justify the costs and the risks of surgery for these patients.

Therefore, we suggest in our algorithm (Figure 3) treating mild cases of anterior epistaxis with traditional and conservative measures (mentioned above).

The management of posterior nasal bleeds will depend on the availability of experienced endoscopists and relevant equipment. The experienced endoscopist may be successful in treating these patients in an emergency setting, therefore avoiding the potential adverse effects of packs insertion and the potential complications and costs of surgery under general anesthesia. ESPAL can always be done after failure of this procedure.

When an endoscopist is not available, medical therapy or warm water irrigation can be attempted before posterior nasal packing. Recurrent cases, or failures of nasal packing, should be referred to an endoscopist for ESPAL. Endovascular embolization can be performed under local anesthesia and can be considered an alternative to ESPAL if patients are poor surgical candidates.

6. Conclusion

The management of epistaxis enjoys a wide range of strategies and treatment options. However, it is important to appreciate when to correctly employ the different individual interventions. It is also important to involve an experienced endoscopist when appropriate who can intervene either with endoscopic control in the emergency department or with ESPAL in the operating room. Recent literature advocates an earlier surgical intervention with ESPAL for such cases due to its simplicity, high success rate, low risks, and cost-effectiveness compared to other treatment modalities such as posterior nasal packing.

Conflict of Interests

The authors declare that there is no conflict of interests regarding the publication of this paper.

References

[1] J. G. Rockey and R. Anand, "A critical audit of the surgical management of intractable epistaxis using sphenopalatine artery ligation/diathermy," *Rhinology*, vol. 40, no. 3, pp. 147–149, 2002.

[2] G. A. Krempl and A. D. Noorily, "Use of oxymetazoline in the management of epistaxis," *Annals of Otology, Rhinology & Laryngology*, vol. 9, part 1, pp. 704–706, 1995.

[3] G. Doo and D. S. Johnson, "Oxymetazoline in the treatment of posterior epistaxis," *Hawaii Medical Journal*, vol. 58, no. 8, pp. 210–212, 1999.

[4] R. Zahed, P. Moharamzadeh, S. AlizadehArasi, A. Ghasemi, and M. Saeedi, "A new and rapid method for epistaxis treatment using injectable form of tranexamic acid topically: a randomized controlled trial," *The American Journal of Emergency Medicine*, vol. 31, no. 9, pp. 1389–1392, 2013.

[5] L. Hilton, "Best evidence topic reports. BET 3: topical intranasal tranexamic acid for spontaneous epistaxis," *Emergency Medicine Journal*, no. 5, pp. 436–437, 2014.

[6] E. Novoa and C. Schlegel-Wagner, "Hot water irrigation as treatment for intractable posterior epistaxis in an out-patient setting," *The Journal of Laryngology & Otology*, vol. 126, no. 1, pp. 58–60, 2012.

[7] S. E. Stangerup, H. Dommerby, C. Siim, L. Kemp, and J. Stage, "New modification of hot-water irrigation in the treatment of posterior epistaxis," *Archives of Otolaryngology—Head and Neck Surgery*, vol. 125, no. 6, pp. 686–690, 1999.

[8] S. E. Stangerup, H. O. Dommerby, and T. Lau, "Hot water irrigation in the treatment of posterior epistaxis," *Ugeskrift For Læger*, vol. 158, no. 27, pp. 3932–3934, 1996.

[9] F. Pond and A. Sizeland, "Epistaxis. Strategies for management," *Australian Family Physician*, vol. 29, no. 10, pp. 933–938, 2000.

[10] J. Shargorodsky, B. S. Bleier, and E. H. Holbrook, "Outcomes analysis in epistaxis management: development of a therapeutic algorithm," *Otolaryngology—Head and Neck Surgery*, vol. 149, no. 3, pp. 390–398, 2013.

[11] P. M. Middleton, "Epistaxis," *Emergency Medicine Australasia*, no. 5-6, pp. 428–440, 2004.

[12] L. E. Pope and C. G. Hobbs, "Epistaxis: an update on current management," *Postgraduate Medical Journal*, vol. 81, no. 955, pp. 309–314, 2005.

[13] A. Ahmed and T. J. Woolford, "Endoscopic bipolar diathermy in the management of epistaxis: an effective and cost-efficient treatment," *Clinical Otolaryngology and Allied Sciences*, vol. 28, no. 3, pp. 273–275, 2003.

[14] M. O'Donnell, G. Robertson, and G. W. McGarry, "A new bipolar diathermy probe for the outpatient management of adult acute epistaxis," *Clinical Otolaryngology and Allied Sciences*, vol. 24, no. 6, pp. 537–541, 1999.

[15] B. Bertrand, P. Eloy, P. Rombaux, C. Lamarque, J. B. Watelet, and S. Collet, "Guidelines to the management of epistaxis," *B-ENT*, vol. 1, supplement 1, pp. 27–43, 2005.

[16] C. J. Kucik and T. Clenney, "Management of epistaxis," *American Family Physician*, vol. 71, no. 2, pp. 305–312, 2005.

[17] V. Srinivasan, I. W. Sherman, and G. O'Sullivan, "Surgical management of intractable epistaxis: audit of results," *Journal of Laryngology and Otology*, vol. 114, no. 9, pp. 697–700, 2000.

[18] D. B. Simmen, U. Raghavan, H. R. Briner, M. Manestar, P. Groscurth, and N. S. Jones, "The anatomy of the sphenopalatine artery for the endoscopic sinus surgeon," *The American Journal of Rhinology*, vol. 20, no. 5, pp. 502–505, 2006.

[19] M. Cassano, M. Longo, E. Fiocca-Matthews, and A. M. D. Giudice, "Endoscopic intraoperative control of epistaxis in nasal surgery," *Auris Nasus Larynx*, vol. 37, no. 2, pp. 178–184, 2010.

[20] A. G. Shah, R. J. Stachler, and J. H. Krouse, "Endoscopic ligation of the sphenopalatine artery as a primary management of severe posterior epistaxis in patients with coagulopathy," *Ear, Nose & Throat Journal*, vol. 84, no. 5, pp. 296–297, 306, 2005.

[21] H. R. Schwartzbauer, M. Shete, and T. A. Tami, "Endoscopic anatomy of the sphenopalatine and posterior nasal arteries: implications for the endoscopic management of epistaxis," *American Journal of Rhinology*, vol. 17, no. 1, pp. 63–66, 2003.

[22] H.-M. Lee, S. H. Lee, and S. J. Hwang, "A giant pyogenic granuloma in the nasal cavity caused by nasal packing," *European Archives of Oto-Rhino-Laryngology*, vol. 259, no. 5, pp. 231–233, 2002.

[23] R. Moorthy, R. Anand, M. Prior, and P. M. Scott, "Inferior turbinate necrosis following endoscopic sphenopalatine artery ligation," *Otolaryngology—Head and Neck Surgery*, vol. 129, no. 1, pp. 159–160, 2003.

[24] O. Edkins, C. T. Nyamarebvu, and D. Lubbe, "Cerebrospinal fluid rhinorrhoea after nasal packing for epistaxis: case report," *The Journal of Laryngology & Otology*, vol. 126, no. 4, pp. 421–423, 2012.

[25] B. Agreda, Á. Urpegui, J. Ignacio Alfonso, and H. Valles, "Ligation of the sphenopalatine artery in posterior epistaxis. Retrospective study of 50 patients," *Acta Otorrinolaringologica Espanola*, vol. 62, no. 3, pp. 194–198, 2011.

[26] B. Schaitkin, M. Strauss, and J. R. Houck, "Epistaxis: medical versus surgical therapy: a comparison of efficacy, complications, and economic considerations," *Laryngoscope*, vol. 97, no. 12, pp. 1392–1396, 1987.

[27] A. Gallo, R. Moi, A. Minni, M. Simonelli, and M. De Vincentiis, "Otorhinolaryngology emergency unit care: the experience of a large university hospital in Italy," *Ear, Nose and Throat Journal*, vol. 79, no. 3, pp. 155–160, 2000.

[28] A. Thakar and C. J. Sharan, "Endoscopic sphenopalatine artery ligation for refractory posterior epistaxis," *Indian Journal of Otolaryngology and Head and Neck Surgery*, vol. 57, no. 3, pp. 215–218, 2005.

[29] J. Sokoloff, I. Wickbom, D. McDonald, F. Brahme, T. C. Goergen, and L. E. Goldberger, "Therapeutic percutaneous embolization in intractable epistaxis," *Radiology*, vol. 111, no. 2, pp. 285–287, 1974.

[30] J. P. Bent III and B. P. Wood, "Complications resulting from treatment of severe posterior epistaxis," *Journal of Laryngology and Otology*, vol. 113, no. 3, pp. 252–254, 1999.

[31] N. P. Christensen, D. S. Smith, S. L. Barnwell, and M. K. Wax, "Arterial embolization in the management of posterior epistaxis," *Otolaryngology—Head and Neck Surgery*, vol. 133, no. 5, pp. 748–753, 2005.

[32] R. L. Voegels, D. C. Thomé, P. P. A. Iturralde, and O. Butugan, "Endoscopic ligature of the sphenopalatine artery for severe posterior epistaxis," *Otolaryngology—Head and Neck Surgery*, vol. 124, no. 4, pp. 464–467, 2001.

[33] S. Seno, M. Arikata, H. Sakurai et al., "Endoscopic ligation of the sphenopalatine artery and the maxillary artery for the treatment of intractable posterior epistaxis," *American Journal of Rhinology and Allergy*, vol. 23, no. 2, pp. 197–199, 2009.

[34] G. C. Isaacson and J. M. Monge, "Arterial ligation for pediatric epistaxis: developmental anatomy," *The American Journal of Rhinology*, vol. 17, no. 2, pp. 75–81, 2003.

[35] D. A. Klotz, M. R. Winkle, J. Richmon, and A. S. Hengerer, "Surgical management of posterior epistaxis: a changing paradigm," *Laryngoscope*, vol. 112, no. 9, pp. 1577–1582, 2002.

[36] R. Budrovich and R. Saetti, "Microscopic and endoscopic ligature of the sphenopalatine artery," *Laryngoscope*, vol. 102, part 1, no. 12, pp. 1391–1394, 1992.

[37] J. R. Chandler and A. J. Serrins, "Transantral ligation of the internal maxillary artery for epistaxis," *Laryngoscope*, vol. 75, pp. 1151–1159, 1965.

[38] B. W. Pearson, R. G. MacKenzie, and W. S. Goodman, "The anatomical basis of transantral ligation of the maxillary artery in severe epistaxis," *The Laryngoscope*, vol. 79, no. 5, pp. 969–984, 1969.

[39] T. Kamani, S. Shaw, A. Ali, G. Manjaly, and M. Jeffree, "Sphenopalatine-sphenopalatine anastomosis: a unique cause of intractable epistaxis, safely treated with microcatheter embolization: a case report," *Journal of Medical Case Reports*, vol. 1, article 125, 2007.

[40] R. Metson and R. Lane, "Internal maxillary artery ligation for epistaxis: an analysis of failures," *Laryngoscope*, vol. 98, no. 7, pp. 760–764, 1988.

[41] P. Spafford and J. S. Durham, "Epistaxis: efficacy of arterial ligation and long-term outcome," *Journal of Otolaryngology*, vol. 21, no. 4, pp. 252–256, 1992.

[42] G. Weddell, R. G. MacBeth, H. S. Sharp, and C. A. Calvert, "The surgical treatment of severe epistaxis in relation to the ethmoidal arteries," *British Journal of Surgery*, vol. 33, no. 132, pp. 387–392, 1946.

[43] B. C. A. Filho, C. D. Pinheiro-Neto, H. F. Ramos, R. L. Voegels, and L. U. Sennes, "Endoscopic ligation of the anterior ethmoidal artery: a cadaver dissection study," *Brazilian Journal of Otorhinolaryngology*, vol. 77, no. 1, pp. 33–38, 2011.

[44] S. R. Floreani, S. B. Nair, M. C. Switajewski, and P.-J. Wormald, "Endoscopic anterior ethmoidal artery ligation: a cadaver study," *Laryngoscope*, vol. 116, no. 7, pp. 1263–1267, 2006.

[45] J. A. Kirchner, E. Yanagisawa, and E. S. Crelin Jr., "Surgical anatomy of the ethmoidal arteries. A laboratory study of 150 orbits," *Archives of Otolaryngology*, vol. 74, pp. 382–386, 1961.

[46] S. Basak, C. Z. Karaman, A. Akdilli, C. Mutlu, O. Odabasi, and G. Erpek, "Evaluation of some important anatomical variations and dangerous areas of the paranasal sinuses by CT for safer endonasal surgery," *Rhinology*, vol. 36, no. 4, pp. 162–167, 1998.

[47] W. C. Lee, P. K. M. Ku, and C. A. van Hasselt, "New guidelines for endoscopic localization of the anterior ethmoidal artery: a cadaveric study," *Laryngoscope*, vol. 110, no. 7, pp. 1173–1178, 2000.

[48] T. J. Woolford and N. S. Jones, "Endoscopic ligation of anterior ethmoidal artery in treatment of epistaxis," *The Journal of Laryngology & Otology*, vol. 114, no. 11, pp. 858–860, 2000.

[49] E. Vis and H. van den Berge, "Treatment of epistaxis without the use of nasal packing, a patient study," *Rhinology*, vol. 49, no. 5, pp. 600–604, 2011.

[50] L. Wang and D. H. Vogel, "Posterior epistaxis: comparison of treatment," *Otolaryngology—Head and Neck Surgery*, vol. 89, no. 6, pp. 1001–1006, 1981.

[51] F. G. M. Pádua and R. L. Voegels, "Severe posterior epistaxis-endoscopic surgical anatomy," *Laryngoscope*, vol. 118, no. 1, pp. 156–161, 2008.

[52] D. D. Pothier, S. MacKeith, and R. Youngs, "Sphenopalatine artery ligation: technical note," *Journal of Laryngology and Otology*, vol. 119, no. 10, pp. 810–812, 2005.

[53] S. A. Nouraei, T. Maani, D. Hajioff, H. A. Saleh, and I. S. Mackay, "Outcome of endoscopic sphenopalatine artery occlusion for intractable epistaxis: a 10-year experience," *Laryngoscope*, vol. 117, no. 8, pp. 1452–1456, 2007.

[54] H. Y. Lee, H.-U. Kim, S.-S. Kim et al., "Surgical anatomy of the sphenopalatine artery in lateral nasal wall," *Laryngoscope*, vol. 112, no. 10, pp. 1813–1818, 2002.

[55] J. M. Prades, A. Asanau, A. P. Timoshenko, M. B. Faye, and C. Martin, "Surgical anatomy of the sphenopalatine foramen and its arterial content," *Surgical and Radiologic Anatomy*, vol. 30, no. 7, pp. 583–587, 2008.

[56] M. J. Wareing and N. D. Padgham, "Osteologic classification of the sphenopalatine foramen," *Laryngoscope*, vol. 108, no. 1, part 1, pp. 125–127, 1998.

[57] S. Kumar, A. Shetty, J. Rockey, and E. Nilssen, "Contemporary surgical treatment of epistaxis. What is the evidence for sphenopalatine artery ligation?" *Clinical Otolaryngology and Allied Sciences*, vol. 28, no. 4, pp. 360–363, 2003.

[58] R. Midilli, M. Orhan, C. Y. Saylam, S. Akyildiz, S. Gode, and B. Karci, "Anatomic variations of sphenopalatine artery and minimally invasive surgical cauterization procedure," *American Journal of Rhinology and Allergy*, vol. 23, no. 6, pp. e38–e41, 2009.

[59] A. Moshaver, J. R. Harris, R. Liu, C. Diamond, and H. Seikaly, "Early operative intervention versus conventional treatment in epistaxis: randomized prospective trial," *Journal of Otolaryngology*, vol. 33, no. 3, pp. 185–188, 2004.

[60] R. C. Dedhia, S. S. Desai, K. J. Smith et al., "Cost-effectiveness of endoscopic sphenopalatine artery ligation versus nasal packing as first-line treatment for posterior epistaxis," *International Forum of Allergy & Rhinology*, vol. 3, no. 7, pp. 563–566, 2013.

[61] L. Rudmik and R. Leung, "Cost-effectiveness analysis of endoscopic sphenopalatine artery ligation vs arterial embolization for intractable epistaxis," *JAMA Otolaryngology—Head & Neck Surgery*, vol. 140, no. 9, pp. 802–808, 2014.

[62] R. M. Leung, T. L. Smith, and L. Rudmik, "Developing a laddered algorithm for the management of intractable epistaxis: a risk analysis," *JAMA Otolaryngology—Head & Neck Surgery*, vol. 141, no. 5, pp. 405–409, 2015.

[63] L. Rudmik and T. L. Smith, "Management of intractable spontaneous epistaxis," *American Journal of Rhinology*, vol. 26, no. 1, pp. 55–60, 2012.

21

More Than One Disease Process in Chronic Sinusitis Based on Mucin Fragmentation Patterns and Amino Acid Analysis

Mahmoud El-Sayed Ali[1,2] and Jeffrey P. Pearson[2]

[1]*Department of Otolaryngology, Mansoura University Hospital, Mansoura University, Mansoura 35516, Egypt*
[2]*Institute for Cell and Molecular Biosciences, Faculty of Medical Sciences, Newcastle University, Newcastle upon Tyne NE2 4HH, UK*

Correspondence should be addressed to Mahmoud El-Sayed Ali; msamomar@yahoo.co.uk

Academic Editor: Ludger Klimek

Objective. To characterise fragmentation patterns and amino acid composition of MUC2 and MUC5AC in chronic sinusitis. *Methods.* Antigenic identity of purified sinus mucins was determined by ELISA. Fragmentation patterns of a MUC5AC rich sample mucin were analysed by Sepharose CL-2B gel chromatography. Samples, divided into one MUC2 rich and one MUC5AC rich group, were subjected to sodium dodecyl sulphate-polyacrylamide gel electrophoresis (SDS-PAGE) and their amino acid contents were analysed. *Results.* Reduction, trypsin digestion, and papain digestion produced progressively smaller mucin species. On SDS-PAGE, digested MUC5AC rich mucin produced four distinct products. Amino acid analysis was characteristic of mucins with high serine, threonine, and proline contents and reduction and proteolysis increased relative proportions of these amino acids. MUC5AC rich mucins contained more protein than MUC2 rich mucins. *Conclusion.* Sinus mucin fragmentation produced mucin subunits and glycopeptide units of smaller molecular sizes which are likely to have lower viscoelastic properties. Applying this in vivo could alter mucus physical properties and biologic functions. Amino acid contents of MUC2 and MUC5AC mucins are different. This could be contributing to biological properties and functions of sinus mucins. These data suggest that there may be different pathological processes occurring at the cellular level on chronic sinusitis.

1. Introduction

Mucin production is controlled by mucin genes (MUCs). To date, 21 human mucin genes (MUCs 1, 2, 3A, 3B, 4, 5AC, 5B, 6–9, 12, 13, and 15–22) have been identified by cDNA cloning [1–4] and all, excluding MUCs 9, 11, 16, and 17, are expressed in airway mucosa [3, 4]. Several studies have shown that the major mucins expressed in chronic sinusitis (CS) are MUC2, MUC5AC, and MUC5B [5–9] and an inverse relationship was found between MUC2 and MUC5AC expression levels and this was strong in the presence of nasal polyps [6].

Mucins represent the major constituent responsible for mucus viscoelastic properties [10] which enables the mucus layer to achieve its protective function for the underlying mucosa. Mucins are highly glycosylated protein molecules of linear and flexible amino acid polymers composed of subunits joined by disulphide bonds [11–13]. Each subunit contains highly glycosylated, proteinase-resistant regions (variable number tandem repeat, VNTR) rich in serine and/or threonine amino acids alternating with sparsely or nonglycosylated (naked), proteinase-sensitive regions [14–16].

As sinus mucus is made up from multiple mucin gene products, it is important to understand the structure and composition of sinus mucins and how their distribution varies in sinus mucus. Alteration of mucus quantity and/or quality could alter mucus viscoelastic properties leading to alterations of the mucociliary clearance. From the clinical point of view, this alteration could aggravate patients' symptoms of mucus rhinorrhea and difficulty in mucus clearance with the development of other nasal, pharyngeal, and laryngeal symptoms. From the pathopharmacological point of view, altered mucus physical and/or biological properties could affect the penetration of mucus by pathogenic and/or therapeutic agents. We studied the sinus mucin fragmentation as this will help in the understanding of the physical and biological properties of sinus mucins in CS and could help to develop therapeutic modalities to alter these properties and facilitate mucus drainage and relieve relevant CS symptoms such as rhinorrhea, chronic cough, and globus pharyngeus.

2. Methods

Sinus mucus was collected from 8 patients undergoing functional endoscopic sinus surgery. Chronic sinusitis is defined as persistence of sinus symptoms (nasal obstruction, discharge, reduced sense of smell, headache, and facial pain) for more than 3 months (with topical steroids used for at least 3 months) [17, 18].

The patients' group included 5 males and 3 females, aged from 19 to 78 years with mean age of 43 years. Mucus samples were collected from the maxillary sinuses through the middle meatal antrostomy (MMA) during functional endoscopic sinus surgery (FESS). Native/polymeric mucins were isolated by 2 rounds of caesium chloride density gradient centrifugation [19] followed by extensive dialysis and freeze-drying. The antigenic identity of sinus mucins was determined by an enzyme linked immunosorbent assay (ELISA) using antibodies for MUC2, MUC5AC, and MUC5B mucins as described elsewhere [6].

2.1. Fragmentation of MUC5AC and MUC2 Mucins. Polymeric sinus mucins were fragmented by reduction with dithiothreitol (DTT) or proteolytic digestion with trypsin or papain.

2.1.1. Reduction. 2 mg of polymeric mucin was incubated with 10 mM DTT, 20 mM tris/HCl, and 6 M guanidinium chloride, pH 8, 37°C, for 5 h. Solid iodoacetamide 25 mM was then added to block the free-SH groups and the incubation continued overnight at room temperature in the dark.

2.1.2. Proteolytic Digestion. 2 mg of mucin from purified sinus mucin sample (S1) rich in MUC5AC mucin was incubated with either porcine trypsin $0.5 \mu g/mg$ of mucin in 100 mM ammonium hydrogen carbonate buffer pH 8.0 at 37°C for 24 h or papain $40 \mu g/mg$ of mucin in 0.1 M sodium phosphate buffer containing 5 mM cysteine HCl, 10 mM EDTA, pH 6.25 at 60°C for 48 h.

After extensive dialysis, polymeric and fragmented mucins were fractionated by gel filtration chromatography using a Sepharose CL-2B column (125 × 1.5 cm) and eluted by upward flow with 0.2 M NaCl and 0.02% (w/v) NaN_3 and 2 mL fractions were collected. Glycoprotein contents were measured by the periodic acid Schiff (PAS) assay. The Kav values were calculated for the glycoprotein rich peaks.

2.2. Sodium Dodecyl Sulphate-Polyacrylamide Gel Electrophoresis (SDS-PAGE). After gel chromatography, polymeric and fragmented mucins were subjected to SDS-PAGE on 4–15% gradient gels. Mucin rich peaks from gel filtration were pooled and dialysed against distilled water for 48 h and then freeze-dried and $1 \mu L$ aliquots of 5 mg/mL mucin solutions in nonreducing loading buffer were applied to the gels. After electrophoresis, gels were stained with PAS and scanned at 555 nm using a Shimadzu dual wavelength chromatoscanner. Sinus mucin samples rich in MUC5AC and MUC2 mucins were subjected to SDS-PAGE.

2.3. Amino Acid Analysis. This was performed by a modified version of the method of Carlton and Morgan [20] which allowed analysis of small amounts of mucins (~10 μg). Norvaline was used as an internal standard and Sigma amino acid mixture was used as an external standard. Samples were vapour-phase-hydrolysed in 6 M HCl for 1 h at 165°C and derivatized with 9-fluorenylmethyl chloroformate prior to analysis with reverse phase high performance liquid chromatography (HPLC) [21]. Amino acid contents were expressed as means ± standard error of the mean (S.E.M.).

3. Results

Four sinus mucin samples had MUC5AC mucin as the major mucin (S1–4) and the other four samples had MUC2 mucin as the major mucin (S5–8).

3.1. Gel Chromatography-Size Distribution of Mucins. Gel filtration was performed on MUC5AC rich sinus mucin sample (S1). The elution profiles are shown in Figure 1. Seventy-five percent of polymeric sinus mucin was excluded (Kav 0) and the remaining 25% spread into the partially included volume as a trailing edge. On reduction, sinus mucin eluted as two peaks: the first, representing 20% of the mucin, was excluded and the other 80% eluted as a partially included broad second peak (Kav 0.28). Trypsin digested mucin eluted as two included peaks. First peak made up 80% of the mucin (Kav 0.47) and the second (20%) constituted a shoulder of smaller size material (Kav 0.69). Papain digested polymeric mucin showed two included, partially separated peaks with Kav 0.57 and 0.78 accounting for 74% and 26% of loaded mucin, respectively.

3.2. SDS-PAGE. Electrophoretic patterns of polymeric and fragmented sinus mucins reflected those noted after gel chromatography. Polymeric mucin remained in the stacking gel phase whereas fragmented mucin migrated into the running gel phase to a distance dependent on its hydrodynamic size with a progressive diminishing of size from reduced to digested conditions (results not shown). Furthermore, SDS-PAGE of a polymeric MUC5AC rich mucin sample without gel chromatography showed that 76% of mucin remained at the point of application and 24% migrated from the point of application compared to 80% excluded and 20% included on gel filtration (results not shown). This indicated that SDS-PAGE can be used as an alternative method to gel chromatography to study sinus mucin fragmentation patterns.

Two sinus mucin samples, one rich in MUC5AC (S1) and one rich in MUC2 (S5) mucins, were subjected to SDS-PAGE. In the 2 samples, polymeric sinus mucins gave similar profiles, with the majority of the mucin at the point of application in the stacking gel and a small amount

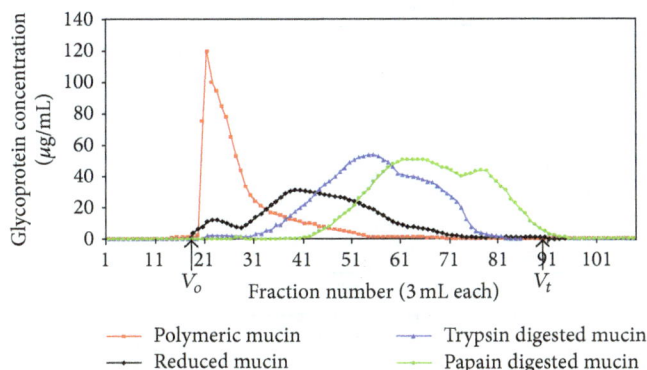

FIGURE 1: Chromatographic profile of the purified fractionated sinus mucin sample (S1). Sepharose CL-2B gel column (125 × 2.5 cm) was eluted by upward flow with 0.2 M sodium chloride containing 0.02% (w/v) sodium azide and flow rate 18 mL/h. Calibration was firstly performed using 1% (w/v) dextran blue solution containing 0.05% (w/v) methyl orange. The glycoprotein content was estimated by the PAS solution assay. V_o and V_t are the void and total volumes, respectively.

migrating to the interface between the stacking and running gels (Figures 2(a) and 2(b)). On reduction the two samples behaved differently. Twenty-four percent of PAS-staining material from MUC5AC rich mucin remained at the loading point and the rest migrated towards and into the running gel. Of this, 45% was located between the origin and the interface between the stacking and running gels and 30% spread from the interface up to 7.5 mm into the running gel (Figure 2(c)). In contrast, MUC2 rich mucin showed little evidence of any material in the running gel with 84% of PAS-staining material remaining at the origin and 16% migrating into the stacking gel (Figure 2(d)). Papain digested MUC5AC rich mucin produced four bands migrating 5.5, 8.5, 10.5, and 13.5 mm into the running gel and constituting 42%, 44%, 10%, and 4% of the total PAS-positive material, respectively (Figure 2(e)). MUC2 rich mucin produced a different profile with 42% of the glycoprotein remaining at the origin, 26% migrating into the stacking gel, and the remaining 32% forming a diffuse staining extending 10 mm in the running gel with no distinct bands (Figure 2(f)). Trypsin digested MUC5AC rich mucin produced four bands migrating into the running gel similar to those produced by papain digestion. However the distribution of staining was different as the second band was relatively smaller. The four bands made up 54%, 24%, 13%, and 9% of glycoprotein, respectively (Figure 2(g)). As papain digestion of the MUC2 rich samples did not give distinct running gel species, SDS-PAGE of trypsin digested MUC2 rich mucins was not performed.

3.3. Amino Acid Analysis of Human Sinus Mucin. Protein content of the mucins varied between 14.2% and 24.8% by weight. MUC5AC rich mucins had higher protein content than the MUC2 rich mucins, 21.1% ± 1.4% and 15.4% ± 0.8%, respectively. The general amino acid composition of sinus mucins showed the characteristic mucin analysis rich in serine, threonine, and proline. Total content of these 3 amino

acids represented 29.7% to 49.6% by weight of the protein core. MUC5AC and MUC2 rich mucins contained total serine, threonine, and proline of 43.6% ± 3.7% and 40.1% ± 3.7%, respectively, the main difference being in serine content which was 7.8 ± 0.5% in MUC5AC rich mucins compared to 16.8 ± 2.1% for the MUC2 rich mucins ($P = 0.02$, paired t-test). Threonine represented 14% ± 0.6% in MUC5AC rich mucins compared to 12.1% ± 1.5% in the MUC2 rich mucins (insignificant difference). The mean serine/threonine ratio was 3 : 5 for MUC5AC rich mucins and 7 : 5 for MUC2 rich mucins. Aspartate and valine amino acids were present in higher levels in MUC5AC rich mucins (Table 1).

Following reduction, a seventh and a fifth of the protein content were lost for the MUC5AC and MUC2 rich mucins, respectively (Table 2). The reduced mucins still contained different amounts of protein (17.9 ± 1.3% and 12.0 ± 1.0% for MUC5AC and MUC2 rich mucins, resp.). The content of serine, threonine, and proline increased on reduction to 39.0 ± 1.6% and 42.5 ± 2.6% for MUC5AC and MUC2 rich mucins, respectively. Reduction did not release protein enriched in any particular amino acids.

Proteolytic digestion of sinus mucins produced a greater loss of protein than reduction with approximately one-third of the protein content lost. Digested mucins still had different protein contents which represented 14.4 ± 1.1% in MUC5AC rich mucin and 10.0 ± 0.9% in MUC2 rich mucin. The content of serine, threonine, and proline increased in both sinus mucin groups after proteolytic digestion to account for almost half the remaining protein, 48.8 ± 1.0% and 48.8 ± 2.3% for MUC5AC and MUC2 rich mucins, respectively. There was a large loss of acidic amino acids on proteolysis, with the MUC5AC rich mucins decreasing from 20% in the polymeric mucins to 8% in the digested mucins and the MUC2 rich mucins decreasing from 15% in the polymeric mucins to 9.5% in the digested mucins (Table 3).

4. Discussion

This study does not include normal sinus mucin as a control. It would be more informative to have such a control to find out if there were differences in its antigenic identity, polymeric structure, and fragmentation behaviour compared to that in chronic sinusitis. There are ethical and technical difficulties to obtain normal sinus mucus for mucin extraction. This would entail an unnecessary invasive procedure to obtain maxillary sinus mucus from healthy sinuses. Furthermore, normal sinus mucus production is extremely small and it would not be possible to do the required biochemical analyses on such small amounts. This would then necessitate pooling different normal sinus mucus samples together to obtain adequate mucin material for these tests. This would not then allow the normal sinus mucin gene profile for each patient to be identified.

Mucins present in paranasal sinus mucus have been identified predominantly as MUC2, MUC5AC, and MUC5B [5, 6, 8, 9]. These are secretory mucins produced by surface epithelium goblet cells and submucosal glands [22, 23]. In this study, MUC5AC rich polymeric mucins were essentially

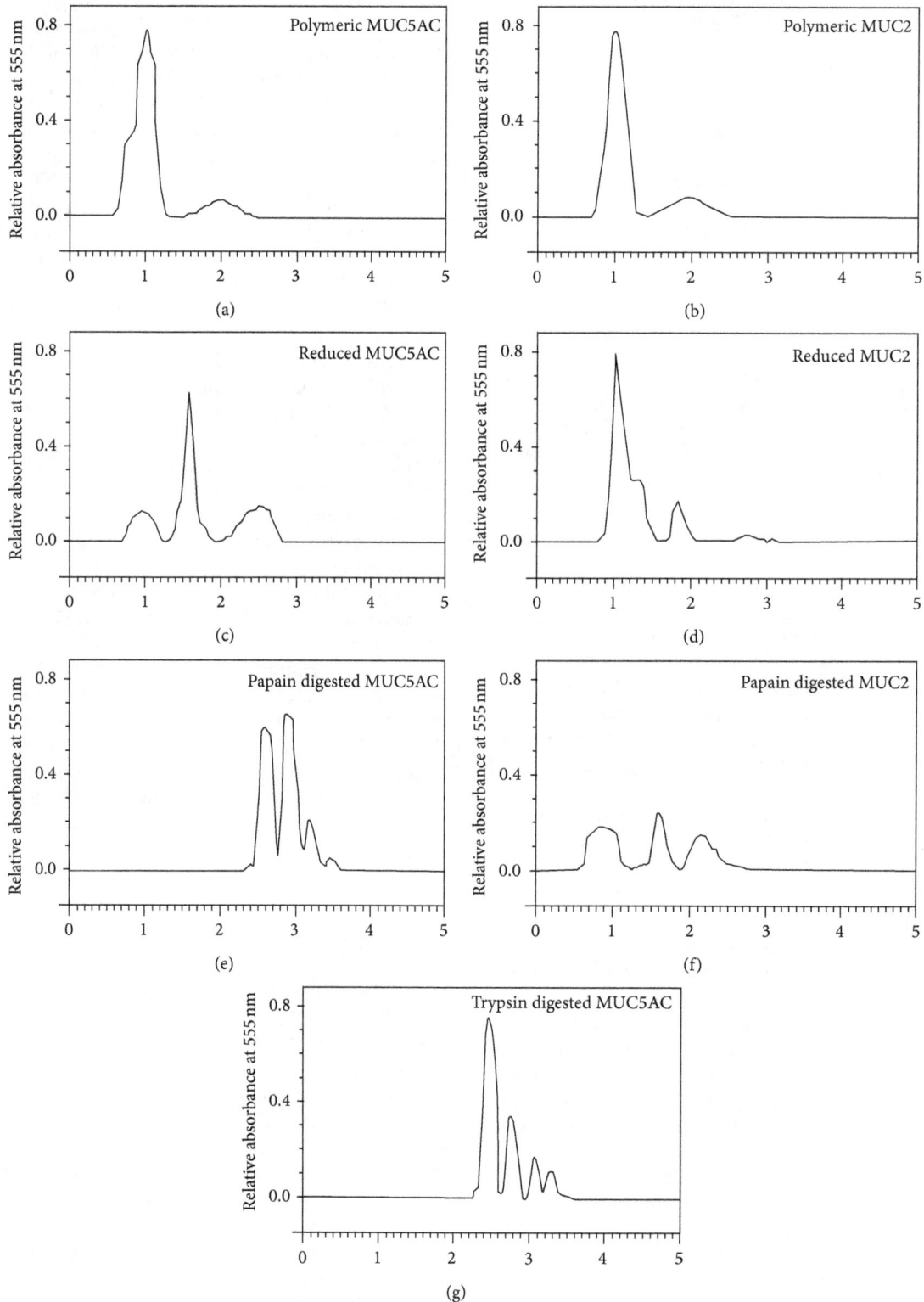

FIGURE 2: Densitometric scans of SDS-PAGE of polymeric and fragmented MUC5AC and MUC2 rich sinus mucins. The x-axis represents the localization of the different PAS-positive peaks relative to the site of application on the stacking gel (1) and the interface between the stacking and migration gel phases (2). The y-axis represents the relative absorbance of the different PAS-positive material (mucins) measured in arbitrary units. For the purpose of comparison of the different electrophoretic patterns, the presented figures were arranged as follows: ((a), (c), (e), and (g)) polymeric, reduced, papain digested, and trypsin digested MUC5AC rich mucins, respectively; ((b), (d), and (f)) polymeric, reduced, and papain digested MUC2 rich mucins, respectively.

TABLE 1: Amino acid composition of native/polymeric chronic sinusitis mucins.

Amino acid	S1	S2	S3	S4	S5	S6	S7	S8
		MUC5AC rich samples				MUC2 rich samples		
		% content of amino acids				% content of amino acids		
His	5.7 ± 0.2	9.9 ± 0.1	6.3 ± 0.7	8.5 ± 0.4	11.0 ± 1.8	1.8 ± 0.4	3.1 ± 0.1	4.1 ± 0.1
Arg	14.9 ± 1.9	16.8 ± 1.8	11.5 ± 1.4	14.6 ± 1.0	6.6 ± 0.6	13.7 ± 1.6	11.2 ± 1.7	24.5 ± 0.5
Ser	14.7 ± 0.2	18.5 ± 1.3	21.0 ± 2.1	12.2 ± 1.3	16.7 ± 2.3	35.7 ± 2.7	27.4 ± 3.5	23.7 ± 0.5
Thr	25.2 ± 0.7	33.2 ± 3.2	35.8 ± 0.8	24.6 ± 0.5	12.1 ± 0.5	25.2 ± 1.1	17.4 ± 1.8	20.1 ± 1.1
Asp	32.3 ± 0.3	19.5 ± 0.3	22.8 ± 0.2	21.3 ± 1.2	12.5 ± 1.5	11.4 ± 0.4	7.3 ± 1.0	6.2 ± 0.2
Glu	23.9 ± 0.4	19.5 ± 1.3	23.5 ± 0.4	12.8 ± 0.9	20.0 ± 1.2	15.6 ± 1.4	7.8 ± 1.2	10.3 ± 0.8
Gly	12.4 ± 0.1	7.8 ± 0.1	13.3 ± 1.2	7.2 ± 0.2	10.3 ± 0.4	3.9 ± 0.9	6.8 ± 0.4	5.3 ± 0.7
Ala	18.1 ± 0.8	23.6 ± 0.6	25.0 ± 0.9	31.0 ± 3.4	12.2 ± 1.4	22.9 ± 2.7	18.0 ± 1.2	19.1 ± 0.1
Pro	21.2. ± 2.8	26.9 ± 1.9	32.3 ± 3.1	27.9 ± 0.1	17.7 ± 0.3	23.1 ± 1.6	15.4 ± 2.3	12.8 ± 0.8
Val	9.5 ± 0.5	12.3 ± 0.3	16.5 ± 0.4	9.7 ± 0.7	7.2 ± 0.7	7.0 ± 0.8	6.6 ± 0.4	3.0 ± 1.1
Ile/Leu/Phe	16.4 ± 0.2	16.6 ± 0.7	23.8 ± 0.1	18.2 ± 0.8	15.0 ± 1.8	11.2 ± 1.3	15.6 ± 1.7	9.7 ± 2.3
Lys	13.0 ± 1.3	11.9 ± 1.8	16.5 ± 1.4	5.0 ± 1.5	11.6 ± 1.5	3.9 ± 0.2	5.8 ± 1.2	4.1 ± 0.9
Calc. ptn	207.3 ± 1.1	216.5 ± 4.5	248.3 ± 5.6	193.0 ± 3.6	152.9 ± 8.3	175.4 ± 14.3	142.2 ± 8.2	142.9 ± 4.0

The values quoted are of the % amino acid contents in polymeric mucins. The samples were arranged according to the proportions of the relevant predominant mucin. In the first 4 samples MUC5AC (S1–S4) was predominant and MUC2 was predominant in the other 4 samples (S5–S8). Amino acid content was calculated in quadruplicate samples and the mean content of amino acid in each sample was calculated. Calc. ptn: calculated total protein in ug/mg of freeze-dried mucin.

TABLE 2: Amino acid composition of reduced chronic sinusitis mucins.

Amino acid	S1	S2	S3	S4	S5	S6	S7	S8
		MUC5AC rich samples				MUC2 rich samples		
		% content of amino acids				% content of amino acids		
His	3.8 ± .0.7	1.6 ± 0.4	2.1 ± 0.1	5.5 ± 0.4	7.8 ± 0.7	2.3 ± 0.3	3.5 ± 0.1	1.5 ± 0.3
Arg	20.4 ± 1.4	13.2 ± 1.7	7.2 ± 0.5	9.7 ± 0.7	4.2 ± 0.2	9.9 ± 1.0	5.9 ± 0.4	7.3 ± 0.7
Ser	27.9 ± 0.1	12.4 ± 1.3	22.5 ± 1.5	14.3 ± 0.7	11.1 ± 1.1	27.8 ± 0.8	25.5 ± 1.6	18.6 ± 1.6
Thr	30.6 ± 0.5	25.4 ± 2.4	32.9 ± 1.2	25.8 ± 2.1	21.2 ± 0.2	19.4 ± 1.2	17.8 ± 0.8	9.4 ± 0.4
Asp	32.4 ± 0.4	19.7 ± 1.6	30.5 ± 2.2	20.6 ± 0.6	11.2 ± 0.3	7.2 ± 0.2	4.9 ± 0.4	20.2 ± 1.6
Glu	9.6 ± 1.4	9.8 ± 0.2	21.2 ± 1.2	11.1 ± 1.0	17.2 ± 0.2	8.2 ± 1.3	8.3 ± 0.3	4.5 ± 0.6
Gly	5.7 ± 1.2	6.8 ± 0.4	17.0 ± 1.3	14.5 ± 0.8	3.4 ± 0.2	6.6 ± 0.6	7.0 ± 0.2	1.0 ± 0.1
Ala	25.2 ± 1.0	22.0 ± 2.2	24.2 ± 1.1	24.2 ± 1.9	5.8 ± 0.8	14.7 ± 1.2	15.4 ± 1.5	10.7 ± 0.1
Pro	26.5 ± 2.7	27.9 ± 0.9	24.8 ± 2.2	16.1 ± 1.7	9.5 ± .0.5	24.2 ± 1.2	11.3 ± 0.2	11.4 ± 0.3
Val	4.6 ± 0.6	3.4 ± 0.6	9.1 ± 0.1	3.7 ± 0.2	2.9 ± 0.3	5.3 ± 0.3	4.6 ± 0.8	1.6 ± 0.4
Ile/Leu/Phe	14.6 ± 1.8	0.9 ± 1.5	11.0 ± 1.1	13.0 ± 1.2	6.9 ± 0.3	15.1 ± 1.3	20.8 ± 0.8	13.7 ± 1.5
Lys	5.4 ± 1.0	5.5 ± 0.4	7.6 ± 1.1	2.6 ± 0.2	8.8 ± 0.2	2.9 ± 0.5	3.6 ± 0.7	00 ± 00
Calc. ptn	206.7 ± 10.2	156.7 ± 9.9	210.0 ± 13.4	161.1 ± 3.8	110.0 ± 2.2	143.6 ± 3.7	128.0 ± 3.4	99.7 ± 7.6

The values quoted are of the % amino acid contents in reduced sinus mucins. The samples were arranged according to the proportions of the relevant predominant mucin. In the first 4 samples MUC5AC (S1–S4) was predominant and MUC2 was predominant in the other 4 samples (S5–S8). Amino acid content was calculated in quadruplicate samples and the mean content of amino acid in each sample was calculated. Calc. ptn: calculated total protein in ug/mg of freeze-dried mucin.

excluded on Sepharose CL-2B giving similar pattern to that of colonic (MUC2 rich) and gastric (MUC5AC rich) mucins [21, 24, 25]. However, the 25% partially included component could represent smaller molecular weight mucin species or possibly products of in vivo mucin fragmentation/degradation and a function of the disease process and this indicates that chronic sinusitis mucin molecules are not of a homogenous size.

Due to limited available amount of mucin which remained after other mucin analyses including mucin identity studies (ELISA), the sinus mucin sample subjected to fragmentation and analysis on gel filtration was rich in MUC5AC. Not enough mucin was available to study gel chromatographic behavior of MUC2 rich samples. However, as the SDS-PAGE distribution of MUC5AC rich polymeric and fragmented mucins mirrored the chromatographic pattern of these mucins on Sepharose 2B gel filtration, SDS-PAGE allowed the study of mucin fragmentation in small quantities of mucin samples. This finding is similar to what was reported in other studies on gastric [25] and cervical [26] and respiratory [27] mucins.

Polymeric MUC5AC and MUC2 rich mucins are of large molecular size with the majority of the sample remaining at the point of application on the polyacrylamide gel. As

TABLE 3: Amino acid composition of papain digested chronic sinusitis mucins.

Amino acid	S1	S2	S3	S4	S5	S6	S7	S8
		MUC5AC rich samples				MUC2 rich samples		
		% content of amino acids				% content of amino acids		
His	2.3 ± 0.2	7.8 ± 0.5	7.4 ± 1.5	2.4 ± 0.3	5.2 ± 1.4	0.0 ± 0.0	3.6 ± 0.1	1.1 ± 0.1
Arg	9.8 ± 0.3	8.4 ± 0.4	6.2 ± 0.7	6.6 ± 2.6	4.1 ± 0.1	7.5 ± 0.1	3.9 ± 0.4	8.3 ± 0.6
Ser	26.2 ± 0.2	32.8 ± 2.8	34.9 ± 1.9	17.2 ± 2.7	14.3 ± 2.0	30.3 ± 0.6	19.8 ± 0.1	22.6 ± 1.6
Thr	17.1 ± 0.5	19.6 ± 1.5	30.3 ± 0.5	16.9 ± 0.9	18.0 ± 0.9	20.3 ± 0.9	12.5 ± 0.5	14.1 ± 1.3
Asp	4.8 ± 0.3	2.8 ± 0.1	4.6 ± 0.6	6.6 ± 1.1	4.9 ± 0.2	3.1 ± 0.1	2.5 ± 0.4	3.1 ± 0.1
Glu	3.9 ± 0.8	3.6 ± 0.3	12.8 ± 0.2	5.6 ± 0.7	9.5 ± 0.2	3.0 ± 0.6	5.6 ± 0.9	4.4 ± 0.5
Gly	00 ± 00	0.0 ± 00	3.4 ± 1.3	0.1 ± 0.1	7.2 ± 0.1	2.2 ± 0.3	7.3 ± 0.3	4.7 ± 0.2
Ala	27.7 ± 2.5	19.6 ± 0.6	22.4 ± 1.4	18.4 ± 3.2	3.6 ± 0.3	28.4 ± 0.3	14.8 ± 1.9	10.3 ± 1.3
Pro	23.1 ± 1.1	18.2 ± 0.3	20.7 ± 1.9	24.1 ± 4.1	5.8 ± 2.0	17.5 ± 2.1	13.2 ± 0.8	8.5 ± 0.1
Val	3.1 ± 0.1	4.2 ± 0.7	4.6 ± 0.1	6.0 ± 1.0	1.9 ± 0.4	2.8 ± 0.1	1.9 ± 0.1	5.6 ± 0.2
Ile/Leu/Phe	23.00 ± 1.5	16.2 ± 1.0	17.8 ± 2.8	12.6 ± 1.0	7.1 ± 0.7	11.4 ± 1.4	4.5 ± 0.2	7.8 ± 0.9
Lys	2.8 ± 0.5	7.0 ± 0.4	6.0 ± 2.4	3.6 ± 0.9	7.4 ± 0.2	0.1 ± 0.1	1.5 ± 0.4	2.5 ± 0.2
Calc. ptn	143.8 ± 2.2	140.2 ± 2.6	171.1 ± 6.9	120.1 ± 0.5	89.0 ± 0.2	126.6 ± 3.3	91.1 ± 2.7	93.0 ± 1.0

The values quoted are of the % amino acid contents in papain digested sinus mucins. The samples were arranged according to the proportions of the relevant predominant mucin. In the first 4 samples MUC5AC (S1–S4) was predominant and MUC2 was predominant in the other 4 samples (S5–S8). Amino acid content was calculated in quadruplicate samples and the mean content of amino acid in each sample was calculated. Calc. ptn: calculated total protein in ug/mg of freeze-dried mucin.

the polymeric structure of MUC2 and MUC5AC mucin molecules is based on disulphide bridges, reduction produced a size change consistent with a subunit structure. However, MUC2 rich mucin showed little change compared to MUC5AC rich mucin. This is similar to previous finding in reduced pig colonic mucin, rich in MUC2, which was largely excluded on Sepharose Cl-2B gel chromatography [21].

Papain digestion of the MUC2 rich mucins did not produce distinct glycosylated units in the running gel whereas MUC5AC rich mucins produced four distinct species in the running gel after papain and trypsin digestion. The antigenic identity of these peaks was not determined but these could reflect different sized glycosylated domains in the MUC5AC molecule that are different in size and/or charge. It is unlikely that these bands represent MUC5B mucin as both the MUC2 and the MUC5AC rich samples contained MUC5B. Furthermore, it has also been reported that MUC5AC may be more susceptible to proteolytic degradation than MUC5B [13]. However the presence of other mucins, besides MUC5AC, that are not present in the MUC2 rich samples cannot be ruled out. These 4 bands could, provisionally, be considered as finger prints for sinus MUC5AC or MUC5AC rich sinus mucins.

The integrity of the polymeric structure is important for the gel-formation character of mucins. The polymeric structure of MUC2 and MUC5AC is based on disulphide bridges between mucin subunits and peptide bonds between mucin glycopeptides [1]. Therefore, disruption of these bonds by reduction or proteolytic digestion splits the mucin molecule polymer into subunits and glycopeptides, respectively, causing solubilisation of the mucus gel. In a pathophysiologic context, biologic agents such as bacteria could produce their pathogenic effect by altering the structure of mucin molecules in the mucus gel and lowering mucus viscosity [24, 25].

On the other hand, a therapeutic effect could be achieved by a mucolytic drug, such as N acetylcysteine, by lowering mucus viscosity [28]. Facilitating mucus clearance and/or penetration by therapeutic agents could contribute to the treatment of chronic airway infections.

Amino acid analysis of the polymeric mucins demonstrated that the two groups of mucins were rich in serine, threonine, and proline similar to reported levels of these amino acids in other well characterized polymeric mucins, that is, human gastric, cervical, respiratory, and middle ear [26, 29, 30]. There were however significant differences between the two mucin groups. MUC5AC rich mucins contained less serine than the MUC2 rich mucins. The proportion of serine/threonine ratio in MUC5AC samples was close to the reported ratio of these amino acids in MUC5AC molecule. However, this proportion was not as would be expected based on the consensus sequence for MUC2 gene and from the amino acid analysis of the insoluble glycoprotein complex from the human colon which consists of human MUC2 mucin where serine : threonine ratio was 1 : 4 [31]. Our mucins are from the sinus and not the colon and contain MUC5B and probably other mucins; that is, it is a mixed secretion and these facts could explain the lack of raised threonine relative to serine in the MUC2 rich samples.

On reduction nearly similar amounts of protein were lost in both groups which meant that the reduced mucin groups still contained different amounts of protein. This amount of protein lost on reduction has previously been shown for pig colonic mucin [21].

Digestion of human sinus mucins results in approximately one-third of the protein content being lost. The proportions of serine, threonine, and proline have increased to almost one-half of the protein core; similar increases have been demonstrated for human middle ear and gastric mucins

[30, 32] and the large loss of acidic amino acids on proteolysis is similar to what has been reported with human gastric and cervical mucins [28].

Detailed characterization of amino acid composition of sinus mucins could help identify potential amino acid sites for reduction and proteolytic activity to break down the mucin molecule and hence reduce its viscosity and facilitate its mucociliary clearance.

5. Conclusion

MUC2 and MUC5AC expressed in chronic sinusitis mucus behave differently on reduction and proteolytic digestion. Proteolytic digestion of MUC5AC rich mucins produced mucin glycopeptides which, on SDS-PAGE, produced 4 distinctive bands which could be used as finger prints for MUC5AC. These mucins have different amino acid composition which, however, is similar to the general amino acid composition profile of known mucins.

Further characterisation of sinus mucins in health and disease conditions could help in the understanding of biological importance of polymeric sinus mucin molecules and its subspecies and might help in the invention of medical treatment modalities for chronic sinusitis.

This study does not include normal sinus mucin as a control. It would be more informative to have such a control to identify the differences in its polymeric structure and fragmentation behaviour compared to that in chronic sinusitis. There are ethical and technical difficulties to obtain normal sinus mucus. Normal nasal mucus might represent an alternative for sinus mucin. However, we have found that nasal and sinus mucin expression are not similar in disease [5] and it is not known if they are similar in health.

Conflict of Interests

The authors declare that there is no conflict of interests regarding the publication of this paper.

References

[1] M. S. Ali and J. P. Pearson, "Upper airway mucin gene expression: a review," *Laryngoscope*, vol. 117, no. 5, pp. 932–938, 2007.

[2] T. Lang, G. C. Hansson, and T. Samuelsson, "Gel-forming mucins appeared early in metazoan evolution," *Proceedings of the National Academy of Sciences of the United States of America*, vol. 104, no. 41, pp. 16209–16214, 2007.

[3] M. E.-S. Ali, "Nasosinus mucin expression in normal and inflammatory conditions," *Current Opinion in Allergy and Clinical Immunology*, vol. 9, no. 1, pp. 10–15, 2009.

[4] M. Hijikata, I. Matsushita, G. Tanaka et al., "Molecular cloning of two novel mucin-like genes in the disease-susceptibility locus for diffuse panbronchiolitis," *Human Genetics*, vol. 129, no. 2, pp. 117–128, 2011.

[5] M. S. Ali, J. A. Wilson, and J. P. Pearson, "Mixed nasal mucus as a model for sinus mucin gene expression studies," *Laryngoscope*, vol. 112, no. 2, pp. 326–331, 2002.

[6] M. S. Ali, D. A. Hutton, J. A. Wilson, and J. P. Pearson, "Major secretory mucin expression in chronic sinusitis," *Otolaryngology—Head and Neck Surgery*, vol. 133, no. 3, pp. 423–428, 2005.

[7] H. Viswanathan, I. A. Brownlee, J. P. Pearson, and S. Carrie, "MUC5B secretion is up-regulated in sinusitis compared with controls," *American Journal of Rhinology*, vol. 20, no. 5, pp. 554–557, 2006.

[8] Q. D. Guo and Q. Z. Chun, "The expression of MUC5AC and MUC5B mucin genes in the mucosa of chronic rhinosinusitis and nasal polyposis," *The American Journal of Rhinology*, vol. 21, no. 3, pp. 359–366, 2007.

[9] H. Xue-Kun, L. Yuan, Y. Jin, L. Peng, and L. Hong, "Expression of MUC2 and MUC5B in ethmoid sinus mucosa of patients with chronic rhinosinusitis," *Scientific Research and Essays*, vol. 5, no. 13, pp. 1690–1696, 2010.

[10] S. Carrie, D. A. Hutton, J. P. Birchall, G. G. Green, and J. P. Pearson, "Otitis media with effusion: components which contribute to the viscous properties," *Acta Oto-Laryngologica*, vol. 112, no. 3, pp. 504–511, 1992.

[11] J. K. Sheehan, D. J. Thornton, M. Somerville, and I. Carlstedt, "Mucin structure: the structure and heterogeneity of respiratory mucus glycoproteins," *The American Review of Respiratory Disease*, vol. 144, no. 3, pp. S4–S9, 1991.

[12] D. J. Thornton, P. L. Devine, C. Hanski, M. Howard, and J. K. Sheehan, "Identification of two major populations of mucins in respiratory secretions," *American Journal of Respiratory and Critical Care Medicine*, vol. 150, no. 3, pp. 823–832, 1994.

[13] J. R. Davies, N. Svitacheva, L. Lannefors, R. Kornfält, and I. Carlstedt, "Identification of MUC5B, MUC5AC and small amounts of MUC2 mucins in cystic fibrosis airway secretions," *Biochemical Journal*, vol. 344, no. 2, pp. 321–330, 1999.

[14] J. F. Forstner and G. G. Forstner, "Gastrointestinal mucus," in *Physiology of the Gastrointestinal Tract*, L. R. Johnson, Ed., pp. 1255–1283, Raven Press, New York, NY, USA, 1994.

[15] V. Shankar, M. S. Gilmore, R. C. Elkins, and G. P. Sachdev, "A novel human airway mucin cDNA encodes a protein with unique tandem-repeat organization," *Biochemical Journal*, vol. 300, no. 2, pp. 295–298, 1994.

[16] S. J. Gendler and A. P. Spicer, "Epithelial mucin genes," *Annual Review of Physiology*, vol. 57, pp. 607–634, 1995.

[17] D. W. Kennedy, "Prognostic factors, outcomes and staging in ethmoid sinus surgery," *The Laryngoscope*, vol. 102, no. 12, pp. 1–18, 1992.

[18] V. J. Lund, H. J. Neijens, P. A. R. Clement, R. Lusk, and H. Stammberger, "The treatment of chronic sinusitis: a controversial issue," *International Journal of Pediatric Otorhinolaryngology*, vol. 32, supplement, pp. S21–S35, 1995.

[19] B. J. Starkey, D. Snary, and A. Allen, "Characterization of gastric mucoproteins isolated by equilibrium density gradient centrifugation in caesium chloride," *Biochemical Journal*, vol. 141, no. 3, pp. 633–639, 1974.

[20] J. E. Carlton and W. T. Morgan, "Simple, economical amino acid analysis based on pre-column derivatisation with 9-fluorenylmethyl chloroformate (FMOC)," in *Techniques in Protein Chemistry*, T. E. Hugli, Ed., pp. 226–270, Academic Press, New York, NY, USA, 1989.

[21] F. J. J. Fogg, D. A. Hutton, K. Jumel, J. P. Pearson, S. E. Harding, and A. Allen, "Characterization of pig colonic mucins," *Biochemical Journal*, vol. 316, no. 3, pp. 937–942, 1996.

[22] D. A. Hutton, L. Guo, J. P. Birchall, T. L. Severn, and J. P. Pearson, "MUC5B expression in middle ear mucosal glands," *Biochemical Society Transactions*, vol. 26, no. 2, article S117, 1998.

[23] J. Shinogi, T. Harada, T. Nonoyama, C. Kishioka, Y. Sakakura, and Y. Majima, "Quantitative analysis of mucin and lectin in maxillary sinus fluids in patients with acute and chrome sinusitis," *Laryngoscope*, vol. 111, no. 2, pp. 240–245, 2001.

[24] B. J. Rankin, E. D. Srivastava, C. O. Record, J. P. Pearson, and A. Allen, "Patients with ulcerative colitis have reduced mucin polymer content in the adherent colonic mucus gel," *Biochemical Society Transactions*, vol. 23, no. 1, p. 104S, 1995.

[25] J. L. Newton, N. Jordan, L. Oliver et al., "*Helicobacter pylori* in vivo causes structural changes in the adherent gastric mucus layer but barrier thickness is not compromised," *Gut*, vol. 43, no. 4, pp. 470–475, 1998.

[26] I. Carlstedt, H. Lindgren, J. K. Sheehan, U. Ulmsten, and L. Wingerup, "Isolation and characterization of human cervical-mucus glycoproteins," *Biochemical Journal*, vol. 211, no. 1, pp. 13–22, 1983.

[27] D. J. Thornton, M. Howard, N. Khan, and J. K. Sheehan, "Identification of two glycoforms of the MUC5B mucin in human respiratory mucus. Evidence for a cysteine-rich sequence repeated within the molecule," *Journal of Biological Chemistry*, vol. 272, no. 14, pp. 9561–9566, 1997.

[28] C. Marriott and I. W. Kellaway, "The effect of tetracyclines on the viscoelastic properties of bronchial mucus," *Biorheology*, vol. 12, no. 6, pp. 391–395, 1975.

[29] D. J. Thornton, I. Carlstedt, M. Howard, P. L. Devine, M. R. Price, and J. K. Sheehan, "Respiratory mucins: identification of core proteins and glycoforms," *Biochemical Journal*, vol. 316, no. 3, pp. 967–975, 1996.

[30] D. A. Hutton, F. J. J. Fogg, H. Kubba, J. P. Birchall, and J. P. Pearson, "Heterogeneity in the protein cores of mucins isolated from human middle ear effusions: evidence for expression of different mucin gene products," *Glycoconjugate Journal*, vol. 15, no. 3, pp. 283–291, 1998.

[31] A. Herrmann, J. R. Davies, G. Lindell et al., "Studies on the 'insoluble' glycoprotein complex from human colon: identification of reduction-insensitive MUC2 oligomers and C-terminal cleavage," *The Journal of Biological Chemistry*, vol. 274, no. 22, pp. 15828–15836, 1999.

[32] J. Dekker, P. H. Aelmans, and G. J. Strous, "The oligomeric structure of rat and human gastric mucins," *Biochemical Journal*, vol. 277, no. 2, pp. 423–427, 1991.

Prediction of Short-Term Outcome in Acute Superior Vestibular Nerve Failure: Three-Dimensional Video-Head-Impulse Test and Caloric Irrigation

Holger A. Rambold[1,2]

[1]Department of Neurology, County Hospitals of Altötting and Burghausen, 84503 Altötting, Germany
[2]Department of Neurology, University of Regensburg, 93053 Regensburg, Germany

Correspondence should be addressed to Holger A. Rambold; h.rambold@krk-aoe.de

Academic Editor: Leonard P. Rybak

This retrospective study examines acute unilateral vestibular failure (up to seven days after onset) with modern vestibular testing (caloric irrigation and video-head-impulse test, vHIT) in 54 patients in order to test if the short-term outcome of the patients depends on the lesion pattern defined by the two tests. Patients were grouped according to a pathological unilateral caloric weakness without a pathological vHIT: group I; additional a pathological vHIT of the lateral semicircular canal (SCC): group II; and an additional pathological vHIT of the anterior SCC: group III. Patients with involvement of the posterior SCC were less frequent and not included in the analysis. Basic parameters, such as age of the subjects, days after symptom onset, gender, side of the lesion, treatment, and dizziness handicap inventory, were not different in groups I to III. The frequency of pathological clinical findings and pathological quantified measurements increased from groups I to III. The outcome parameter "days spent in the hospital" was significantly higher in group III compared to group I. The analysis shows that differential vestibular testing predicts short-term outcome of the patients and might be in future important to treat and coach patients with vestibular failure.

1. Introduction

Acute unilateral vestibular failure (UVF) is diagnosed by an acute persistent vertigo, spontaneous nystagmus (SPN), and a unilateral vestibular hypofunction of one lateral semicircular canal (SCC) without auditory symptoms [1]. Technically the clinical diagnosis is confirmed by a unilateral pathological head-impulse test (HIT) and/or a unilateral weakness in caloric bithermal irrigation [2]. Modern vestibular techniques using the video-HIT (vHIT) could measure not only the lateral but also, selectively, the vertical (anterior and posterior) SCCs [3, 4]. In addition, the otoliths function could be measured using the cervical and ocular vestibular-evoked potentials (VEMPs) [5]. These modern tests enable us to differentiate lesion patterns, which resemble the innervations pattern of the ampullary nerves and are referred to as inferior, superior, or total vestibular failure [6]. Different lesion

pattern classifications have been proposed in recent years based on the results of vHIT and VEMPs [7, 8].

The clinical relevance of the differential vestibular testing with the vHIT is not clear so far. The long-term outcome in various studies is very heterogeneous and it is unclear which parameters might be critical for prognosis and patient management. In recent studies based on a classification of six different lesion patterns, it was shown that the one-year outcome of patients with a lesion pattern of the superior or total vestibular nerve was worse [9]. The short-term outcome of patients with a vestibular neuritis is even more unclear and the time course is scattered [2]. One study showed that an inferior vestibular neuritis had a better prognosis in the time to remission compared to superior or a complete vestibular neuritis form [10].

In previous work we observed that unilateral weakness (UW) of caloric irrigation and vHIT did measure different functions of the VOR [2, 11, 12]. Based on this concept, we retrospectively studied a group of inpatients diagnosed with UVF and analyzed the time of hospitalization and short-term outcome with respect to a classification based on the caloric irrigation and progressively more pathological SCCs identified by the three-dimensional vHIT. We will show that the short-term outcome is worse in more extended lesions of the superior vestibular nerve identified by caloric and vHIT.

2. Methods

This is a retrospective study of patients diagnosed with a first-time acute UVF in a time window of up to seven days after symptom onset [1]. Patients exhibiting a hearing loss, signs and symptoms of another peripheral vestibular or brainstem disease (e.g., Menière's disease, horizontal benign paroxysmal positioning vertigo, bilateral vestibular neuritis, and central vestibular disease), or a premedical history of repetitive vertigo were excluded from the study. Patients were included in the analysis if they had a unilateral weakness (UW) over 25% and/or a pathological vHIT. The patients were grouped according *to caloric irrigation and vHIT*: group I, an isolated UW without a pathological vHIT; group II, a unilateral pathological vHIT of the lateral SCC in addition to the pathological UW; group III, a combined pathological vHIT of the lateral and anterior SCCs in addition to the pathological UW; group IV, a pathological vHIT of the lateral and posterior and/or anterior SCC in addition to the pathological UW; and group V, a pathological vHIT of the posterior SCC only. As we found three cases in groups IV and V, they were not included in the analysis.

Patients were routinely examined at the county hospital and underwent a detailed clinical history and standard clinical neurological, oculomotor, and neurovestibular testing performed by the same experienced observer (Holger A. Rambold) [12]. Eye movements were recorded with a commercial binocular video-oculography system (Vestlab 7.1, GN Otometrics, Taastrup, Denmark) to measure the horizontal eye movements; and caloric bithermal testing was performed. UW in the caloric response was quantified according to Jongkees' formula. A value greater than or equal to 25% was pathological according to our normative data. Additionally, the directional preponderance (DP) was measured, which was normal below a value of 30% [12].

The subjective visual vertical (SVV) was measured with the "bucket method" (normative values: ±2°) [13] and the ocular torsion (OT) with a nonmydriatic fundus camera in the two eyes (Topcon TRC NW300; normative values: −2° incyclotorsion to 13.5° excyclotorsion). VEMPs were not elicited or tested in all patients and therefore not analyzed in this paper.

The vHIT (ICS Impulse, GN Otometrics, Taastrup, Denmark, http://www.icsimpulse.com/) was used to test the function of all SCCs. A pathological vHIT was defined as a combination of pathological gain values and correcting saccades for each of the six SCCs [3]. Side difference of the gain was calculated as the ratio of right to left gain difference to right/left gain sum. Additionally the dizziness

handicap inventory (DHI) in the German version was used as a subjective parameter [14].

2.1. Patients. From August 2012 until December 2014, we selected 59 patients (aged 59 ± 17 years, 34 males, 25 females) diagnosed with UVF (31 right-sided, 28 left-sided), with the first examination up to seven days after symptom onset (3.0 ± 2.2 days). Of these patients four have been published before in [12] and 23 in [11] with respect to the horizontal vHIT and caloric irrigation. In addition to the clinical examination, the testing always included a three-dimensional vHIT and a caloric bithermal irrigation, a VOG-testing (SPN in the dark in sitting position), the SVV, and a fundus photography on the same day. All patients were treated after the vestibular testing with dimenhydrinate to relieve autonomous symptoms, with oral corticoids, prednisolone, one mg/kg of body weight if necessary [15], and with physiotherapy according to a standardized protocol. Clinical details and basic measurements at first examination are shown in Table 1.

Patients were dismissed from the hospital if they were able to ambulate independently without falling during clinical gait test with eyes open on a firm floor. At the same time, they were routinely asked if they still had symptoms, such as dizziness, vertigo, unsteadiness, or oscillopsia with fast head movements or if they were symptom-free.

2.2. Statistical Design. As our data could not be described by a normal distribution we used the Kruskal-Wallis test for the group comparison of quantitative data (Table 2) and Fisher's exact test for the group comparison of qualitative data (Table 1). Linear correlation analysis of the form out(t) = intercept + slope $* t$ was performed and the correlation coefficient of determination (r^2) used. Significant difference of the slope from zero was tested by the t-test (Matlab, The Mathworks Inc., USA).

3. Results

3.1. Basic Parameters. Groups I to III were not different in the basic parameters such as age of subjects, days of admission after symptom onset (Table 2), gender, side of the lesion, and prednisolone and dimenhydrinate treatment (Tables 1(a) and 1(c)). The initial DHI was not significantly different between the three groups, but there was an increasing trend from groups I to III (Table 2). The frequency of *clinically* observed spontaneous and head shaking nystagmus (nystagmus after 20 s of horizontal head shaking with eye closed) and of pathological Romberg test increased from groups I to III (Table 1). Similarly, but with less significance, the frequency of the pathological Fukuda-Stepping test increased from groups I to III (s.Table 1(b)). A clinically observed gait disturbance was very similar in groups I to III.

3.2. Vestibular Tests. Vestibular tests coded as pathological were expressed as frequency per group and compared (Table 1(d)). The frequency of pathological SVV and OT increased from groups I to III. Quantified values of the vestibular tests are presented for the three groups in Table 2.

TABLE 1: Qualitative data.

(a) Frequency of basic parameters

| | % | % | % | p Fisher's exact | | |
	Group I	Group II	Group III	I versus II	I versus III	II versus III
Males	50	61	67	0.721	0.492	0.754
Comorbidity	50	50	13	1.000	**0.023**	**0.016**
Lesion right side	35	61	54	0.285	0.328	0.757

(b) Frequency of pathological clinical signs

| | % | % | % | p Fisher's exact | | |
	Group I	Group II	Group III	I versus II	I versus III	II versus III
HSN	43	87	100	**0.021**	**0.000**	0.167
SPN	21	65	87	**0.029**	**0.000**	0.134
Romberg test	14	33	71	0.390	**0.002**	**0.041**
Fukuda-Stepping test	54	87	95	0.096	**0.010**	0.571
Gait disturbance	64	88	91	0.198	0.084	1.000

(c) Frequency of treatment

| | % | % | % | p Fisher's exact | | |
	Group I	Group II	Group III	I versus II	I versus III	II versus III
Prednisolone	15	22	29	1.000	0.446	0.731
Dimenhydrinate	31	38	30	0.507	0.658	0.79

(d) Frequency of pathological tests

| | % | % | % | p Fisher's exact | | |
	Group I	Group II	Group III	I versus II	I versus III	II versus III
UW %	100	100	100	1.000	1.000	1.000
vHIT LC %	0	100	100	**0.000**	**0.000**	1.000
vHIT AC %	0	0	100	1.000	**0.000**	**0.000**
vHIT PC %	0	0	0	1.000	1.000	1.000
SVV %	31	75	79	**0.027**	**0.006**	1.000
OT %	10	50	77	0.087	**0.001**	0.098

(e) Frequency of symptoms at discharge

| % | % | % | p Fisher's exact | | |
Group I	Group II	Group III	I versus II	I versus III	II versus III
71	72	83	1.000	0.433	0.462

Frequency per group is given in percentage and p values of Fisher's exact probability test obtained by intergroup comparison. Significant different p values are indicated in bold numbers.
HSN: head shaking nystagmus, SPN: spontaneous nystagmus in the dark, UW: unilateral weakness of caloric irrigation, DP: directional preponderance of caloric irrigation, vHIT: video-head-impulse test, LC: lateral SCC, AC: anterior SCC, PC: posterior SCC, SVV: subjective visual vertical, OT: ocular torsion.

There was an increase in the value of the SVV, OT, and slow-phase velocity of SPN from groups I to III, with a statistical significance between groups I and III. The value of UW was increased in group III compared to groups I and II. The DP was significantly increased from groups I to III, comparable to the increase in SPN.

The vHIT gain values of the contralesional SCC were within normal limits. Ipsilesional vHIT gains of the lateral SCC were reduced in groups II and III and gains of the anterior SCC in group III, as expected. There were no differences in stimulus velocities of the vHIT to the contra- and ipsilesional side and in the three groups for the lateral

and posterior SCC. The vHIT of the anterior SCC had slightly higher stimulus velocity in group II for the ipsilesional side. Nevertheless, the obtained velocity values are within realistic clinical limits (head peak velocities during lateral SCC stimulation was 200–230°/s and during vertical SCC stimulation 123–158°/s; Table 2). Frequency of overt and covert saccades for the lateral vHIT was not different in group II versus III.

3.3. Outcome. The short-term outcome parameter, days spent in the hospital, was significantly higher in group III (6.0 ± 1.5 days) compared to group I (3.6 ± 1.5 days). Group II

TABLE 2: Quantitative data.

Variable		Group I mean ± std	Group II mean ± std	Group III mean ± std	Significant differences I versus II	I versus III	II versus III
Basic							
Age [years]		64 ± 17	63 ± 17	53 ± 16			
Days to admission		2.6 ± 2.0	3.2 ± 2.6	2.7 ± 1.9			
Days in clinic		3.6 ± 1.5	5.1 ± 3.0	6.0 ± 1.5		×	
DHI		32 ± 20	39 ± 29	50 ± 27			
Tests							
SVV [°]		0.3 ± 1.65	3.3 ± 5.2	7.1 ± 5.3		×	
OT [°]	ipsi	7.5 ± 2.9	13.2 ± 7.1	15.8 ± 7.6		×	
OT [°]	contra	6.6 ± 4.3	1.1 ± 8.8	−3.5 ± 6.2		×	
SPN [°/s]		−0.6 ± 3.5	−3.3 ± 4.2	−6.4 ± 5.7		×	
Caloric							
UW [%]		41 ± 20	48 ± 16	63 ± 25		×	
DP [%]		34 ± 39	83 ± 61	152 ± 82		×	
vHIT							
Gain LC	ipsi	0.97 ± 0.16	0.65 ± 0.29	0.36 ± 0.18	×		×
Gain LC	contra	0.96 ± 0,12	1.03 ± 0.23	0.87 ± 0.17			
Gain AC	ipsi	0.93 ± 0.15	1.02 ± 0.21	0.53 ± 0.18	×		×
Gain AC	contra	1.03 ± 0.20	0.99 ± 0.25	1.02 ± 0.20			
Gain PC	ipsi	1.05 ± 0.28	1.05 ± 0.28	1.03 ± 0.19			
Gain PC	contra	1.05 ± 0.19	1.04 ± 0.29	0.97 ± 0.25			
SD LC		0.07 ± 0.05	0.27 ± 0.05	0.47 ± 0.16		×	×
SD AC		0.08 ± 0.04	0.11 ± 0.05	0.34 ± 0.15		×	×
SD PC		0.13 ± 0.10	0.11 ± 0.09	0.16 ± 0.10			
LC Vel [°/s]	ipsi	218 ± 37	216 ± 39	232 ± 35			
LC Vel [°/s]	contra	205 ± 39	224 ± 40	218 ± 39			
AC Vel [°/s]	ipsi	129 ± 27	123 ± 27	158 ± 31			×
AC Vel [°/s]	contra	133 ± 25	137 ± 26	137 ± 29			
PC Vel [°/s]	ipsi	125 ± 26	128 ± 29	138 ± 26			
PC Vel [°/s]	contra	127 ± 26	131 ± 28	138 ± 31			

Quantified data are shown for groups I to III as mean standard deviation (std). To the right the significant differences ($p < 0.05$, Kruskal-Wallis test) of intergroup comparison are indicated by an ×.
DHI: dizziness handicap inventory, SVV: subjective visual vertical, OT: ocular torsion, SPN: slow phase velocity of the SPN in the dark, UW: unilateral weakness of caloric irrigation, DP: directional preponderance of caloric irrigation, vHIT: video-head-impulse test; LC: lateral SCC, AC: anterior SCC, PC: posterior SCC, Vel: maximal stimulus velocity applied during the vHIT, SD: side difference of the vHIT. The measurement side is given in respect to the lesion side (ipsi: ipsilesional, contra: contralesional).

(5.1 ± 3.0 days) was not different from groups I and III (Table 2). Most patients had symptoms at dismissal (75%). Frequencies of symptoms at dismissal were lower in groups I (71%) and II (72%) compared to group III (83%), but without any statistical significance (Table 1(e)). We did not find any significant linear correlation between the outcome parameter "days spent in the hospital" and the quantified parameters of vestibular function as, for example, SPN, OT, SVV, UW, and DP, indicating that those parameters do not predict the outcome in our data.

4. Discussion

Patients with different lesion patterns based on caloric irrigation and three-dimensional vHIT predict a different short-term outcome defined by the time of hospitalization.

Patients without symptoms at dismissal were statistically not different between the groups but showed a trend towards less symptoms in groups I and II compared to group III.

We are aware that our results on the short-term outcome could be influenced by different parameters, for example, the social and cultural background of the patients and the general nursing and management of the ward in our hospital, which could not be controlled. Nevertheless, in our consistent setting with standardized treatment algorithms we could show an effect of the extent of the lesion on the parameter, days the patients spend in hospital, in this retrospective analysis. This might be economically important to plan and manage patients on the ward.

4.1. Limitations. There are some limitations, as in every retrospective study. This study includes routine patient data and might have a selection bias due to the health system organization and the patients sent to our specialized vertigo clinic. In this study, we were careful that the vHIT glasses did not slip on the patient's head and that traces with artifacts as blinks were excluded. The vHIT is sensitive to the examiner. In particular the maximal stimulus velocity applied is critical. Our data shows that we reached high enough stimulation velocities around 200–230°/s horizontally and 125–158°/s vertically to be within the recommended range [3]. Indeed, higher stimulus velocities might show more pathological values, but often such velocities could not be reached in the routine examination.

4.2. Comparison to Previous Studies. In contrast to previous studies, we focused on the short-term outcome and on a group of patients with a superior vestibular nerve lesion pattern. Vestibular loss consistent with a lesion pattern of the inferior and total vestibular nerve was not included in the study due to insufficient patient numbers. In another study a very similar analysis was performed in Japan which compared the superior, inferior, and total vestibular lesion pattern in vestibular neuritis (VN) [10], showing that the latter had a longer time to remission. They showed a trend for the time of hospitalization increasing from inferior to superior to total VN, which was not significant. For the superior nerve pattern, we had slightly shorter but comparable data of hospitalization. This is in line with worse short-term and long-term outcome with increasing lesion load [8, 10].

4.3. Lesion Load. The frequency of pathological clinical signs and the increase in pathological vestibular assessments was increased from groups I to III indicating an increase in the extent of the vestibular lesion pattern as reported before [11, 12]. The gain of the vHIT of the lateral SCC decreased from groups I to III, with pathological gain values in groups II and III. Similarly we found signs of static vestibular imbalance measured as SVV and OT and of dynamic imbalance measured as SPN, HSN, or DP which increased from groups I to III, very similar to a previous publication [11, 12]. This supports an increasing lesion load from groups I to III.

If the different lesion patterns (groups I to III) resemble different etiologies or disease remains unclear. The etiology of acute vestibular failure is controversial and might be caused by a viral or vascular genesis [1]. By clinical means, we excluded all other peripheral, central, and repetitive vestibular diseases. Group I was diagnosed based on a unilateral weakness in caloric testing in the acute stage. This group is not of central origin by clinical means and actual diagnostic standards.

The difference of caloric irrigation and vHIT has been discussed in previous papers before [2, 12] and is still under debate. It is known from previous studies that pathological lateral (v)HITs were observed with a UW higher than 43% [12, 16]. This is consistent with presented data here with an average of 41% UW in group I (caloric only) and higher values in groups II (48%) and III (63%). In recent studies on Ménière's disease (MD) it was hypothesized that the dissociation of a pathological caloric and normal vHIT

might be a consequence of the physical enlargement of the membranous duct in the hydropic labyrinths [17]. According to clinical criteria we excluded patients with MD, but an isolated endolymphatic hydrops in the labyrinth could be possible.

5. Conclusion

The extent of the lesion measured by caloric irrigation and vHIT has a direct impact on time of hospitalization. Caloric only lesion and additional lesion of the lateral SCC have a better short-term outcome than similar lesions with anterior canal involvement.

Disclosure

Holger A. Rambold is beta-tester of the Otosuite vHIT system but has no financial interest in the product. He received honorary from Hennig-Arzneimittel, GN Otometrics, and Actelion.

Conflict of Interests

The author declares that there is no conflict of interests regarding the publication of this paper.

Acknowledgments

The author thanks B. Blümel and U. Goetz for technical assistance and W. Benning for copyediting the paper.

References

[1] T. Brandt, *Vertigo: Its Multisensory Syndromes*, Springer, London, UK, 2nd edition, 2003.

[2] S. Zellhuber, A. Mahringer, and H. A. Rambold, "Relation of video-head-impulse test and caloric irrigation: a study on the recovery in unilateral vestibular neuritis," *European Archives of Oto-Rhino-Laryngology*, vol. 271, no. 9, pp. 2375–2383, 2014.

[3] H. G. MacDougall, L. A. McGarvie, G. M. Halmagyi, I. S. Curthoys, and K. P. Weber, "Application of the video head impulse test to detect vertical semicircular canal dysfunction," *Otology and Neurotology*, vol. 34, no. 6, pp. 974–979, 2013.

[4] K. P. Weber, S. T. Aw, M. J. Todd, L. A. McGarvie, I. S. Curthoys, and G. M. Halmagyi, "Horizontal head impulse test detects gentamicin vestibulotoxicity," *Neurology*, vol. 72, no. 16, pp. 1417–1424, 2009.

[5] I. S. Curthoys, L. Manzari, Y. E. Smulders, and A. M. Burgess, "A review of the scientific basis and practical application of a new test of utricular function—ocular vestibular-evoked myogenic potentials to bone-conducted vibration," *Acta Otorhinolaryngologica Italica*, vol. 29, no. 4, pp. 179–186, 2009.

[6] S. T. Aw, M. Fetter, P. D. Cremer, M. Karlberg, and G. M. Halmagyi, "Individual semicircular canal function in superior and inferior vestibular neuritis," *Neurology*, vol. 57, no. 5, pp. 768–774, 2001.

[7] L. E. Walther and A. Blödow, "Ocular vestibular evoked myogenic potential to air conducted sound stimulation and video head impulse test in acute vestibular neuritis," *Otology & Neurotology*, vol. 34, no. 6, pp. 1084–1089, 2013.

[8] G. Magliulo, S. Gagliardi, M. C. Appiani, G. Iannella, and M. Re, "Vestibular neurolabyrinthitis: a follow-up study with cervical and ocular vestibular evoked myogenic potentials and the video head impulse test," *The Annals of Otology, Rhinology and Laryngology*, vol. 123, no. 3, pp. 162–173, 2014.

[9] G. Magliulo, G. Iannella, S. Gagliardi, and M. Re, "A 1-year follow-up study with C-VEMPs, O-VEMPs and video head impulse testing in vestibular neuritis," *European Archives of Oto-Rhino-Laryngology*, vol. 272, no. 11, pp. 3277–3281, 2015.

[10] Y. Chihara, S. Iwasaki, T. Murofushi et al., "Clinical characteristics of inferior vestibular neuritis," *Acta Oto-Laryngologica*, vol. 132, no. 12, pp. 1288–1294, 2012.

[11] HA. Rambold and HA. Rambold, "Economic management of vertigo/dizziness disease in a county hospital: video-head-impulse test vs. Caloric irrigation," *European Archives of Oto-Rhino-Laryngology*, vol. 272, no. 10, pp. 2621–2628, 2014.

[12] A. Mahringer and H. A. Rambold, "Caloric test and video-head-impulse: a study of vertigo/dizziness patients in a community hospital," *European Archives of Oto-Rhino-Laryngology*, vol. 271, no. 3, pp. 463–472, 2014.

[13] A. Zwergal, N. Rettinger, C. Frenzel, M. Dieterich, T. Brandt, and M. Strupp, "A bucket of static vestibular function," *Neurology*, vol. 72, no. 19, pp. 1689–1692, 2009.

[14] A. Kurre, C. J. A. W. van Gool, C. H. G. Bastiaenen, T. Gloor-Juzi, D. Straumann, and E. D. de Bruin, "Translation, cross-cultural adaptation and reliability of the German version of the dizziness handicap inventory," *Otology & Neurotology*, vol. 30, no. 3, pp. 359–367, 2009.

[15] M. Strupp, V. C. Zingler, V. Arbusow et al., "Methylprednisolone, valacyclovir, or the combination for vestibular neuritis," *The New England Journal of Medicine*, vol. 351, no. 4, pp. 354–361, 2004.

[16] N. Perez and J. Rama-Lopez, "Head-impulse and caloric tests in patients with dizziness," *Otology & Neurotology*, vol. 24, no. 6, pp. 913–917, 2003.

[17] L. A. McGarvie, I. S. Curthoys, H. G. MacDougall, and G. M. Halmagyi, "What does the dissociation between the results of video head impulse versus caloric testing reveal about the vestibular dysfunction in Ménière's disease?" *Acta Oto-Laryngologica*, vol. 135, no. 9, pp. 859–865, 2015.

Efficacy of Epley's Maneuver in Treating BPPV Patients: A Prospective Observational Study

Sushil Gaur, Sanjeev Kumar Awasthi, Sunil Kumar Singh Bhadouriya, Rohit Saxena, Vivek Kumar Pathak, and Mamta Bisht

Department of E.N.T. and Head & Neck Surgery, School of Medical Science & Research, Greater Noida 201306, India

Correspondence should be addressed to Sunil Kumar Singh Bhadouriya; drsunil7121@gmail.com

Academic Editor: Leonard P. Rybak

Vertigo and balance disorders are among the most common symptoms encountered in patients who visit ENT outpatient department. This is associated with risk of falling and is compounded in elderly persons with other neurologic deficits and chronic medical problems. BPPV is the most common cause of peripheral vertigo. BPPV is a common vestibular disorder leading to significant morbidity, psychosocial impact, and medical costs. The objective of Epley's maneuver, which is noninvasive, inexpensive, and easily administered, is to move the canaliths out of the canal to the utricle where they no longer affect the canal dynamics. Our study aims to analyze the response to Epley's maneuver in a series of patients with posterior canal BPPV and compares the results with those treated exclusively by medical management alone. Even though many studies have been conducted to prove the efficacy of this maneuver, this study reinforces the validity of Epley's maneuver by comparison with the medical management.

1. Introduction

BPPV was first described by Barany in 1921, and he attributed the disorder to otolith disease [1]. The clinical diagnosis of this disorder was not well defined until Dix and Hallpike described the classic positioning which causes a characteristic nystagmus [2]. Benign paroxysmal positioning vertigo is a disorder characterized by brief attacks of vertigo, with associated nystagmus, precipitated by certain changes in head position with respect to gravity [3]. BPPV is the most common cause of vertigo in patients seen by the otolaryngologist. The incidence is difficult to estimate because of the benign, typically self-limited course of the disease. It is thought to range from 10.7 per 100,000 to 17.3 per 100,000 population in Japan [4] and has been reported as 64 per 100,000 in a population study from Minnesota [5]. The mean age at onset is in the fourth and fifth decades, but BPPV also may occur in childhood. Overall, the incidence increases with age. Symptoms occur suddenly and last on the order of seconds but never in excess of a minute. The subjective impression of attack reported by the patient frequently is longer. In most cases of BPPV, no specific etiologic disorder can be identified. The most common known cause was closed head injury, followed by vestibular neuritis. BPPV will eventually develop in nearly 15% of patients suffering from vestibular neuritis. Other cited predisposing events include infections and certain surgical procedures, including stapedectomy and insertion of a cochlear implant [6]. Prolonged bed rest and Meniere's disease [7] also are predisposing factors. Schuknecht observed granular deposits on the cupula of the posterior semicircular canal in temporal bone specimens and proposed the "cupulolithiasis" theory to explain the pathophysiology. This theory provides a basis for understanding the disorder, although more recent work has shown that the disorder is more commonly due to free-floating particles in the semicircular canal ("canalithiasis"), rather than cupulolithiasis. The suggestion that the mechanism of BPPV could result from deflection of the posterior canal cupula by the movement of debris in the posterior canal was revisited by Hall and colleagues [8]. The posterior semicircular canal was affected in the majority of cases of BPPV (93% of cases), with 85% being unilateral and 8% affecting the PSC on both sides. The horizontal semicircular canal was affected in 5% of cases. Involvement of anterior canal is rare. The positioning examination (Dix-Hallpike test) is important for identifying BPPV. A Dix-Hallpike maneuver produces transient vertigo

TABLE 1: Age profile.

Variables	Category	Case (n = 25)		Control (n = 25)		Total (N = 50)
		n	%	n	%	n
	Mean	53 ± 15		53 ± 11		53 ± 13
Age	<40	6	24	4	16	10
	40–60	11	44	14	56	25
	>60	8	32	7	28	15

TABLE 2: Gender profile.

Variables	Category	Case (n = 25)		Control (n = 25)		Total (N = 50)	
		n	%	n	%	n	%
Gender	Female	15	60	15	60	30	60
	Male	10	40	10	40	20	40

and nystagmus and is diagnostic. The bedside Dix-Hallpike test combined with an appropriate history is key in making the diagnosis [2]. Standard electrooculography and the many videonystagmography devices do not record the torsional eye movements associated with BPPV. It was noted that the disease could be cured by a chemical labyrinthectomy and eighth nerve section. Gacek proposed transection of only the posterior ampullary nerve for relief of BPPV, confirming the posterior canal origin. In most patients, however, Epley's canalith repositioning maneuver is adequate treatment [9], and no surgery is required. First-line therapy for BPPV is organized around repositioning maneuvers. For posterior canal BPPV, the maneuver developed by Epley is particularly effective [10].

2. Materials and Method

This prospective observational study was conducted among patients attending the Department of ENT, Sharda Hospital, School of Medical Sciences and Research, Greater Noida, for a period of two years from June 2013 to June 2015. The clinical case patients above 18 years of age with posterior semicircular canal benign positional paroxysmal vertigo were included in this study. Informed written consent was taken from all the patients included in the study. The patients with cervical spondylosis, ongoing CNS disease (stroke or TIA), and cardiovascular disease and pregnant women beyond 24 weeks were excluded from this study. 50 study participants with positive positional test were divided into two groups each consisting of 25 patients. One group of 25 patients who received medical therapy with Epley's maneuver were considered as the cases and the other group of 25 patients who received only medical therapy were considered as the controls. Epley's maneuver will be repeated until symptomatic relief. The results were classified after treatment with and without the Epley maneuver into resolution of vertigo, presence of nonpositional vertigo, partial resolution, and same or worse. The maneuver begins with placement of the head into the Dix-Hallpike position, to evoke vertigo. The posterior canal on the affected side is in the earth vertical plane with the head in this position. After the initial nystagmus subsides,

a 180-degree roll of the head to the position in which the offending ear is up is performed. The patient is then brought to the sitting upright position. The maneuver is likely to be successful when nystagmus of the same direction continues to be elicited in each of the new positions. The maneuver is repeated until no nystagmus is elicited. The patients were given concomitantly both the drugs betahistine 16 mg thrice daily and cinnarizine 25 mg twice daily, till the patient had complete resolution of symptoms. We collected baseline information and clinical history and documented the procedures and treatment assigned to the study participants. We followed the patients for one year with review visit at the 1st week, 4 weeks, 3 months, 6 months, and at the end of one year. The followup process was explained to the patients and they were followed up throughout the study period. Response rate was 100%. The identification forms were separated from data collection instruments and kept under lock and key. Preprocedural and postprocedural instructions were given to all the patients who undergo Epley maneuver. The study protocol was approved by Institute Ethical Committee. Chi square test was used to test the significance of association in the observed data.

3. Results

The median age of the participants was 55 years and mean age was 53 years with standard deviation of 13 years. Table 1 compares the age profile of study and control group. The age distribution of patients was comparable between the two groups with no significance in age distribution between the two groups ($p = 0.500$), implying that there is no age related factors in the incidence of adverse events.

Among all participants, 30 participants (60%) were female. Gender ratio was comparable between two groups of patients with no significant difference (Table 2).

The cases and controls were studied for the associated symptoms which may be variable factor among the two groups influencing the results. 19 (38%) patients had associated symptoms of nausea and vomiting. The incidence of the associated symptoms was comparable among the two groups (Table 3).

TABLE 3: Associated symptoms.

Variables	Category	Case (n = 25)		Control (n = 25)		Total (N = 50)	
		n	%	n	%	n	%
Associated symptoms	Tinnitus	1	4	2	8	3	6
	Nausea and vomiting	11	44	8	32	19	38
	Nausea, vomiting, and tinnitus	1	4	0	0	1	2

TABLE 4: Presence of associated clinical illnesses.

Variables	Category	Case (n = 25)		Control (n = 25)		Total (N = 50)	
		n	%	n	%	n	%
Systemic diseases	Diabetes	12	48	6	24	18	36
	Hypertension	12	48	6	24	18	36
	CAD and others	3	12	3	12	6	12

TABLE 5: Dose response relationship between Epley's maneuver and controls among BPPV patients.

Level	Followup	Cases	Control	Total	Odds of Exp.	OR	Mantel-Haenszel chi square for linear trend	p value
1st course		18	3	21	6	1		
2nd course	1st	5	10	15	0.5	0.08		
3rd course	2nd	1	6	7	0.17	0.03	16.82	0.00004115
4th course	3rd	1	6	7	0.17	0.03		
Total		25	25	50				

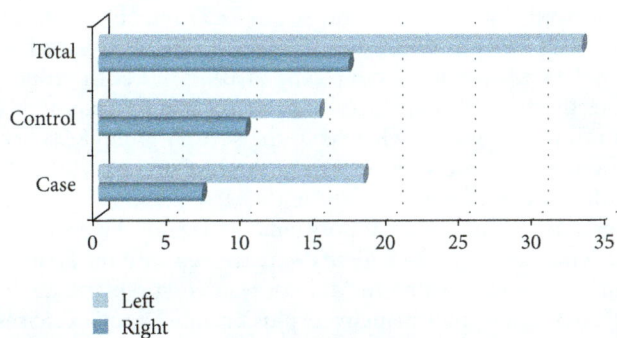

FIGURE 1: Side of BPPV.

Hypertension and diabetes were found among 18 (36%) participants (Table 4). This variable may influence the results of the observation of study.

The side of BPPV between the cases and controls was compared. 28% of cases and 40% of controls had right-sided and 72% of cases and 60% of controls had left-sided BPPV (Figure 1).

Among 25 case patients, 18 (72%) recovered from vertigo immediately after the Epley maneuver and 23 (92%) patients recovered from vertigo at first week of followup. The remaining 2 case patients recovered from vertigo during the second and third follow-up visits, whereas, among 25 control patients, 3 (12%) recovered from vertigo at first followup and 19 (76%) participants recovered from the vertigo at third followup. In dose response analysis, control patients needed 2 more visits than case patients; chi square for linear trend

was 16.82 and it was significant (p value: 0.00004) (Table 5). Case patients were 6 times more likely to recover than control patients (RR: 5.95, 95% CI: 3.85–8.78) and it is statistically significant ($p < 0.005$). The recovery was attributed to Epley maneuver among 67% (95% CI: 43%–81%) of case patients (Table 6).

In regression analysis, preexisting hypertension and diabetes mellitus were confounding the result of Epley maneuver which is evidenced by differing stratum odds ratio (OR: 70.5, Adjusted OR: 55.4, 95% CI: 10.5–457.5, p value: <0.05) (Table 7). When controlling the past history, current medications, and associated symptoms, the case patients showed protective Cox proportional hazard ratio of 0.18 (95% CI: 0.06–0.4, p value: 0.0007) and it is statistically significant.

4. Discussion

BPPV affects all age groups, though it appears to be more common in the elderly. This condition seems to have a predilection for the older population. In our study, the median age of the participants was 55 years and mean age was 53 years with standard deviation of 13 years correlating with the literature [5, 11].

The sex distribution seems to indicate a predilection for women. Among all participants, 30 participants (60%) were female; this is similar to other published reports [5]. Predilection to side was found as left side was affected among 33 (66%) participants. On the other hand some researchers have found that BPPV affects predominantly the right labyrinth [12].

TABLE 6: Efficacy of Epley's maneuver based on person time among benign paroxysmal positional vertigo patients.

Type	Point estimates		95% confidence interval		p value
	Value		Lower	Upper	
Conditional maximum likelihood estimate of RR (CMLE)	3.071		1.69	5.57	
Rate in the exposed	5.95		3.85	8.78	
Rate in the unexposed	1.93		1.25	2.86	0.00018
Rate difference	4.01		1.56	6.46	
Attributable fraction in exposed	67.44%		43.30%	81.30%	
Attributable fraction in population	33.72%		15.80%	51.63%	

TABLE 7: Factors affecting the efficacy of Epley's maneuver among BPPV patients.

Variables	Response	Case	Control	OR		95% CI		p value
				Crude	Adjusted	Lower	Upper	
Hypertension	Yes	11	1	70.5	55.4	10.5	457.5	<0.005
Diabetes mellitus	Yes	11	1	70.5	55.4	10.5	457.5	<0.005
Past H/o giddiness	Yes	3	0	70.5	107.04	14.17	2846.17	<0.005
On medication	Yes	1	0	70.5	46.4	8.4	410.07	<0.005

Hypertension and diabetes were found among 18 (36%) participants. Diabetes was found to be unusually prevalent in BPPV patients in a study done by Cohen et al. [13].

In the present study, we found that up to 92% of patients reported benefit after the first follow-up period of one week. In a randomised study, 90% of patients were either improved or cured after a single session with either Semont's or Epley maneuver [14]. Epley himself reported a success rate of more than 90% following a single treatment session. Among 25 case patients, 18 (72%) recovered from vertigo immediately after the Epley maneuver and 23 (92%) patients recovered from vertigo at first week of followup. The remaining 2 case patients recovered from vertigo during second and third follow-up visits, whereas, among 25 control patients, 3 (12%) recovered from vertigo at first followup and 19 (76%) participants recovered from the vertigo at third followup. This clearly indicates the efficacy of Epley maneuver in treatment of BPPV against the medical therapy. In our study labyrinthine sedatives were used in both case and control groups. In the control group of 25 patients, labyrinthine sedatives were given from the time of first visit to the period when patient is symptom-free. Labyrinthine sedatives failed to control the symptoms of BPPV even after a prolonged use, although they may provide minimal relief for some patients.

A review of the literature revealed the extremely good results of the Epley maneuver. In one study, the success rate after 1 week was 63.6%, which increased to 72.7% after 2 weeks [15]. One Brazilian study also revealed similar results [16]. A meta-analysis done by Prim-Espada et al. on the efficacy of Epley's maneuver in benign paroxysmal positional vertigo using a critical review of the medical literature concluded that the patients on whom Epley's maneuver was performed had six and half times more chance of their clinical symptoms improving compared to the control group of patients (OR = 6.52; 95% CI, 4.17–10.20) [17]. The efficacy of Epley's

maneuver in the treatment of BPPV was assessed in a study of 62 patients conducted by Khatri et al. Patients were selected based on symptoms of positional vertigo and positive Dix-Hallpike's test. At the end of 1 month patients were assessed subjectively by visual analogue scale (VAS) and objectively by Dix-Hallpike's positional test. On VAS, 85.7% of patients had complete resolution of symptoms of BPPV in both groups. Objectively 88.2% did not have positional nystagmus after 1 month in first group, whereas in the second group 86% had complete response at the end of 1 month of therapy [18].

In a study of four hundred and twelve patients with unilateral benign paroxysmal positional vertigo of the posterior semicircular canal, the patients were treated with the Semont maneuver and if symptoms did not resolve, successive application of three Epley maneuvers plus Brandt-Daroff exercises was given. The study concluded that, in unilateral benign paroxysmal positional vertigo of the posterior semicircular canal, the above treatment protocol cured 98% of patients [19]. In a prospective study liberatory maneuver-betahistine and Brandt-Daroff-betahistine groups did significantly better than liberatory maneuver and Brandt and Daroff groups (p < 0.05). This study signifies the added efficiency of betahistine with particle repositioning maneuver in treating BPPV [20]. However there are very few studies which have compared the medical therapy with the particle repositioning maneuver.

5. Conclusion

BPPV is common among the elderly with a sex predilection for women and affecting the left side in majority of patients. Comorbid conditions do have a role in causative factors. In our study, Epley's maneuver was more effective than medicines alone not only in treating the condition but also in preventing the recurrence. This maneuver gave recovery among majority of the case patients during their first visit itself. Those who were treated with medicines alone needed more number of visits than those who were treated with Epley's maneuver and medicines. Epley maneuver can be considered safe and effective procedure to treat benign paroxysmal positional vertigo in majority of patients as a bedside maneuver. After controlling the confounders, Epley maneuver with medicines was found more effective than medicines alone.

Conflict of Interests

The authors declare that there is no conflict of interests regarding the publication of this paper.

References

[1] E. Bárány, "Diagnose yon krankheitserscheinungen im bereiche des otolithenapparates," *Acta Oto-Laryngologica*, vol. 2, no. 3, pp. 434–437, 1920.

[2] M. R. Dix and C. S. Hallpike, "The pathology, symptomatology and diagnosis of certain common disorders of the vestibular system," *Annals of Otology, Rhinology & Laryngology*, vol. 61, no. 4, pp. 987–1016, 1952.

[3] L. S. Parnes, S. K. Agrawal, and J. Atlas, "Diagnosis and management of benign paroxysmal positional vertigo (BPPV)," *Canadian Medical Association Journal*, vol. 169, no. 7, pp. 681–693, 2003.

[4] D. A. Froehling, M. D. Silverstein, D. N. Mohr, C. W. Beatty, K. P. Offord, and D. J. Ballard, "Benign positional vertigo: incidence and prognosis in a population-based study in Olmsted County, Minnesota," *Mayo Clinic Proceedings*, vol. 66, no. 6, pp. 596–601, 1991.

[5] R. W. Baloh, V. Honrubia, and K. Jacobson, "Benign positional vertigo: clinical and oculographic features in 240 cases," *Neurology*, vol. 37, no. 3, pp. 371–378, 1987.

[6] M. Viccaro, P. Mancini, R. La Gamma, E. De Seta, E. Covelli, and R. Filipo, "Positional vertigo and cochlear implantation," *Otology & Neurotology*, vol. 28, no. 6, pp. 764–767, 2007.

[7] E. M. Gross, B. D. Ress, E. S. Viirre, J. R. Nelson, and J. P. Harris, "Intractable benign paroxysmal positional vertigo in patients with Meniere's disease," *Laryngoscope*, vol. 110, no. 4, pp. 655–659, 2000.

[8] S. F. Hall, R. R. F. Ruby, and J. A. McClure, "The mechanics of benign paroxysmal vertigo," *Journal of Otolaryngology*, vol. 8, no. 2, pp. 151–158, 1979.

[9] J. M. Epley, "The canalith repositioning procedure: for treatment of benign paroxysmal positional vertigo," *Journal of Otolaryngology—Head & Neck Surgery*, vol. 107, no. 3, pp. 399–404, 1992.

[10] M. Wolf, T. Hertanu, I. Novikov, and J. Kronenberg, "Epley's manoeuvre for benign paroxysmal positional vertigo: a prospective study," *Clinical Otolaryngology and Allied Sciences*, vol. 24, no. 1, pp. 43–46, 1999.

[11] E. Marciano and V. Marcelli, "Postural restrictions in labyrintholithiasis," *European Archives of Oto-Rhino-Laryngology*, vol. 259, no. 5, pp. 262–265, 2002.

[12] M. Von Brevern, T. Seelig, H. Neuhauser, and T. Lempert, "Benign paroxysmal positional vertigo predominantly affects the right labyrinth," *Journal of Neurology, Neurosurgery & Psychiatry*, vol. 75, no. 10, pp. 1487–1488, 2004.

[13] H. S. Cohen, K. T. Kimball, and M. G. Stewart, "Benign paroxysmal positional vertigo and comorbid conditions," *ORL*, vol. 66, no. 1, pp. 11–15, 2004.

[14] S. J. Herdman, R. J. Tusa, D. S. Zee, L. R. Proctor, and D. E. Mattox, "Single treatment approaches to benign paroxysmal positional vertigo," *Archives of Otolaryngology: Head and Neck Surgery*, vol. 119, no. 4, pp. 450–454, 1993.

[15] S. S. U. Waleem, S. M. Malik, S. Ullah, and Z. ul Hassan, "Office management of benign paroxysmal positional vertigo with Epley's maneuver," *Journal of Ayub Medical College, Abbottabad*, vol. 20, no. 1, pp. 77–79, 2008.

[16] L. J. Teixeira and J. N. P. Machado, "Manoeuvres for the treatment of benign positional paroxysmal vertigo: a systematic review," *Brazilian Journal of Otorhinolaryngology*, vol. 72, no. 1, pp. 130–139, 2006.

[17] M. P. Prim-Espada, J. I. De Diego-Sastre, and E. Pérez-Fernández, "Meta-analysis on the efficacy of Epley's manoeuvre in benign paroxysmal positional vertigo," *Neurologia*, vol. 25, no. 5, pp. 295–299, 2010.

[18] M. Khatri, R. M. Raizada, and M. P. Puttewar, "Epley's canalith-repositioning manoeuvre for benign paroxysmal positional vertigo," *Indian Journal of Otolaryngology and Head and Neck Surgery*, vol. 57, no. 4, pp. 315–319, 2005.

[19] A. Soto-Varela, M. Rossi-Izquierdo, G. Martínez-Capoccioni, T. Labella-Caballero, and S. Santos-Pérez, "Benign paroxysmal positional vertigo of the posterior semicircular canal: efficacy of Santiago treatment protocol, long-term follow up and analysis of recurrence," *Journal of Laryngology and Otology*, vol. 126, no. 4, pp. 363–371, 2012.

[20] M. Cavaliere, G. Mottola, and M. Iemma, "Benign paroxysmal positional vertigo: a study of two manoeuvres with and without betahistine," *Acta Otorhinolaryngologica Italica*, vol. 25, no. 2, pp. 107–112, 2005.

Hearing Preservation in Cochlear Implant Surgery

**Priscila Carvalho Miranda,[1] André Luiz Lopes Sampaio,[1,2]
Rafaela Aquino Fernandes Lopes,[1] Alessandra Ramos Venosa,[1,2]
and Carlos Augusto Costa Pires de Oliveira[1,2]**

[1] *Brasília University Hospital, Hospital Universitário de Brasília-HUB, SGAN 605, Avenida L2 Norte, 70830-200 Brasília, DF, Brazil*
[2] *Universidade de Brasília (UnB), Campus Universitário Darcy Ribeiro, 70910-900 Brasília, DF, Brazil*

Correspondence should be addressed to Priscila Carvalho Miranda; pritcp@gmail.com

Academic Editor: David W. Eisele

In the past, it was thought that hearing loss patients with residual low-frequency hearing would not be good candidates for cochlear implantation since insertion was expected to induce inner ear trauma. Recent advances in electrode design and surgical techniques have made the preservation of residual low-frequency hearing achievable and desirable. The importance of preserving residual low-frequency hearing cannot be underestimated in light of the added benefit of hearing in noisy atmospheres and in music quality. The concept of electrical and acoustic stimulation involves electrically stimulating the nonfunctional, high-frequency region of the cochlea with a cochlear implant and applying a hearing aid in the low-frequency range. The principle of preserving low-frequency hearing by a "soft surgery" cochlear implantation could also be useful to the population of children who might profit from regenerative hair cell therapy in the future. Main aspects of low-frequency hearing preservation surgery are discussed in this review: its brief history, electrode design, principles and advantages of electric-acoustic stimulation, surgical technique, and further implications of this new treatment possibility for hearing impaired patients.

1. Introduction

In the past three decades, cochlear implantation has evolved from an experimental procedure to represent the standard of care for deaf patients. Advances in processing strategies, implant design, and patient selection criteria have significantly improved implant users' performance. Nowadays, the current frontiers in implantation involve strategies to preserve residual acoustic hearing and the development of algorithms to combine electrical and acoustic hearing. Moreover, it is important to keep in mind that, by preserving apical organ of Corti structures, it is possible to take advantage of new technologies that may lead to regeneration of the inner ear in the future [1].

Cochlear implantation with a standard-length electrode has been a reality in treating patients who have profound deafness. However, the loss of residual acoustic hearing following cochlear implantation is an important clinical consideration when determining the most appropriate options for patients with severe hearing losses [2]. There are some patients with substantial low-frequency acoustic hearing up to 1500 Hz and severe to profound high-frequency hearing loss that do poorly with bilateral amplification who have not been considered as candidates for implantation using standard criteria [3].

High frequencies report information about vocal vibration (like the ability to distinguish between "s" and "z"), whereas lower frequencies apprise information regarding the vocal formants and spectral patterns (such as the difference between "b" and "g") [4]. Patients with high-frequency losses are able to distinguish loudness and speech pattern (due to their low-frequency acoustic hearing), but they cannot interpret spectral patterns well (which erodes their capacity to distinguish between the different consonant sounds and thus their word discrimination scores) [5].

The loss of low-frequency hearing during cochlear implantation is the result of the technique used to create the cochleostomy and its size combined with the characteristics of the electrode design (diameter, stiffness, and length) since it may induce substantial damage to the basilar membrane and cochlear hair cells as it advances into the scala tympani [1, 2].

2. Electric-Acoustic Stimulation (EAS)

2.1. Shortened Electrodes. It is known that cochlear implantation with a standard-length electrode and standard surgical technique in patients with some residual hearing results in complete loss of the remaining acoustic hearing [6, 7]. Nevertheless, since Hodges et al. [8] presented a series of patients who had undergone implantation and had preserved residual hearing, many studies have demonstrated the ability to retain residual low-frequency hearing in standard-length electrode implantation [9, 10].

The idea of acoustic plus electric hearing means a cochlear implant aided by an ipsilateral hearing aid, to benefit from the residual low-frequency hearing of an individual. This idea of electric-acoustic stimulation (EAS) first emerged from the work of two independent groups, one from Iowa, USA, and the other from Frankfurt, Germany. In 1995, the University of Iowa Cochlear Implant research team along with the Cochlear Corporation (Lane Cove, Australia) developed a shortened electrode array called the Hybrid S. It was designed to be inserted only into the lower basal turn of the cochlea and thus stimulate the missing areas of high frequency for those specific patients with preserved low-frequency thresholds [2]. The Hybrid S electrode has a smaller diameter than the standard electrode (0.2 mm × 0.4 mm) and initially, it was 6 mm in length and it contained 6 electrodes. Because some patients reported a very high-pitched sound [11], it was then lengthened to 10 mm, still with 6 electrodes. The ideal insertion depth is at approximately 195° of the basal turn of the cochlea [12].

In 2003, Gantz and Turner [11] reported the first 6 patients implanted with the Hybrid S electrode, three of which received the 6 mm electrode and the other three received the 10 mm electrode. Patients who received the 6 mm electrode improved their consonant recognition scores by 10%, whereas those who received the 10 mm electrode improved by 40%. Also, patients who received the 10 mm electrode did better in the combined mode (cochlear implant + bilateral hearing aids) than those who received the 6 mm electrode [13]. A larger multicenter phase 1 FDA trial was conducted for the Hybrid S 10 mm electrode with 87 patients from 13 centers, and preliminary data was published in 2009 [14]. Two patients lost all residual hearing within 1 month of implantation (initial hearing preservation rate (IHPR) of 98%). Between 3 and 24 months after activation, 6 more patients lost residual hearing (IHPR of 91%). Over time, 30% of the patients had a low-frequency threshold drop of more than 30 decibels (dB). A duration of deafness of over 40 years and low preoperative consonant-nucleus-consonant (CNC) word scores were found to have a negative impact on functional outcomes [14].

Another short electrode named Hybrid L24 has been developed in conjunction with the Cochlear Corporation. It contains 22 electrodes that are 16 mm long and its optimal insertion is 250° of the basal turn of the cochlea. It would still preserve the residual hearing from the apical portions of the cochlea and if the low-frequency hearing is lost, it can be used as a traditional electric device since it has 22 electrodes, similar to a standard one. The FDA trial for the Hybrid L has not been published yet, but the preliminary results from the European clinical trial [15] demonstrated the ability to preserve residual hearing. Thirty-two patients were enrolled, 24 of whom were hybrid candidates and 8 long-electrode candidates. In 96% of the subjects, hearing was preserved within 30 dB of preoperative thresholds and in 68% within 15 dB. These results were stable over time and there was a significant improvement in word scores between the 6-month and 12-month marks, demonstrating, as in the Hybrid S trial, that there is a learning period for patients with short electrodes [16].

The Med-El Corporation has also developed a shortened electrode called M, which is 22 mm long with an ideal insertion of 360° from the basal turn of the cochlea. It has a very flexible tip and a significantly reduced diameter in the distal portion. This Flex^{EAS} electrode can be used for both round window insertion and cochleostomy techniques [17]. Much of the data regarding Flex^{EAS} involves mixed cohorts of patients. Gstoettner et al. in 2008 [18] reported a series of 18 patients implanted with the M electrode. Twelve of the 18 (68%) had low-frequency hearing preservation that could be usefully amplified. Three of the patients had some residual low-frequency hearing but did not find amplification useful. Three of the 18 (16%) lost all residual hearing. Interestingly, the loss of the residual hearing was not immediate, but delayed by 3 to 6 months after hybrid activation.

2.2. Standard-Length Electrodes. An alternative strategy for preserving the low-frequency hearing was developed with standard-length electrodes, but limiting the depth of insertion. Kiefer et al. [7] implanted 14 patients with the Med-El Combi40+ electrode, limiting the length of insertion to less than 24 mm (full insertion is 31.5 mm) and using a "soft insertion" technique. In 12 out of the 14 patients (85%), useful low-frequency hearing (less than 20 dB drop in thresholds) was maintained, with 2 patients losing all residual hearing. Using a standard-length electrode and modified surgical techniques, other authors have reported rates from 67% to 89% of hearing preserved within 20 dB of preoperative thresholds [7, 19–22]. Nevertheless, not all of these patients maintain the ability to discriminate. Balkany et al. reported that although patients experienced only a 15 dB drop in the low frequencies, the average acoustic CNC postoperative word score was 0% [9].

2.3. Discussion. There is controversy in the literature about the preferred electrode length. There is a higher rate of reduced thresholds and anacusis with the long electrodes. Some authors defend this reason for its use, so if residual hearing is lost, the patient can have the full-length electrode to benefit from its electric-only listening mode, which would not happen with a short electrode. Since the short electrode is 10 mm long, it accesses only the 2800 to 4700 Hz range according to the Greenwood frequency placement map of the basilar membrane. Even though this was thought to be a tonotopic mismatch, which could impair discrimination, Hybrid S electrode users in electric-only mode showed similar performance as long-electrode users on consonant recognition tasks [23]. Improved performance with the Hybrid S electrode appears to require a longer time (over 12 months) than the long-electrode (usually 6 to 12 months to adapt to electric hearing) [16, 23].

One argument in favor of long electrode used to be the likelihood of progressive low-frequency hearing loss. However, Yao et al. [24] demonstrated a loss of only 1.05 dB in low-frequency hearing (up to 2000 Hz) per year in Hybrid S users, regardless of their age. It seems that low-frequency hearing is relatively stable over time. If it can be preserved at the time of implantation, it is likely that the patient will have minimal further hearing loss in the long term [24].

Another concern regarding Hybrid or EAS studies is the progression of hearing loss after activation. At the time of implantation, very few patients lose all their residual low-frequency hearing. In the phase 1 Hybrid S10 trial [14], 2% of the patients lost their residual low-frequency hearing, and within 3 months of activation, 10% of the initial number of patients had a 30 dB drop from their preoperative thresholds up to 500 Hz. The cause of this loss is still unknown; some hypotheses suggest an immune reaction to the electrode, loss of afferent spiral ganglion neuron synapses at the hair cell related to the combination of acoustic amplification and electrical stimulation, or even an initial injury from noise-induced hearing loss [25].

Steroids have been shown to reduce noise-induced cochlear damage and hearing loss and to increase recovery after noise trauma. However, their efficacy has been controversially discussed due to a lack of adequate clinical trials [1]. Also, there is controversy regarding drug application methods, be it systemic or local, either via diffusion from the middle ear space through the round window membrane or by direct instillation into the perilymphatic space. A single-shot intracochlear glucocorticoid application appears to be a promising method for reducing progressive hearing loss caused by electrode insertion trauma due its long-term effects, such as reduction of inflammatory processes [1]. Further in vitro studies with otoprotective drugs believed to bring new perspectives on an improved rate of hearing preservation are promising [1, 26, 27].

3. Indication Guidelines for EAS

In the initial studies, the indication was closer to standard cochlear implantation for thresholds above 65 dB in the low frequencies between 125 and 500 Hz [28]. After encouraging results from these studies, the criteria were gradually expanded to normal low-frequency hearing in the frequencies up to 1500 Hz (partial deafness cochlear implantation) [29].

Actual guidelines determine that pure tone audiometry scores for both ears have to be greater than 60 dB between

125 and 500 Hz and below 70 dB at 1500. In addition, monosyllables tested at a 10 dB signal-to-noise ratio (SNR) should not exceed a score of 40% in the best aided condition [1]. Further, these patients must have substantial CNC word scores in the best aided condition, with between 10% and 60% correct in the worse hearing ear and up to 80% correct in the best hearing ear.

4. Surgical Technique for Hearing Preservation

Wright and Roland in 2005 [30] first described a "soft surgery" technique, which was later modified by other authors [7, 12, 13]. When developing new strategies, the most import factors that contribute to possible cochlear damage during or after the surgery must be kept in mind [1]:

(i) mechanical damage during electrode insertion (fractures of the osseous spiral lamina, disruption of the basilar membrane, tearing of the lateral spiral ligament, and leakage of traumatized blood vessels),

(ii) shock waves in the perilymph fluid due to implantation,

(iii) acoustic trauma due to drilling,

(iv) loss of perilymph and disruption of inner ear fluid homeostasis,

(v) potential bacterial infection,

(vi) secondary intracochlear fibrous tissue formation.

The technique used at the University of Iowa for implantation of the cochlear Hybrid S and L devices is described in this review.

A standard mastoidectomy is performed through a post-auricular incision. A portion of the superior margin of the mastoid cortex is left in place and a suture is passed through the cortex to anchor the electrode before placing it in the cochlea. The objective of this suture is to reduce the spring of the electrode and to prevent movement of the electrode during placement in the scala tympani (ST). A bonny well for the internal processor is also created in the same manner used for a standard cochlear receiver/stimulator. A ridge of bone between the mastoid cavity and the well is left so the implant does not later slide. A subperiosteal pocket is created deeply to the temporalis muscle and pericranium. The facial recess is opened widely, and the round window niche is totally exposed by removing the bone overlying and anterior to the facial nerve. With a 1 mm diamond burr, the bony overhang of the round window niche is drilled away to expose the entire round window membrane.

Before creating the cochleostomy, the surgical field must be extensively irrigated and meticulous hemostasis must be done in order to prevent bone chips and blood debris from entering into the cochlea upon opening. The cochleostomy is created in the inferior-posterior quadrant of a box created by drawing a line at the superior margin of the round window and a perpendicular line at the inferior margin of the round window [2]. Entering into the scala tympani in this specific location prevents damage to the basilar membrane and avoids injury to inner ear structures by facilitating insertion of the electrodes in the correct trajectory [3]. Although in the United States a cochleostomy is the preferred strategy for placing the electrode, many European surgeons usually prefer the round window approach [3]. The round window technique may result in a conductive hearing loss [15] and it predisposes to fracturing the osseous spiral lamina, according to some studies [30, 31]. A recent systematic review [32], however, did not show any benefit of one surgical approach over the other regarding the preservation of residual hearing.

The electrode and processor must be seated in position before opening the endosteum of the cochleostomy. Two holes are drilled into the tegmen tympani, which allow a 2-0 or 4-0 nylon suture to be passed through the bone in order to secure the Hybrid S and L electrode array (not the ground electrode). Once the processor and electrode are seated and secured, a temporalis fascia "washer" with a 1.5 mm × 1.5 mm diameter is harvested and flattened in a fascial tissue press. It is then punctured with a straight needle and the electrode is inserted through the fascia up to the Dacron collar in order to seal the scala tympani at the cochleostomy. Opening the endosteum into the scala tympani with a 0.2 mm footplate hook must be the final act of the procedure to reduce the time the cochlea is open. The electrode is advanced slowly into the scala tympani (over 1 to 2 minutes) in order to minimize insertional trauma and to allow perilymph displacement.

There are some intraoperative tests described in order to further improve the safety of hearing preservation surgery, such as the measure of cochlear microphonics [1] and auditory brainstem response (ABR) during electrode insertion [3]. Likewise, Oghalai et al. [33] used auditory steady-state response audiometry to access hearing thresholds during regular cochlear implantation and draw the surgeon's attention to the critical moments of the insertion procedure. The surgeon must pause during the insertion to allow data for these tests to be collected.

The middle ear is not packed with muscle or fascia. The periosteum should then be closed completely over the receiver/stimulator and the electrode. Soft tissues are then closed in the standard way.

Helbig et al. [34] recently reported a series of 3 patients in whom revision surgery for cochlear implantation was required. Reimplantation was possible in these patients who had previously undergone EAS surgery with the preservation of low-frequency hearing and without losing the residual hearing function. Also, a reduced insertion depth at the initial surgery could be followed by deeper insertion into the cochlea without any deterioration of residual hearing [34].

5. Benefits of Acoustic and Electric Processing

Current literature has already reported several discrete advantages to both modalities, but the full benefits of an EAS of the ipsilateral cochlea are still under investigation.

5.1. Speech Perception with EAS. Patients with preserved low-frequency hearing show significant improvements in their discrimination scores. Hybrid S electrode users continue to improve on CNC scores over 1 to 2 years after activation. In the Hybrid S trial [14], 48% of the patients showed improvement in both SRT and CNC scores. Improvement on CNC testing ranged from 10% to 70% over preoperative scores for 73% of the patients with long-term followups [14]. For those implanted with the Hybrid L24, word recognition scores improved by 21% on average; one single patient had improvement from 5% to 95% on the Freiburg monosyllabic word test (FMT) [15].

Exceptional improvement in speech understanding is possible for patients in the combined mode with all electrodes activated: some patients score more than 90% on the CNC monosyllabic word test. Flex^{EAS} users had preoperatively open-set sentence recognition of 24% and after 12 months of use, scores averaged 71%. Monosyllable recognition also improved from 16% to 44% on average.

Improvements in discrimination tasks have also been observed in long-electrode users with preserved acoustic hearing. Patients who received the Med-El Combi40+ with 19 to 24 mm of insertion scored 75% on monosyllabic tests after 1 year, an important improvement from the 9% preoperative scores.

5.2. Hearing in Noisy Backgrounds. Distinguishing the correct words in a background of competing talkers is a challenging test for traditional cochlear implant users. Normal-hearing listeners have a signal-to-noise ratio (SNR) of -30 dB and -15 dB for competing talkers [35]. The average SNR of a long-electrode user is $+3$ dB for unmodulated background noise and $+8$ for multitalker babble (MTB), which means the talker has to speak 3 dB louder than the competing noise or 8 dB louder than MTB.

Hybrid S users do better than traditional cochlear implant patients, but not as well as normal-hearing listeners in noisy backgrounds. In a subgroup of 27 Hybrid S patients with at least 12 months of activation, SNRs ranged from -12 to $+17$ dB (average -9 dB) [14]. Patients who had a drop greater than 30 dB in their low-frequency hearing experienced a worse SNR.

Hybrid L electrode patients also improved their SNR preoperatively from 12.1 dB to 2.1 dB postoperatively [15]. Those with the Flex^{EAS} electrode changed their preoperative open-set sentence scores with a SNR of $+10$ dB from 14% to 60% after 1 year of activation [18].

Long-electrode users with preserved hearing in low frequencies also benefit when listening in noise. Med-El Combi40+ users with a low-frequency threshold of <80 dB scored better than patients with a cochlear implant and no residual hearing with a SNR of $+5$ dB [19]. Gstoettner et al. showed an increase in understanding scores from 13.1% preoperatively to 75% in the electric-acoustic stimulation condition [22].

5.3. EAS and Music Perception. It is known that traditional cochlear implant users have difficulties identifying and enjoying music because of the extremely complex encoded spectral information. They can usually distinguish lyrics to a certain degree but have significant trouble with pitch, timbre, and melody recognition [35, 36].

Music appreciation has been a part of the research protocol for the Hybrid S/L trials. Patients with preserved acoustic hearing have a distinct advantage over traditional cochlear implant users regarding pitch, lyrics, melody, and timbre of the instruments. When Hybrid users were provided with excerpts of easily recognizable American songs, they were able to correctly identify the songs 65%–100% of the time, similar to normal-hearing listeners. In tasks regarding pitch recognition and melody without lyrics, the Hybrid users still scored better than the traditional cochlear implant patients, but not as well as normal-hearing listeners did [36, 37].

Brockmeier et al. [38] studied music testing in EAS patients with long-electrode insertion (Med-El Combi40+). Thirteen EAS patients were compared with long-electrode users with no residual hearing and normal-hearing listeners. Subjects were matched by age and musical experience. EAS patients did as well as normal-hearing listeners on pitch discrimination and better than traditional cochlear implant users. However, EAS patients' scores in melody discrimination, instrument detection, and instrument identification were not significantly different from those of traditional cochlear implant users.

6. Future of Hybrid-Type Cochlear Implantation

Apical cochlear preservation may become a significant issue in the future. It is possible that treatments will emerge that require naïve cochlear tissue (i.e., hair cell generation or tissue transfer). This concern is relevant for families weighing the risks and benefits of bilateral cochlear implantation for deaf children. The Iowa CI research team has recently reported a series of 9 children with bilateral implants: one ear with a standard long electrode and the other with Hybrid S12 research electrode [39]. The children were only 12 to 24 months old at the time of implantation and they scored an average of 80 in Preschool Language Scale-3 (PLS-3), whereas the average score in the same test for children with bilateral standard electrodes is 83. A long-term followup is necessary to determine whether the trends of the preliminary data are long-lasting; a larger-scale study is being carried out.

7. Conclusion

Although hearing preservation in cochlear implantation is technically challenging, the importance of preserving residual low-frequency hearing cannot be underestimated in light of the added benefit of hearing in noisy atmospheres and music quality for EAS users. Electrode designs and processor technology are constantly being improved. Nowadays, patients undergoing hearing preservation surgery can expect a long-term low-frequency hearing preservation rate of 50–70%. Although surgeons have largely modified the initially described "soft surgery" technique over the years, there is not a unique protocol to be followed.

Few would have imagined the progress that has been made in the past 30 years regarding aiding deafened patients, and the future promises to be equally exciting. The potential EAS advantages highlight the value of the endeavors to preserve low-frequency hearing in the implanted ear and to continue amplification where appropriate. Further research is also needed to maximize outcomes for recipients with different degrees of hearing loss who use devices that combine electric and acoustic stimulation.

Conflict of Interests

The authors declare that there is no conflict of interests regarding the publication of this paper.

References

[1] C. A. von Ilberg, U. Baumann, J. Kiefer, J. Tillein, and O. F. Adunka, "Electric-acoustic stimulation of the auditory system: a review of the first decade," *Audiology and Neurotology*, vol. 16, supplement 2, pp. 1–30, 2011.

[2] B. J. Gantz, C. Turner, K. E. Gfeller, and M. W. Lowder, "Preservation of hearing in cochlear implant surgery: advantages of combined electrical and acoustical speech processing," *Laryngoscope*, vol. 115, no. 5, pp. 796–802, 2005.

[3] S. E. Mowry, E. Woodson, and B. J. Gantz, "New frontiers in cochlear implantation: acoustic plus electric hearing, hearing preservation, and more," *Otolaryngologic Clinics of North America*, vol. 45, no. 1, pp. 187–203, 2012.

[4] C. W. Turner, B. J. Gantz, S. Karsten, J. Fowler, and L. A. Reiss, "Impact of hair cell preservation in cochlear implantation: combined electric and acoustic hearing," *Otology and Neurotology*, vol. 31, no. 8, pp. 1227–1232, 2010.

[5] C. A. Hogan and C. W. Turner, "High-frequency audibility: benefits for hearing-impaired listeners," *Journal of the Acoustical Society of America*, vol. 104, no. 1, pp. 432–441, 1998.

[6] F. M. Rizer, P. N. Arkis, W. H. Lippy, and A. G. Schuring, "A postoperative audiometric evaluation of cochlear implant patients," *Otolaryngology: Head and Neck Surgery*, vol. 98, no. 3, pp. 203–206, 1988.

[7] J. Kiefer, W. Gstoettner, W. Baumgartner et al., "Conservation of low-frequency hearing in cochlear implantation," *Acta Oto-Laryngologica*, vol. 124, no. 3, pp. 272–280, 2004.

[8] A. V. Hodges, J. Schloffman, and T. Balkany, "Conservation of residual hearing with cochlear implantation," *The American Journal of Otology*, vol. 18, no. 2, pp. 179–183, 1997.

[9] T. J. Balkany, S. S. Connell, A. V. Hodges et al., "Conservation of residual acoustic hearing after cochlear implantation," *Otology and Neurotology*, vol. 27, no. 8, pp. 1083–1088, 2006.

[10] C. von Ilberg, J. Kiefer, J. Tillein et al., "Electric-acoustic stimulation of the auditory system. New technology for severe hearing loss," *ORL*, vol. 61, no. 6, pp. 334–340, 1999.

[11] B. J. Gantz and C. W. Turner, "Combining acoustic and electrical hearing," *Laryngoscope*, vol. 113, no. 10, pp. 1726–1730, 2003.

[12] J. T. Roland Jr., D. M. Zeitler, D. Jethanamest, and T. C. Huang, "Evaluation of the short hybrid electrode in human temporal bones," *Otology and Neurotology*, vol. 29, no. 4, pp. 482–488, 2008.

[13] B. J. Gantz and C. Turner, "Combining acoustic and electrical speech processing: iowa/nucleus hybrid implant," *Acta Oto-Laryngologica*, vol. 124, no. 4, pp. 344–347, 2004.

[14] B. J. Gantz, M. R. Hansen, C. W. Turner et al., "Hybrid 10 clinical trial," *Audiology and Neurotology*, vol. 14, supplement 1, pp. 32–38, 2009.

[15] T. Lenarz, T. Stöver, A. Buechner, A. Lesinski-Schiedat, J. Patrick, and J. Pesch, "Hearing conservation surgery using the hybrid-L electrode: results from the first clinical trial at the Medical University of Hannover," *Audiology and Neurotology*, vol. 14, no. 1, pp. 22–31, 2009.

[16] L. A. J. Reiss, C. W. Turner, S. R. Erenberg, and B. J. Gantz, "Changes in pitch with a cochlear implant over time," *Journal of the Association for Research in Otolaryngology*, vol. 8, no. 2, pp. 241–257, 2007.

[17] I. Hochmair, P. Nopp, C. Jolly et al., "MED-EL cochlear implants: state of the art and a glimpse into the future," *Trends in Amplification*, vol. 10, no. 4, pp. 201–220, 2006.

[18] W. K. Gstoettner, P. van de Heyning, A. Fitzgerald O'Connor et al., "Electric acoustic stimulation of the auditory system: results of a multi-centre investigation," *Acta Oto-Laryngologica*, vol. 128, no. 9, pp. 968–975, 2008.

[19] B. Fraysse, Á. R. Macías, O. Sterkers et al., "Residual hearing conservation and electroacoustic stimulation with the nucleus 24 contour advance cochlear implant," *Otology and Neurotology*, vol. 27, no. 5, pp. 624–633, 2006.

[20] L. Garcia-Ibanez, A. R. MacIas, C. Morera et al., "An evaluation of the preservation of residual hearing with the Nucleus Contour Advance electrode," *Acta Oto-Laryngologica*, vol. 129, no. 6, pp. 651–664, 2009.

[21] W. di Nardo, I. Cantore, P. Melilo et al., "Residual hearing in cochlear implant patients," *European Archives of Oto-Rhino-Laryngology*, vol. 264, no. 8, pp. 855–860, 2007.

[22] W. K. Gstoettner, S. Heibig, N. Maier, J. Kiefer, A. Radeloff, and O. F. Adunka, "Ipsilateral electric acoustic stimulation of the auditory system: results of long-term hearing preservation," *Audiology and Neurotology*, vol. 11, no. 1, pp. 49–56, 2006.

[23] L. A. J. Reiss, B. J. Gantz, and C. W. Turner, "Cochlear implant speech processor frequency allocations may influence pitch perception," *Otology and Neurotology*, vol. 29, no. 2, pp. 160–167, 2008.

[24] W. N. Yao, C. W. Turner, and B. J. Gantz, "Stability of low-frequency residual hearing in patients who are candidates for combined acoustic plus electric hearing," *Journal of Speech, Language, and Hearing Research*, vol. 49, no. 5, pp. 1085–1090, 2006.

[25] J.-L. Puel, J. Ruel, C. Gervais D'Aldin, and R. Pujol, "Excitotoxicity and repair of cochlear synapses after noise- trauma induced hearing loss," *NeuroReport*, vol. 9, no. 9, pp. 2109–2114, 1998.

[26] U. Scarpidis, D. Madnani, C. Shoemaker et al., "Arrest of apoptosis in auditory neurons: implications for sensorineural preservation in cochlear implantation," *Otology and Neurotology*, vol. 24, no. 3, pp. 409–417, 2003.

[27] H. Staecker, D. E. Brough, M. Praetorius, and K. Baker, "Drug delivery to the inner ear using gene therapy," *Otolaryngologic Clinics of North America*, vol. 37, no. 5, pp. 1091–1108, 2004.

[28] C. Von Ilberg, J. Kiefer, J. Tillein et al., "Electric-acoustic stimulation of the auditory system. New technology for severe hearing loss," *ORL*, vol. 61, no. 6, pp. 334–340, 1999.

[29] H. Skarzynski, A. Lorens, A. Piotrowska, and I. Anderson, "Preservation of low frequency hearing in partial deafness cochlear implantation (PDCI) using the round window surgical approach," *Acta Oto-Laryngologica*, vol. 127, no. 1, pp. 41–48, 2007.

[30] C. G. Wright and P. S. Roland, "Temporal bone microdissection for anatomic study of cochlear implant electrodes," *Cochlear Implants International*, vol. 6, no. 4, pp. 159–168, 2005.

[31] R. J. S. Briggs, M. Tykocinski, K. Stidham, and J. B. Roberson, "Cochleostomy site: implications for electrode placement and hearing preservation," *Acta Oto-Laryngologica*, vol. 125, no. 8, pp. 870–876, 2005.

[32] S. Havenith, M. J. W. Lammers, R. A. Tange et al., "Hearing preservation surgery: cochleostomy or round window approach? A systematic review," *Otology and Neurotology*, vol. 34, no. 4, pp. 667–674, 2013.

[33] J. S. Oghalai, R. Tonini, J. Rasmus et al., "Intra-operative monitoring of cochlear function during cochlear implantation," *Cochlear Implants International*, vol. 10, no. 1, pp. 1–18, 2009.

[34] S. Helbig, G. P. Rajan, T. Stöver, M. Lockley, J. Kuthubutheen, and K. M. Green, "Hearing preservation after cochlear reimplantation," *Otology and Neurotology*, vol. 34, no. 1, pp. 61–65, 2013.

[35] C. W. Turner, B. J. Gantz, C. Vidal, A. Behrens, and B. A. Henry, "Speech recognition in noise for cochlear implant listeners: benefits of residual acoustic hearing," *Journal of the Acoustical Society of America*, vol. 115, no. 4, pp. 1729–1735, 2004.

[36] K. E. Gfeller, C. Olszewski, C. Turner, B. Gantz, and J. Oleson, "Music perception with cochlear implants and residual hearing," *Audiology and Neurotology*, vol. 11, supplement 1, pp. 12–15, 2006.

[37] K. Gfeller, C. Turner, J. Oleson et al., "Accuracy of cochlear implant recipients on pitch perception, melody recognition, and speech reception in noise," *Ear and Hearing*, vol. 28, no. 3, pp. 412–423, 2007.

[38] S. J. Brockmeier, M. Peterreins, A. Lorens et al., "Music perception in electric acoustic stimulation users as assessed by the Mu.S.I.C. test," *Advances in Oto-Rhino-Laryngology*, vol. 67, pp. 70–80, 2010.

[39] B. J. Gantz, C. C. Dunn, E. A. Walker et al., "Bilateral cochlear implants in infants: a new approach-nucleus hybrid S12 project," *Otology and Neurotology*, vol. 31, no. 8, pp. 1300–1309, 2010.

The Complications of Sinusitis in a Tertiary Care Hospital: Types, Patient Characteristics, and Outcomes

Saisawat Chaiyasate,[1] Supranee Fooanant,[1] Niramon Navacharoen,[1] Kannika Roongrotwattanasiri,[1] Pongsakorn Tantilipikorn,[2] and Jayanton Patumanond[3,4]

[1]*Department of Otolaryngology, Faculty of Medicine, Chiang Mai University, Chiang Mai 50000, Thailand*
[2]*Department of Otorhinolaryngology, Faculty of Medicine, Siriraj Hospital, Mahidol University, Bangkok 10700, Thailand*
[3]*Division of Clinical Epidemiology, Department of Community Medicine, Faculty of Medicine, Chiang Mai University, Chiang Mai 50000, Thailand*
[4]*Clinical Research Center, Faculty of Medicine, Thammasat University, Pathum Thani 12120, Thailand*

Correspondence should be addressed to Saisawat Chaiyasate; saisawat.c@cmu.ac.th

Academic Editor: Leonard P. Rybak

Objective. To study the complications of sinusitis in a referral hospital and the outcome of the treatment according to the type of complication. *Methods.* A retrospective study was performed on patients with sinusitis who were admitted to a referral hospital from 2003 to 2012. The data for the sinusitis patients who had complications were reviewed. *Results and Discussion.* Eighty-five patients were included in the study, of whom 50 were male (58.8%). Fourteen of the cases were less than 15 years old, and 27 of the patients (31.7%) had more than one type of complication. The most common complication was of the orbital type (100% in the children, 38% in the adults). After the treatment, all of the children and 45 of the adults (63.4%) recovered, eight of the adult patients died (11.3%), and 18 of the adults were cured with morbidity (25.3%). The patients with more numerous complications had poorer outcomes. When the types of complications were compared (adjusted for age, gender, and comorbidities), the intracranial complication was the only one that was statistically significant for mortality. *Conclusion.* The outcomes of the treatment depended on the number and type of complications, with the poorest results achieved in cases of intracranial complications.

1. Introduction

Sinusitis, which is a common ear, nose, and throat disease, develops after a viral upper respiratory tract infection in 0.5–2% of patients [1]. However, its complications are unusual. The complication rates of the patients admitted with acute sinusitis varied from 3.7 to 20% [2].

Generally, the complications of sinusitis are classified into three types: local (osseous), orbital, and intracranial complications [2, 3]. The most common complication is the orbital type (60–75%), followed by the intracranial (15–20%) and the local type (5–10%). Many studies have reported cranial nerve(s) palsy in the posterior ethmoid or sphenoiditis, which did not occur with the orbital or intracranial type [4–7]. However, optic neuropathy alone has been included in the complications of chronic sinusitis [2]. In a 1997–2002 study

of Thai patients by the senior author, 8.2% of the admitted sinusitis patients had complications, but the frontal sinus was not a common cause of the intracranial complications, and cranial neuropathies did not occur with either meningitis or brain abscesses in these patients [8]. The objective of the current study was to determine the complications of sinusitis in a referral hospital and the outcome of the treatments according to the type of the complication.

2. Materials and Methods

A retrospective study was performed on sinusitis patients admitted to Chiang Mai University Hospital from 2003 to 2012. The data for the sinusitis patients with complications and their operative schedules were reviewed, gathered, and grouped as follows.

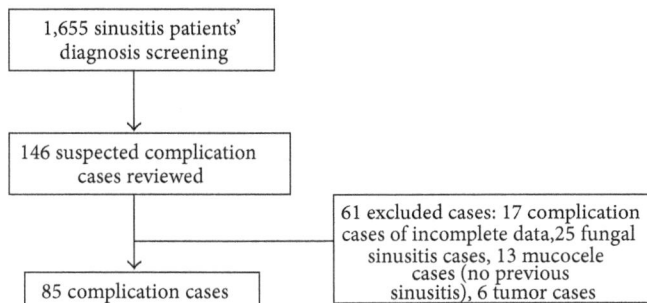

FIGURE 1: Study flow.

(1) The local complications [2] included facial cellulitis, facial abscesses, osteomyelitis, and mucocele/mucopyocele that occurred either after the sinus surgery or following a previous history of sinusitis.

(2) The orbital complications were classified into five groups: inflammatory oedema, orbital cellulitis, subperiosteal abscesses, orbital abscesses, and cavernous sinus thrombosis [2, 3].

(3) The intracranial complications (IC) were classified into meningitis, brain abscesses (e.g., epidural and subdural), intracerebral abscesses, and dural sinus thrombosis (e.g., cavernous sinus and superior sagittal sinus) [3].

(4) The authors classified cranial nerve (CN) palsy as a separate type of complication.

The data for the patients' characteristics, the organisms involved, and the outcomes of treatment were gathered. Anaerobic cultures were not available in the routine emergency setting of the hospital.

2.1. Statistical Analysis. The data were analysed using the STATA program version 11.0 (Stata Corporation, Texas, USA). The exact probability test was used for the proportion of the complications between the age groups, and multinomial logistic regression was used for the outcomes.

The Research Ethics Committee of the Faculty of Medicine of Chiang Mai University approved the study protocol.

3. Results

There were 146 suspected cases of complications in the 1,655 admitted sinusitis patients. The remainder of the patients had been admitted for sinus surgery due the failure to medically control their sinusitis. After reviewing the patients' histories, 85 patients (5.1%) were included in the study. Figure 1 shows the 61 excluded cases, including 17 cases with incomplete data (five cases of mucocele, eight of orbital complications, one case of meningitis with an orbital complication, one of cavernous sinus thrombosis, one case with intracranial (IC) and orbital complications, and one of cerebellar abscess with a cavernous sinus thrombosis), 25 cases of fungal sinusitis, 13 cases of mucocele without a history of sinusitis (four cases

had a history of a head injury and nine had no previous nasal complaints), and six tumour cases. The diagnoses of the complications were made based on the clinical findings and CT scans. Lumbar punctures and CSF examinations were performed on the patients suspected of having meningitis. All of the cases were treated empirically with intravenous antibiotics according to the organisms determined to be involved. Surgical drainage of the involved sinus, with or without the area of complication, was performed for all but one adult case with meningitis that improved with medical treatment alone.

Fifty males (58.8%) and 35 females (35%) were included in the study. Fourteen of the patients were children younger than 15 years (16.5%), and 71 were adults (83.5%). The mean age was 43.5 (±23.3), ranging from one month to 81 years. Overall, 27 of the patients had more than one type of complication (Table 1). Twenty-five of the patients (29.4%) had at least one known underlying condition that had the potential to affect their immune status and outcomes: diabetes mellitus (18.8%), chronic renal failure (8.2%), malignancy (5.9%), chronic liver disease (3.5%), and HIV infection (2.4%). The most common type of complication was orbital in nature (Table 1).

There were 15 cases of CN palsy without other types of complications. Nine of the patients had isolated unilateral or bilateral sphenoiditis, four patients had pansinusitis that also involved the sphenoid sinus, one patient had ethmoiditis, and one patient had both maxillary sinusitis and frontal sinusitis.

Of the 29 cases with local complications, facial cellulitis or an abscess was the most common complication (15 cases), followed by mucocele (12 cases) and osteomyelitis (two cases). All of the local complications except for the mucocele included the maxillary sinus with or without other sinus involvements.

In the orbital complications group (41 cases), a subperiosteal abscess was the most common complication (16 cases), followed by orbital cellulitis (10 cases), periorbital cellulitis (eight cases), cavernous sinus thrombosis (six cases), and orbital abscess (one case).

In the 24 cases of intracranial (IC) complications, five of the patients had more than one intracranial complication. The incidences of intracranial (IC) complication included 13 cases of meningitis, five brain abscesses (temporal, frontal, midbrain and pons, epidural, and along the superior sagittal sinus), and eleven cases with dural venous sinus thrombosis (eight cases of cavernous sinus thrombosis, two cases of transverse sinus and sigmoid sinus thrombosis, and one superior sagittal sinus). There were also other uncommon ICN findings, such as internal carotid artery (ICA) thrombosis, intraventricular hemorrhaging, and hydrocephalous.

The most common sinus involvement in the IC complications was the sphenoid sinus, either isolated (10 cases) or combined with the posterior ethmoid sinus (four cases). There were six cases of pansinusitis in this type of complication, three of which involved the frontal sinus alone or in combination with the ethmoid sinus and one case in which data were unavailable on the sinus involvement. Other systemic findings included sepsis, disseminated intravascular coagulation (DIC), acute respiratory failure, and liver failure.

TABLE 1: Type of complication from sinusitis.

Type(s) of complication	Patients (%)	Details

1	58 (68.3%)	Local: 14
		  9 cases of mucocele, 2 cases of facial cellulitis, 2 cases of facial abscess, and 1 case of osteomyelitis
		Orbital: 16
		  5 cases of periorbital cellulitis, 5 cases of orbital cellulitis, and 6 cases of subperiosteal abscess (SPOA)
		Intracranial: 13
		  5 cases of meningitis, 2 cases of meningitis with frontal abscess, 1 case of temporal abscess, 1 case of midbrain abscess and CN VII palsy (UMNL), and 4 cases of meningitis with other complications*
		Cranial nerve (CN) palsy: 15
		  2 CN II cases
		  4 CN III cases
		  1 CN IV case
		  3 CN VI cases
		  1 CN III, CN IV case
		  1 CN III, CN VI case
		  3 CN III, CN IV, and CN VI cases

2	17 (20%)	3 mucocele cases
		  2 with SPOA and 1 with optic neuropathy
		8 SPOA cases
		  4 with CN palsy (limitation of EOM all directions, visual loss)
		  3 with facial cellulitis/abscess
		  1 with osteomyelitis
		4 periorbital/orbital cellulitis cases with facial cellulitis/abscess
		1 orbital cellulitis and superior ophthalmic vein thrombosis with meningitis
		1 transverse and sigmoid sinus thrombosis with bilateral CN VI palsy

3	8 (9.4%)	6 cavernous thrombosis cases
		  3 CN II, CN III, CN IV, and CN VI cases
		  1 CN II, VI case
		  1 CN III, VI case
		  1 CN II, VII case
		1 orbital and facial abscess case with blindness
		1 orbital cellulitis, scalp abscess, lid abscess, and superior sagittal sinus thrombosis case

4	2 (3%)	2 cases of cavernous sinus thrombosis with facial abscess or cellulitis

SPOA: subperiosteal abscess; UMNL: upper motor neuron lesion; CN: cranial nerve; EOM: extraocular movement.
*Hydrocephalus, DIC, sepsis, prevertebral abscess, and transverse and sigmoid sinus thrombosis.

TABLE 2: Types of complication classified by age groups.

Types of complication	Age <15 year (14 patients)	Age ≥15 year (71 patients)	P value*
Local (29 patients)	5 (35.7%)	24 (33.8%)	1.000
Orbital (41 patients)	14 (100%)	27 (38.0%)	<0.001
ICN (24 patients)	1 (7.1%)	23 (32.4%)	0.100
CN palsy (30 patients)	3 (21.4%)	27 (38.0%)	0.360

*Exact probability test.
ICN: intracranial; CN: cranial nerve.

With regard to age, all of the children had orbital complications: three with local complications and one with meningitis (Table 2).

After treatment, all of the 14 children (100%) and 45 of the adults (63.4%) fully recovered. Eight of the adult patients died (11.3%), and 18 of the adults were cured with residual morbidity (25.3%) upon hospital discharge. Of all of the cases of morbidity, those with limitations in extraocular movements recovered within two months of the follow-up period (eight cases), but the visual impairment (five cases), facial deformity/weakness (two cases) and hemiparesis (three cases) did not recover. Seven of the eight cases of mortality had intracranial complications, such as venous sinus thrombosis and meningitis with sepsis, and the other case had orbital cellulitis and sepsis. The results of the blood cultures were available for five of the eight deaths, two of which did not identify an organism and three in which the identified organisms were *Chryseobacterium indologenes*, *Staphylococcus aureus* (MRSA), and micrococcus spp.

Multinomial logistic regression was used for the analysis of the outcomes according to the number and type of complications and adjusted for age group, gender and comorbidities such as diabetes, liver disease, chronic renal disease, malignancy and HIV infection. The cases with more numerous types of complications had poorer outcomes (Table 3). Among the different types of complications,

TABLE 3: Risk (odds ratio and 95% confidence interval) of poor clinical outcomes (recovery with morbidity or death) from the total number of complication types*, analysed by multinomial logistic regression.

Poor clinical outcomes	OR	95% CI		P value
Recovery with morbidity	2.49	1.15,	5.37	**0.020**
Death	3.27	1.24,	8.63	**0.017**

Total number of complication types*: combined number of any type of sinusitis complication (local, orbital, intracranial complications, and cranial nerve palsy), ranging from 1 to 4.
Adjusted for age, gender, and comorbidities: diabetes, liver disease, chronic renal disease, malignancy, and HIV infection.

the IC complication alone had both significant morbidity ($P = 0.042$) and mortality ($P = 0.020$) (Table 4).

The pus culture reports were successfully obtained for 60 of the cases (70.1%), 24 of which showed no organisms. In the 36 cases with positive specimens, the organisms were either single or multiple, including seven cases of coagulase negative *Staphylococcus* (11.7%), five cases of *S. aureus* (8.3%), one case of methicillin-resistant *Staphylococcus aureus* (MRSA) (1.7%), seven cases of *Streptococcus* spp. (11.7%), five cases of *Pseudomonas aeruginosa* (8.3%), five cases of *Klebsiella* species (8.3%), three cases of *Enterococcus* spp. (5%), three cases of *Enterobacter* spp. (5%), three cases of *Diphtheroid bacilli* (5%), and four *Acinetobacter* spp. (6.7%), in addition to others, including *Haemophilus influenza*, *Neisseria* spp., *Corynebacterium* spp., *Pasteurella* spp., *E coli*, *Citrobacter koseri*, *Proteus* spp., *Aeromonas hydrophila*, and *Burkholderia pseudomallei*.

4. Discussion

Complications of sinusitis continue to occur despite the worldwide availability of antibiotics and do not always result in a complete recovery.

The results shown in Tables 1 and 2 demonstrate that the most common complication was the orbital complication, which is in accordance with the findings of the previous studies [9–12]. However, in our hospital, orbital cellulitis and subperiosteal abscesses were more commonly found than the periorbital cellulitis previously reported. This may be the result of the response to the antibiotics used in periorbital cellulitis, which improved the disease and did not require a surgical referral from other hospitals. Furthermore, in the comparison of the types of complications in the different age groups, the orbital complication was significantly more common in the children ($P < 0.001$), Table 2.

The second most common complication in this study was cranial nerve(s) palsy, followed by local complications. Other previous studies, however, have reported IC complications to be the second most common complication [2, 3]. This difference in findings may be explained by the high proportion of adults in this study, the severity of the disease, and the sinus cases that required surgical referrals, as at the beginning of our study, sphenoid sinus surgery was not performed in the other local hospitals. Table 1 shows the 15 cases that presented with CN palsy either alone or in combination with other

TABLE 4: Risk (odds ratio and 95% confidence interval) of poor clinical outcomes (recovery with morbidity or death) from sinusitis, classified by types of sinusitis complication, analysed by multinomial logistic regression.

Poor clinical outcomes and types of complication	OR	95% CI		P value
Recovery with morbidity				
Local	1.67	0.33,	8.40	0.534
Orbital	1.58	0.42,	5.97	0.466
IC	4.61	1.06,	20.08	**0.042**
CN palsy	3.55	0.85,	14.82	0.082
Death				
Local	1.02	0.04,	28.18	0.990
Orbital	4.82	0.15,	156.26	0.376
IC	106.55	2.06,	5512.16	**0.020**
CN palsy	0.75	0.02,	23.94	0.872

CN: cranial nerve; IC: intracranial.
Adjusted for age, gender, and comorbidities: diabetes, liver disease, chronic renal disease, malignancy, and HIV infections.

types of complications. Potential explanations for this result may include poor hygiene, ethnicity, and the differences in the craniofacial complex and cranial base orientation, for example, the large cranial base angle in the Asian population [13–16]. As the basicranium influences the cranial shape [13], it may also affect the bone thickness and the configuration of the neurocranium as well as the facial appearance. In turn, these features may also affect the pathway for the spread of the infection and inflammation to the vasculature, bone, and cranial nerves. This suggestion is supported by the fact that sphenoid sinusitis, which has a prevalence of 1–2.7% according to the literature, is commonly observed in Asian practice, as well as in this study [5–7, 17–20]. Moreover, as in a previous study [8], the sphenoid sinus rather than the frontal sinus is the most common source of IC complications in the Thai population.

In one study in the literature, the results of treatment have been reported to vary according to the complications: 6% of the patients with IC complications died (ranging from 0 to 16%) and 23% were disabled (ranging from 0 to 46%) [21]. In our study, the overall death rate was 11.3%, while 29% of the patients with IC complications died. These higher rates may be the result of the occurrence of systemic complications such as sepsis or from the severity of the IC complication, both of which would bear monitoring and improvements with medical care.

When the types of complications were compared (adjusted for age, gender, and comorbidities), the IC complication was the only complication that was statistically significant in its poor clinical outcomes, recovery with morbidity ($P = 0.042$), and death ($P = 0.020$) (Table 4). These findings confirm those of other previous studies and should be targeted to improve the treatment outcomes in patients with complications of sinusitis.

5. Conclusion

The orbital complication was the most common complication in both children and adults. Additionally, in adult patients, CN palsy occurred either alone or in combination with other types of complications.

The outcomes of the treatment depended on the number and types of the complications, with the poorest results occurring in the cases with IC complications.

Conflict of Interests

The authors declare that there is no conflict of interests regarding the publication of this paper.

References

[1] R. M. Rosenfeld, D. Andes, N. Bhattacharyya et al., "Clinical practice guideline: adult sinusitis," *Journal of Otolaryngology—Head & Neck Surgery*, vol. 137, no. 3, supplement, pp. S1–S31, 2007.

[2] W. J. Fokkens, V. J. Lund, J. Mullol et al., "EPOS 2012: European position paper on rhinosinusitis and nasal polyps 2012. A summary for otorhinolaryngologists," *Rhinology*, vol. 50, no. 1, pp. 1–12, 2012.

[3] V. A. Epstein and R. C. Kern, "Invasive fungal sinusitis and complications of rhinosinusitis," *Otolaryngologic Clinics of North America*, vol. 41, no. 3, pp. 497–524, 2008.

[4] A. Friedman, P. S. Batra, S. Fakhri, M. J. Citardi, and D. C. Lanza, "Isolated sphenoid sinus disease: etiology and management," *Otolaryngology—Head and Neck Surgery*, vol. 133, no. 4, pp. 544–550, 2005.

[5] M. G. Güvenç, A. Kaytaz, G. Ozbilen Acar, and M. Ada, "Current management of isolated sphenoiditis," *European Archives of Oto-Rhino-Laryngology*, vol. 266, no. 7, pp. 987–992, 2009.

[6] Y. A. Nour, A. Al-Madani, A. El-Daly, and A. Gaafar, "Isolated sphenoid sinus pathology: spectrum of diagnostic and treatment modalities," *Auris Nasus Larynx*, vol. 35, no. 4, pp. 500–508, 2008.

[7] D. S. Sethi, "Isolated sphenoid lesions: diagnosis and management," *Otolaryngology: Head and Neck Surgery*, vol. 120, no. 5, pp. 730–736, 1999.

[8] S. Fooanant, "Complications of sinusitis," in *Proceedings of the 14th ASIAN Research Symposium in Rhinology (ARSR '10)*, Ho Chi Minh City, Vietnam, March 2010.

[9] F. S. Hansen, R. Hoffmans, C. Georgalas, and W. J. Fokkens, "Complications of acute rhinosinusitis in The Netherlands," *Family Practice*, vol. 29, no. 2, pp. 147–153, 2012.

[10] K. D. Schlemmer and S. K. Naidoo, "Complicated sinusitis in a developing country, a retrospective review," *International Journal of Pediatric Otorhinolaryngology*, vol. 77, no. 7, pp. 1174–1178, 2013.

[11] V. Siedek, A. Kremer, C. S. Betz, U. Tschiesner, A. Berghaus, and A. Leunig, "Management of orbital complications due to rhinosinusitis," *European Archives of Oto-Rhino-Laryngology*, vol. 267, no. 12, pp. 1881–1886, 2010.

[12] M. Sultész, Z. Csákányi, T. Majoros, Z. Farkas, and G. Katona, "Acute bacterial rhinosinusitis and its complications in our pediatric otolaryngological department between 1997 and 2006," *International Journal of Pediatric Otorhinolaryngology*, vol. 73, no. 11, pp. 1507–1512, 2009.

[13] D. E. Lieberman, O. M. Pearson, and K. M. Mowbray, "Basicranial influence on overall cranial shape," *Journal of Human Evolution*, vol. 38, no. 2, pp. 291–315, 2000.

[14] M. Hubbe, T. Hanihara, and K. Harvati, "Climate signatures in the morphological differentiation of worldwide modern human populations," *Anatomical Record*, vol. 292, no. 11, pp. 1720–1733, 2009.

[15] S. B. Sholts, P. L. Walker, S. C. Kuzminsky, K. W. P. Miller, and S. K. T. S. Wärmländer, "Identification of group affinity from cross-sectional contours of the human midfacial skeleton using digital morphometrics and 3D laser scanning technology," *Journal of Forensic Sciences*, vol. 56, no. 2, pp. 333–338, 2011.

[16] K. Kuroe, A. Rosas, and T. Molleson, "Variation in the cranial base orientation and facial skeleton in dry skulls sampled from three major populations," *European Journal of Orthodontics*, vol. 26, no. 2, pp. 201–207, 2004.

[17] J. A. Socher, M. Cassano, C. A. Filheiro, P. Cassano, and A. Felippu, "Diagnosis and treatment of isolated sphenoid sinus disease: a review of 109 cases," *Acta Oto-Laryngologica*, vol. 128, no. 9, pp. 1004–1010, 2008.

[18] Z. M. Wang, N. Kanoh, C. F. Dai et al., "Isolated sphenoid sinus disease: an analysis of 122 cases," *Annals of Otology, Rhinology & Laryngology*, vol. 111, pp. 323–327, 2002.

[19] D. Lew, F. S. Southwick, W. W. Montgomery, A. L. Weber, and A. S. Baker, "Sphenoid sinusitis. A review of 30 cases," *The New England Journal of Medicine*, vol. 309, no. 19, pp. 1149–1154, 1983.

[20] D. Gilony, Y. P. Talmi, L. Bedrin, Y. Ben-Shosan, and J. Kronenberg, "The clinical behavior of isolated sphenoid sinusitis," *Otolaryngology—Head and Neck Surgery*, vol. 136, no. 4, pp. 610–615, 2007.

[21] E. Bayonne, R. Kania, P. Tran, B. Huy, and P. Herman, "Intracranial complications of rhinosinusitis. A review, typical imaging data and algorithm of management," *Rhinology*, vol. 47, no. 1, pp. 59–65, 2009.

26

The Correlation of the Tinnitus Handicap Inventory with Depression and Anxiety in Veterans with Tinnitus

Jinwei Hu,[1,2] **Jane Xu,**[3] **Matthew Streelman,**[3] **Helen Xu,**[1,2] **and O'neil Guthrie**[1,2,4]

[1]*Department of Otolaryngology and Head & Neck Surgery, Loma Linda University Medical Center, Loma Linda, CA, USA*
[2]*Loma Linda Veterans Affairs Medical Center, Loma Linda, CA, USA*
[3]*Loma Linda University Medical School, Loma Linda, CA, USA*
[4]*Cell & Molecular Pathology Laboratory, Department of Communication Sciences and Disorders,*
 Northern Arizona University, Flagstaff, AZ, USA

Correspondence should be addressed to Jinwei Hu; jhu@llu.edu

Academic Editor: Sergio Motta

Objective. The mechanisms of tinnitus are known to alter neuronal circuits in the brainstem and cortex, which are common to several comorbid conditions. This study examines the relationship between tinnitus and anxiety/depression. *Subjects and Methods.* Ninety-one male veterans with subjective tinnitus were enrolled in a Veterans Affairs Tinnitus Clinic. The Tinnitus Handicap Inventory (THI) was used to assess tinnitus severity. ICD-9 codes for anxiety/depression were used to determine their prevalence. Pure tone averages (PTA) were used to assess hearing status. *Results.* Descriptive analyses revealed that 79.1% of the 91 tinnitus sufferers had a diagnosis of anxiety, 59.3% had depression, and 58.2% suffered from both anxiety/depression. Patients with anxiety had elevated total THI scores as compared to patients without anxiety ($p < 0.05$). Patients with anxiety or depression had significantly increased Functional and Emotional THI scores, but not Catastrophic THI score. Significant positive correlations were illustrated between the degree of tinnitus and anxiety/depression ($p < 0.05$). There were no differences in PTA among groups. *Conclusions.* A majority of patients with tinnitus exhibited anxiety and depression. These patients suffered more severe tinnitus than did patients without anxiety and depression. The data support the need for multidisciplinary intervention of veterans with tinnitus.

1. Introduction

Subjective tinnitus is an acoustic sensation perceived in the absence of an auditory stimulus. The sounds heard by tinnitus sufferers can be a ringing, buzzing, chirping, roaring, and/or a large variety of other types of sounds. The sound may be intermittent or constant and may localize to the right ear, left ear, either ear, or neither ear but instead may be perceived in the head. Epidemiology studies report that 15%–20% of the adult populations experience some form of tinnitus, either temporarily or permanently [1]. Many people can cope with chronic tinnitus, but for 1-2% of the population, it is a severe handicap significantly impairing their quality of life [2]. According to the American Tinnitus Association, fifty million Americans suffer with tinnitus and tinnitus is the most prevalent service connected disability among veterans (exceeding posttraumatic stress disorder and traumatic brain injury). The Department of Veterans Affairs (VA) has reported that tinnitus disability claims have exceeded 840,000 and the cost to compensate veterans for tinnitus is over $1.28 billion annually. A wide variety of therapies exist for tinnitus, but none have been consistent in providing relief. This is due, in part, to the fact that tinnitus patients have not been clustered in such a way that determines the best treatment approach for individual patients.

Tinnitus is believed to be a sign of dysfunctional auditory neurons [3]. For instance, loud noise exposure is the most prevalent and direct cause of tinnitus and loud noise exposure can induce primary neuropathy of the VIIIth craniofacial nerve (primary auditory neurons) whether the hearing loss recovers or not [4]. Additionally, tinnitus is an early warning sign of auditory neoplastic neuromas [5]. Furthermore, patients with normal hearing and tinnitus reveal deafferentation of high threshold VIIIth nerve fibers with normal low and mid threshold fibers, indicating that only a subset of neurons may drive tinnitus [3]. These and other evidences demonstrate that tinnitus is a signal for the presence of dysfunctional auditory neurons. However, not all auditory neuronal dysfunctions lead to tinnitus and therefore tinnitus may represent a specific type of dysfunction among a specific population of neurons.

Tinnitus may start within the VIIIth nerve but the generating loci may shift with time to more central (brainstem and cortex) regions [6]. This suggests that the particular auditory neuronal dysfunction that drives tinnitus will also affect the central nervous system. This is plausible, given that certain lesions to the VIIIth nerve result in the reorganization of tonotopic maps in the cortex and more important for tinnitus, results in an increase in neuronal excitability from the brainstem to the cortex [7]. Recent literature has shown that up to 77% of the tinnitus population may present with psychiatric comorbidities [2, 8, 9]. Among those psychiatric disorders, anxious and depressive symptoms seem to be the most common complications with tinnitus [10], with a lifetime prevalence of depression and anxiety significantly higher in tinnitus patients than in the general population [9].

When considering psychological comorbidities such as anxiety/depression with tinnitus, the disease may be further categorized into compensated versus decompensated tinnitus. In compensated tinnitus, the patient copes well with the tinnitus and there is little or no psychological strain. On the other hand, in decompensated tinnitus, the tinnitus perception is considered uncontrollable and interferes with the patient's quality of life, causing associated emotional and psychological distress [10].

In compensated tinnitus patients, the perception of auditory sounds is normally extinguished in a short time through the "habituation" mechanism: the superior brain (involving the frontal gyri, cingulate gyrus, and parietal cortices) activates thalamic filters to "switch off" the signal, often independently of the resolution of the dysfunction that generated the tinnitus (peripheral auditory nerve dysfunction and neural changes of the central auditory system). This mechanism was initially identified by Dehaene and Changeux as components a "global neuronal workspace" that is activated by normal hearing subjects when required to consciously process task stimuli and make behavioral responses [11]. It has recently been proposed that engagement of the global workspace is essential for the conscious experience of a tinnitus sound [12]. In other words, the perception of tinnitus requires active awareness of the sensation, and shifting attention extinguishes the perception of the sounds. This understanding plays a significant role in medical therapy for tinnitus, as is evidenced in the use of "masking" techniques.

In decompensated tinnitus, there is usually a negative emotional reaction such as fear, anxiety, or tension associated with the perception of the sounds. Psychology literature illustrates that negative appraisals of events and situations produce distorted misinterpretations of the events, leading to memory and attention strategies that recall negative elements in the environment during the event [13, 14]. Based on this model, Fagelson proposed that the individual suffering from tinnitus could develop emotional disorders such as

anxiety and depression that were triggered or heightened by an inappropriate interpretation of a sensory event [13]. While Fagelson studied a cohort who also suffered from PTSD (posttraumatic stress disorder) and this disorder was not included in our patient population, the finding of these investigators can only be compared with ours with qualification. In this context, negative emotional reinforcement may interfere with the habituation mechanism by drawing more attention to the perception and prolonging the event. Although current literature is still inconclusive on whether tinnitus leads to anxiety and depression or vice versa, substantial physiological evidence through PET and fMRI studies suggests that negative emotions and continued perception of tinnitus are amplified in a vicious negative feedback loop. The model proposed by Georgiewa et al. [15] and Hazell and Jastreboff [16] describes continued perception of tinnitus as being supported by the amygdala, which is also activated by negative emotions. When tinnitus and negative emotions are present together, there is amplification (via increased neuronal excitability) and chronification (via neural plasticity mechanism) of signals, resulting in persistence of both emotional and tinnitus symptoms.

Because of the strong association of tinnitus with psychiatric disorders and indications that veterans are particularly vulnerable to experiencing tinnitus, anxiety, and depression [17], this study aimed to further evaluate comorbid anxiety and depression associated with tinnitus in a veteran population.

2. Subjects and Method

Ninety-one male veterans who reported subjective tinnitus were enrolled in a VAMC Tinnitus Clinic from 2010 to 2013. A retrospective chart review of case history, audiometric thresholds, self-assessment of tinnitus handicap, and ICD-9 codes was conducted on all patients. The Institutional Review Board (IRB) at the VAMC approved all protocols.

Data from the medical records included demographic information, tinnitus case history, audiologic case history, pure-tone thresholds, and information contained in self-assessment inventories. The Tinnitus Handicap Inventory (THI) [18] was used to assess tinnitus severity. The diagnoses of anxiety and depression were established through screening and intake examinations conducted by the Behavioral Medicine Service at the VAMC. ICD-9 codes for anxiety and depression were used to identify patients with these diagnoses and were recorded as categorical data for analysis (e.g., 1 = anxiety, 0 = no anxiety). Pure-tone averages (PTAs) at 500, 1000, and 2000 Hz were used to assess hearing status.

3. Statistics

For the purpose of analyzing the effect of anxiety and depression on tinnitus, the patients were divided into five groups: tinnitus with anxiety, tinnitus without anxiety, tinnitus with depression, tinnitus without depression, and tinnitus with both anxiety and depression (see Table 1). SPSS (version 21;

TABLE 1: The median age, standard deviations, and age ranges of veterans with tinnitus with/without anxiety and depression ($n = 91$).

Age parameters	Anxiety	No anxiety	Depression	No depression	Both	Neither
Median	62.5	61	64	65	65	64
SD	10.04	11.40	10.18	11.76	10.18	9.99
Range	31–73	51–80	31–79	31–84	39–79	51–84

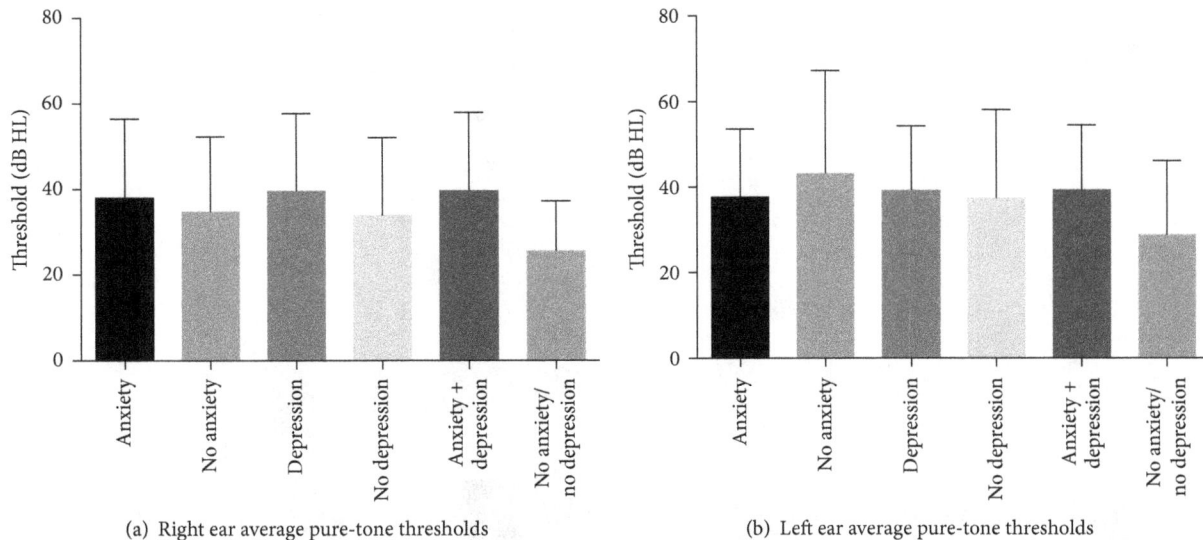

(a) Right ear average pure-tone thresholds

(b) Left ear average pure-tone thresholds

FIGURE 1: The pure-tone average (500, 1000, and 2000 Hz) of both ears among tinnitus patients with and without anxiety and depression.

IBM Corporation, Armonk, NY) was used for statistical analysis. p value was considered significant when $p < 0.05$.

4. Results

4.1. Demographic Information.

Among the 91 male veterans with subjective tinnitus, 72/91 (79.1%) were diagnosed with anxiety; 19/91 (20.9%) were without anxiety; 54/91 (59.3%) were diagnosed with depression; 37/91 (40.6%) were without depression; and 53/91 (58.2%) were diagnosed with both anxiety and depression. Table 1 lists the median age, standard deviations, and age ranges among five groups. There is no significant age difference among the five groups, with the median age being 64.

4.2. Hearing Loss and Tinnitus.

The mean PTAs showed no differences among the five groups or between ears ($p > 0.05$). The average hearing loss was around 38 dB HL among all the groups (Figure 1). A bivariate plot of the PTAs and the THI scores was performed and indicated that both the PTAs and THI scores displayed substantial variability, and the comparison of means demonstrated that self-assessed handicap between the groups was independent of auditory thresholds (data no shown).

4.3. Anxiety, Depression, and Tinnitus.

Tinnitus severity was assessed with the THI. The THI is a 25-item self-report questionnaire that has functional, emotional, and catastrophic subscales. Figure 2(a) shows that patients with anxiety had elevated total THI scores as compared to patients without anxiety ($p < 0.01$). Patients with both anxiety and depression had elevated total THI scores as compared to patients without anxiety ($p < 0.01$). However, there was no significant difference between patients with or without depression ($p > 0.05$). Figure 2(b) shows that patients with either anxiety or depression had significantly increased functional THI scores ($p < 0.01$). Similar to the functional subscale, patients with either anxiety or depression had significantly increased emotional THI scores ($p < 0.01$) (Figure 2(c)). However, there was no statistical difference among the five groups in the catastrophic THI subscale ($p > 0.05$) (Figure 2(d)). Interestingly, patients with both anxiety and depression do not have worsening subscale scores as compared to patients with either condition (Figure 2). There is no significant difference between patients with neither anxiety nor depression versus patients with no anxiety or no depression only in terms of THI and subscale scores (Figure 2).

4.4. Correlations between the Degree of Tinnitus and Anxiety/Depression.

Pearson correlation analysis was performed between scores for tinnitus and anxiety or depression. These are reported in Tables 2(a) and 2(b). Functional THI scores had the strongest correlation with both anxiety and depression, followed by emotional scores. The data also demonstrated that anxiety has higher correlation to more severe tinnitus in terms of total THI score than depression.

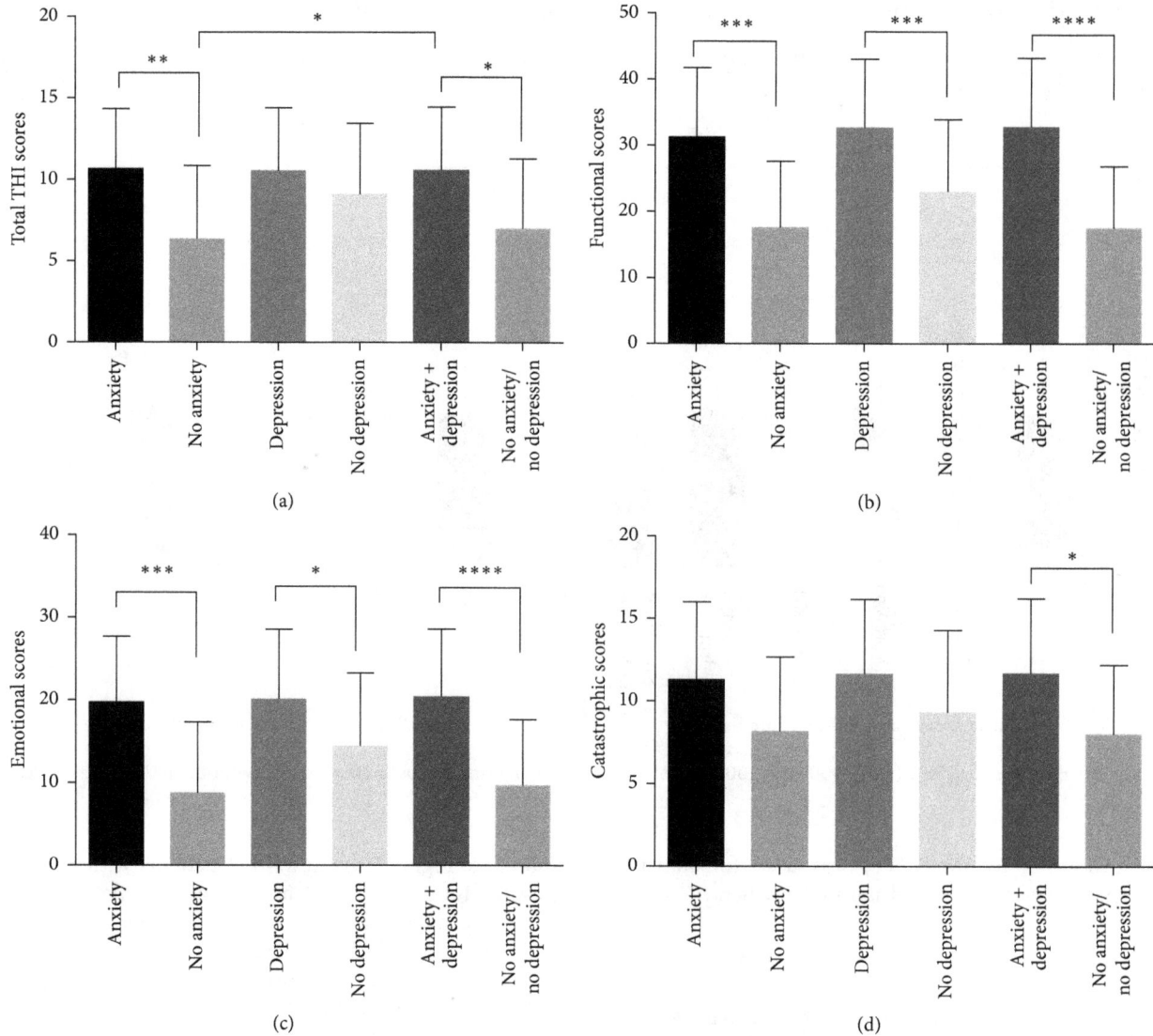

FIGURE 2: Tinnitus severity presented with total THI (a) and functional (b), emotional, (c) and catastrophic subscales (d) among tinnitus patients with and without anxiety and depression. $^*P < 0.05$; $^{**}P < 0.01$; $^{***}P < 0.001$; and $^{****}P < 0.0001$.

4.5. Association between Tinnitus Characteristics and Comorbid Anxiety/Depression.

Tinnitus characteristics such as occurrence (e.g., intermittent and persistent), lateralization (unilateral and bilateral), and years of suffering were evaluated among patients with and without anxiety/depression (see Table 3). The prevalence of anxiety was higher among patients with intermittent tinnitus relative to those who suffer with persistent tinnitus. However, depression was more prevalent among those who suffered with persistent tinnitus relative to intermittent tinnitus. The prevalence of anxiety was higher among patients who suffered with unilateral tinnitus relative to those with bilateral tinnitus. In contrast, the prevalence of depression was higher among patients with bilateral tinnitus compared with patients with unilateral tinnitus. Interestingly, both anxiety and depression tend to be more prevalent after 10 years of suffering with tinnitus. These results suggest that the characteristics of the tinnitus perception may be associated with comorbid conditions.

5. Discussion

5.1. Association of Tinnitus with Anxiety/Depression.

Subjective tinnitus, as opposed to objective tinnitus with a physical stimulation generator within the body, is by far the more common type of tinnitus experienced by patients. Various studies have shown a positive correlation between the severity of tinnitus and quantitative measures of anxiety and depression. Unterrainer et al. showed that comorbid depression was one of the best predictors for perceived severity of tinnitus, greater than duration, pitch, locus of control, or the perception of tinnitus as an illness [19]. According to Zöger et al., increased severity of anxiety and depression is associated with more severe tinnitus [20]. This finding was replicated by Zeman et al. using the THI questionnaire, underscoring the usefulness of the THI as a screening instrument for comorbid depression and anxiety [21]. The same study also found that 15 out of the 25 items of the THI are significantly related to the Beck

TABLE 2: (a) Correlations between the degree of tinnitus and anxiety. (b) Correlations between the degree of tinnitus and depression.

(a)

	Pearson correlation	Significance (2-tailed)
Total THI score * anxiety	0.401	0.000
Functional THI score * anxiety	0.474	0.000
Emotional THI score * anxiety	0.473	0.000
Catastrophic THI score * anxiety	0.279	0.006

(b)

	Pearson correlation	Significance (2-tailed)
Total THI score * depression	0.205	0.044
Functional THI score * depression	0.429	0.000
Emotional THI score * depression	0.331	0.001
Catastrophic THI score * depression	0.271	0.007

Depression Inventory (BDI) and explain more variance of BDI than the total THI score, although the authors suggest the THI should still be considered a one-factor instrument in explaining quality of life. Similar to the above studies, we demonstrated positive correlations between the severity of tinnitus and anxiety or depression in a VA population. Furthermore, tinnitus patients presented with anxiety (79.1%) and depression (59.3%) were considerably higher than the civilian population [2, 8, 9, 22]. This finding might suggest that veterans with tinnitus present with a higher prevalence of anxiety and depression than the general population; however more extensive analysis of larger veterans cohorts will likely be needed to clarify such a predilection.

When comparing anxiety against depression, Granjeiro et al. showed that patients with depression had milder tinnitus symptoms while patients with anxiety had more moderate tinnitus symptoms, and patient with both anxiety and depression together had the most severe tinnitus symptoms [22]. The same study also showed that higher anxiety and depression scores correlated with higher tinnitus severity scores [22]. In addition, our study showed that anxiety has higher correlation to more severe tinnitus than depression, consisting with Granjeiro et al.'s study [22]. However, our study showed that patients with both anxiety and depression do not exhibit worsening tinnitus symptoms as compared to patients with anxiety or depression alone, which was different from the above study [22].

Interestingly, Folmer et al. found no correlation between depression and loudness of perceived tinnitus, but there was a positive correlation with severity of tinnitus [23]. This finding is in line with the model that the severity of tinnitus as elucidated by the questionnaires as well as associated emotional distress is less related to the causes of the condition and more to the cognitive factors of perception and reaction to tinnitus [20, 24]. When looking at the reverse effects of tinnitus on anxiety and depression, Gomaa et al. found that the duration of tinnitus had positive correlation on

both severity of depression and severity of anxiety, but the severity of tinnitus did not affect severity of anxiety and depression [25]. In contrast to most literature, Ooms et al. found no correlation between depression and tinnitus and proposed that high correlations between the THI and BDI scores were due to significant content overlap [26]. The THI was validated against the BDI in its original development, and Langguth et al. further countered Ooms's argument with a study using quality of life measurements that indicated high THI scores reflecting a significant impairment in quality of life, independent of potential overlap in single items between the THI and BDI [27].

Our results showed that there were no differences in the mean PTAs among the five groups or in between ears in all the groups. The average hearing loss was around 38 dB HL. The lack of association between the PTA results and anxiety or depression suggests that these variables are independent in our veteran population. This finding was consistent with the study of Gomaa et al., demonstrating that hearing loss is not the dominant cause of anxiety/depression [25].

5.2. Mechanisms Associated with Anxiety/Depression and Tinnitus. Subjective tinnitus has been assumed to be caused by or associated with damage to the auditory system, both peripherally and centrally [28]. Early theories of tinnitus neural mechanisms suggested a peripheral generation model, where the origin of the phantom sound resides in the inner ear. The idea was based on the fact that cochlear damage from traumatizing sounds and ototoxic agents induced both hearing loss and tinnitus [29]. However, this idea was countered when bilateral auditory nerve sectioning did not always eliminate tinnitus [30]. Current measurements with magnetoencephalography (MEG) show increased spontaneous firing rate (SFR) of neurons in several auditory structures including the dorsal and ventral cochlear nucleus, the inferior colliculus, and auditory cortices, but no signals were seen in peripheral nerve fibers [28]. This evidence points to a central generation model, where all forms of tinnitus, even those triggered by cochlear damage, have origin in the central auditory system (CAS). The connection between peripheral damage and central auditory changes is explained as an alteration in the normal balance between excitatory and inhibitory nerve transmission brought about by loss of inhibition, which leads to increased firing rate [28, 31]. Auditory regions of the cerebral cortex have also been studied in relation to the Tonotopic Reorganization Model of tinnitus. The auditory cortex is organized tonotopically with specific anatomical sites relating to specific frequencies. According to Salvi et al., a lack of afferent signals from a specific region of the cochlea due to hearing loss leads to a rapid reduction in activity within the corresponding section of the auditory cortex, and neural plasticity allows new connections to adjacent cortical fields [32]. As a consequence of this reorganization, a disproportionately large number of neurons become sensitive to lower or high frequencies bordering on the area of hearing reduction. The spontaneous activity seen in this field may be perceived as tinnitus noise.

TABLE 3: Tinnitus characteristics and duration.

Tinnitus character (Total)	Anxiety Total (%)	No anxiety Total (%)	Depression Total (%)	No depression Total (%)	Both Total (%)	Neither Total (%)
Intermittent (35)	28 (80)	4 (11.4)	18 (51.4)	14 (40)	18 (51.4)	4 (11.4)
Persistent (55)	37 (67.3)	10 (18.2)	33 (60)	16 (29.1)	30 (54.5)	9 (16.4)
Bilateral (84)	60 (71.4)	15 (17.9)	49 (58.3)	28 (33.3)	46 (54.8)	14 (16.7)
Unilateral (7)	6 (85.7)	1 (14.3)	4 (57.1)	3 (42.9)	3 (42.9)	0 (0)
More than 10 yrs. (45)	31 (15.6)	7 (15.6)	22 (48.9)	17 (37.8)	21 (46.7)	7 (15.6)
Less than 10 yrs. (21)	13 (19)	4 (19)	10 (47.6)	9 (42.9)	8 (38.1)	4 (19)

Functional MRI have shown increased signals in the middle and superior frontal gyri, the cingulate gyrus, the precuneus, and the parietal cortices in tinnitus patients, verified by EEG and MEG studies. The nonauditory structures are evidenced to play the greatest role in understanding the reaction to tinnitus, the subjective reporting of tinnitus severity, persistence of tinnitus perception, and physiological relationship to comorbid psychological factors such as anxiety and depression. Functional imaging studies show that the subgenual anterior cingulate cortex (sgACC) plays an important role in both coping styles [33] and depression [34]. The most recent study by Vanneste et al. showed that tinnitus patients using a maladaptive coping style show increased scores on the BDI and THI and experienced louder sounds and more distress in comparison to tinnitus patients using adaptive coping styles [35]. The sgACC and ventromedial prefrontal cortex are considered central dysfunction nodes in depression. The dorsolateral prefrontal cortex has been found to play an important role in anxiety [36]. These evidences further suggest why tinnitus can be associated with major depression, anxiety, and other psychosomatic and/or psychological disturbances.

5.3. Treatment of Tinnitus in Patients with Anxiety/Depression. Standard care of subjective tinnitus involves education/ counseling, sound therapy (either hearing aids or sound generators), and intervention to reduce the distress (relaxation therapy or cognitive behavioral therapy (CBT) or both) [37]. The approach to using CBT for tinnitus patients follows the theory that relaxation and cognitive restructuring of thoughts may promote improved and habituated responses to the phantom noise, thus decreasing the distress level and perceived severity of tinnitus. The Cochrane Collaboration in 2007 reviewed 6 trials of CBT for tinnitus with 285 participants. Although the data analysis did not demonstrate any significant effect in the subjective loudness of tinnitus or comorbid depression, there was a significant improvement in quality of life, as assessed by the THI. This outcome further supports the idea that anxiety and depression are comorbidities that affect the perception and response to tinnitus [38].

At present no specific therapy for tinnitus is acknowledged to be satisfactory for all patients. Due to the high comorbidity of tinnitus and psychiatric illnesses [39], a wide range of pharmacological agents, including anticonvulsants, benzodiazepines, tricyclic antidepressants (including amitriptyline, imipramine, and nortriptyline), and selective serotonin reuptake inhibitors (SSRIs), have been used. However, there is debate about whether psychoactive drugs act on the central auditory system and reduce tinnitus directly, whether they act by treating concomitant psychological illnesses, or whether they have a simultaneous effect of both the psychological disturbance and tinnitus [40]. The Cochrane Study in 2012 evaluated six trials involving 610 patients with the object of assessing the effectiveness of antidepressants in the treatment of tinnitus and whether any benefit is due to a direct tinnitus effect or a secondary effect due to treatment of concomitant depressive states. They concluded that all trials assessing tricyclic antidepressants showed slight improvement in tinnitus, but the effects may have been attributed to methodological bias. The SSRI drug trial showed possible benefit for the subgroup that received higher doses of SSRIs, and the observation merits further investigation. The trial investigating trazodone showed an improvement in tinnitus intensity and quality of life, but it did not reach statistical significance. Overall, the Cochrane Collaboration concluded that further research is required because only one of the studies they reviewed met the high quality standard [41].

In conclusion, this study verified that strong correlations exist between the degree of tinnitus and anxiety and depression in a veteran population. Although tinnitus and anxiety/depression involve distinct perceptual events, they may share many mechanisms of the central nerve system, particularly those comprising the auditory cortical pathways and limbic system. A multidisciplinary team comprising psychiatrists and audiologists is needed to evaluate and manage the tinnitus patients with psychiatric comorbidity. There are still numerous uncertainties relating to tinnitus assessment, diagnosis, and treatment. We will further determine mechanisms of tinnitus, including whether particular neuronal dysfunction that drives tinnitus may also lower the threshold of susceptibility for anxiety/depression or vice versa.

Conflict of Interests

The authors declare that there is no conflict of interests regarding the publication of this paper.

References

[1] A. J. Heller, "Classification and epidemiology of tinnitus," *Otolaryngologic Clinics of North America*, vol. 36, no. 2, pp. 239–248, 2003.

[2] M. Salviati, F. S. Bersani, S. Terlizzi et al., "Tinnitus: clinical experience of the psychosomatic connection," *Neuropsychiatric Disease and Treatment*, vol. 10, pp. 267–275, 2014.

[3] R. Schaette and D. McAlpine, "Tinnitus with a normal audiogram: physiological evidence for hidden hearing loss and computational model," *The Journal of Neuroscience*, vol. 31, no. 38, pp. 13452–13457, 2011.

[4] H.-B. Liu, J.-P. Fan, S.-Z. Lin, S.-W. Zhao, and Z. Lin, "Botox transient treatment of tinnitus due to stapedius myoclonus: case report," *Clinical Neurology and Neurosurgery*, vol. 113, no. 1, pp. 57–58, 2011.

[5] C. Fahy, T. P. Nikolopoulos, and G. M. O'Donoghue, "Acoustic neuroma surgery and tinnitus," *European Archives of Oto-Rhino-Laryngology*, vol. 259, no. 6, pp. 299–301, 2002.

[6] W. H. A. M. Mulders and D. Robertson, "Progressive centralization of midbrain hyperactivity after acoustic trauma," *Neuroscience*, vol. 192, pp. 753–760, 2011.

[7] R. J. Salvi, J. Wang, and D. Ding, "Auditory plasticity and hyperactivity following cochlear damage," *Hearing Research*, vol. 147, no. 1-2, pp. 261–274, 2000.

[8] E. Marciano, L. Carrabba, P. Giannini et al., "Psychiatric comorbidity in a population of outpatients affected by tinnitus," *International Journal of Audiology*, vol. 42, no. 1, pp. 4–9, 2003.

[9] J. Harrop-Griffiths, W. Katon, R. Dobie, C. Sakai, and J. Russo, "Chronic tinnitus: association with psychiatric diagnoses," *Journal of Psychosomatic Research*, vol. 31, no. 5, pp. 613–621, 1987.

[10] C. Stobik, R. K. Weber, T. F. Münte, M. Walter, and J. Frommer, "Evidence of psychosomatic influences in compensated and decompensated tinnitus," *International Journal of Audiology*, vol. 44, no. 6, pp. 370–378, 2005.

[11] S. Dehaene and J.-P. Changeux, "Experimental and theoretical approaches to conscious processing," *Neuron*, vol. 70, no. 2, pp. 200–227, 2011.

[12] D. De Ridder, A. B. Elgoyhen, R. Romo, and B. Langguth, "Phantom percepts: tinnitus and pain as persisting aversive memory networks," *Proceedings of the National Academy of Sciences of the United States of America*, vol. 108, no. 20, pp. 8075–8080, 2011.

[13] M. A. Fagelson, "The association between tinnitus and posttraumatic stress disorder," *American Journal of Audiology*, vol. 16, no. 2, pp. 107–117, 2007.

[14] R. L. Folmer, "Long-term reductions in tinnitus severity," *BMC Ear, Nose and Throat Disorders*, vol. 2, article 3, 2002.

[15] P. Georgiewa, B. F. Klapp, F. Fischer et al., "An integrative model of developing tinnitus based on recent neurobiological findings," *Medical Hypotheses*, vol. 66, no. 3, pp. 592–600, 2006.

[16] J. W. P. Hazell and P. J. Jastreboff, "Tinnitus. I: auditory mechanisms: a model for tinnitus and hearing impairment," *The Journal of Otolaryngology*, vol. 19, no. 1, pp. 1–5, 1990.

[17] R. Lampert, "Veterans of Combat: still at risk when the battle is over," *Circulation*, vol. 129, no. 18, pp. 1797–1798, 2014.

[18] C. W. Newman, S. A. Sandridge, and G. P. Jacobson, "Psychometric adequacy of the Tinnitus Handicap Inventory (THI) for evaluating treatment outcome," *Journal of the American Academy of Audiology*, vol. 9, no. 2, pp. 153–160, 1998.

[19] J. Unterrainer, K. V. Greimel, M. Leibetseder, and T. Koller, "Experiencing tinnitus: which factors are important for perceived severity of the symptom?" *The International Tinnitus Journal*, vol. 9, no. 2, pp. 130–133, 2003.

[20] S. Zöger, J. Svedlund, and K.-M. Holgers, "Relationship between tinnitus severity and psychiatric disorders," *Psychosomatics*, vol. 47, no. 4, pp. 282–288, 2006.

[21] F. Zeman, M. Koller, B. Langguth et al., "Which tinnitus-related aspects are relevant for quality of life and depression: results from a large international multicentre sample," *Health and Quality of Life Outcomes*, vol. 12, article 7, 2014.

[22] R. C. Granjeiro, H. M. Kehrle, T. S. C. de Oliveira, A. L. Sampaio, and C. A. C. P. De Oliveira, "Is the degree of discomfort caused by tinnitus in normal-hearing individuals correlated with psychiatric disorders?" *Otolaryngology—Head and Neck Surgery*, vol. 148, no. 4, pp. 658–663, 2013.

[23] R. L. Folmer, S. E. Griest, M. B. Meikle, and W. H. Martin, "Tinnitus severity, loudness, and depression," *Otolaryngology: Head and Neck Surgery*, vol. 121, no. 1, pp. 48–51, 1999.

[24] W. Hiller and G. Goebel, "When tinnitus loudness and annoyance are discrepant: audiological characteristics and psychological profile," *Audiology & Neurotology*, vol. 12, no. 6, pp. 391–400, 2007.

[25] M. A. M. Gomaa, M. H. A. Elmagd, M. M. Elbadry, and R. M. A. Kader, "Depression, anxiety and stress scale in patients with tinnitus and hearing loss," *European Archives of Oto-Rhino-Laryngology*, vol. 271, no. 8, pp. 2177–2184, 2014.

[26] E. Ooms, R. Meganck, S. Vanheule, B. Vinck, J.-B. Watelet, and I. Dhooge, "Tinnitus severity and the relation to depressive symptoms: a critical study," *Otolaryngology—Head and Neck Surgery*, vol. 145, no. 2, pp. 276–281, 2011.

[27] B. Langguth, T. Kleinjung, and M. Landgrebe, "Severe tinnitus and depressive symptoms: a complex interaction," *Otolaryngology—Head and Neck Surgery*, vol. 145, no. 3, pp. 519–520, 2011.

[28] L. E. Roberts, J. J. Eggermont, D. M. Caspary, S. E. Shore, J. R. Melcher, and J. A. Kaltenbach, "Ringing ears: the neuroscience of tinnitus," *The Journal of Neuroscience*, vol. 30, no. 45, pp. 14972–14979, 2010.

[29] N. Y. Kiang, E. C. Moxon, and R. A. Levine, "Auditory-nerve activity in cats with normal and abnormal cochleas," in *Sensorineural Hearing Loss. Ciba Foundation Symposium*, pp. 241–273, Churchill Livingstone, London, UK, 1970.

[30] D. M. Baguley, P. Axon, I. M. Winter, and D. A. Moffat, "The effect of vestibular nerve section upon tinnitus," *Clinical Otolaryngology and Allied Sciences*, vol. 27, no. 4, pp. 219–226, 2002.

[31] H. Wang, T. J. Brozoski, and D. M. Caspary, "Inhibitory neurotransmission in animal models of tinnitus: maladaptive plasticity," *Hearing Research*, vol. 279, no. 1-2, pp. 111–117, 2011.

[32] R. J. Salvi, A. H. Lockwood, and R. Burkard, *Neural Plasticity and Tinnitus*, Singular, San Diego, Calif, USA, 2000.

[33] E. Kross, M. Davidson, J. Weber, and K. Ochsner, "Coping with emotions past: the neural bases of regulating affect associated with negative autobiographical memories," *Biological Psychiatry*, vol. 65, no. 5, pp. 361–366, 2009.

[34] W. C. Drevets, J. L. Price, and M. L. Furey, "Brain structural and functional abnormalities in mood disorders: implications for neurocircuitry models of depression," *Brain Structure & Function*, vol. 213, no. 1-2, pp. 93–118, 2008.

[35] S. Vanneste, K. Joos, B. Langguth, W. T. To, and D. De Ridder, "Neuronal correlates of maladaptive coping: an EEG-study in tinnitus patients," *PLoS ONE*, vol. 9, no. 2, Article ID e88253, 2014.

[36] F. Fregni, R. Marcondes, P. S. Boggio et al., "Transient tinnitus suppression induced by repetitive transcranial magnetic stimulation and transcranial direct current stimulation," *European Journal of Neurology*, vol. 13, no. 9, pp. 996–1001, 2006.

[37] D. Baguley, D. McFerran, and D. Hall, "Tinnitus," *The Lancet*, vol. 382, no. 9904, pp. 1600–1607, 2013.

[38] P. Martinez Devesa, A. Waddell, R. Perera, and M. Theodoulou, "Cognitive behavioural therapy for tinnitus," *The Cochrane Database of Systematic Reviews*, no. 9, Article ID CD005233, 2007.

[39] L. McKenna, R. S. Hallam, and R. Hinchcliffe, "The prevalence of psychological disturbance in neurotology outpatients," *Clinical Otolaryngology and Allied Sciences*, vol. 16, no. 5, pp. 452–456, 1991.

[40] D. J. McFerran and D. M. Baguley, "Is psychology really the best treatment for tinnitus?" *Clinical Otolaryngology*, vol. 34, no. 2, pp. 99–102, 2009.

[41] P. Baldo, C. Doree, P. Molin, D. McFerran, and S. Cecco, "Antidepressants for patients with tinnitus," *The Cochrane Database of Systematic Reviews*, vol. 9, Article ID CD003853, 2012.

27

The Epworth Sleepiness Scale in the Assessment of Sleep Disturbance in Veterans with Tinnitus

Yuan F. Liu,[1] **Jinwei Hu,**[1] **Matthew Streelman,**[2] **and O'neil W. Guthrie**[1,2,3]

[1]*Department of Otolaryngology-Head and Neck Surgery, Loma Linda University Medical Center, 11234 Anderson Street, Loma Linda, CA 92354, USA*
[2]*Loma Linda University School of Medicine, 11175 Campus Street, Loma Linda, CA 92350, USA*
[3]*Loma Linda Veterans Affairs Medical Center, 11201 Benton Street, Loma Linda, CA 92357, USA*

Correspondence should be addressed to Yuan F. Liu; yfangl09@gmail.com

Academic Editor: Leonard P. Rybak

Purpose. Tinnitus and sleep disturbance are prevalent in veterans, and a better understanding of their relationship can help with tinnitus treatment. *Materials and Methods.* Retrospective chart review of 94 veterans seen in audiology clinic between 2010 and 2013 is presented. *Results.* The mean age was 62 years, and 93 of 94 veterans were males. The majority (96%) had hearing loss. The positive predictive value of the ESS for sleep disorder was 97% and the negative predictive value was 100%. Veterans with a Tinnitus Handicap Inventory (THI) score ≥38 had significantly higher Epworth Sleepiness Scale (ESS) scores compared to those with THI score <38 ($P = 0.006$). The former had a significantly higher incidence of PTSD, anxiety, and sleep disorder. A subgroup of patients had normal sleep despite rising THI scores. Bilateral tinnitus, vertigo, and anxiety were found to be predictors of sleep disturbance. *Conclusions.* The ESS can be used as a tool in the initial assessment of sleep disorders in veterans with tinnitus. Higher tinnitus handicap severity is significantly associated with greater sleep disturbance. Optimal management of tinnitus may require concomitant treatment of sleep disorder, PTSD, anxiety, and depression.

1. Introduction

Tinnitus, defined as the perception of sound without an external source, affects an estimated 35 to 50 million Americans or 5 to 15% of the general population [1–5]. Although the majority of those affected by tinnitus habituate to the condition and do not seek treatment, 10–20% experience tinnitus as a severe handicap [6].

Those who live with tinnitus may be burdened by comorbid stressors such as sleep disorders, depression, anxiety disorder, and suicidal ideation [7–9]. These conditions negatively impact many aspects of daily life, causing impairments in work and memory and reducing quality of life [7, 8, 10].

Sleep disturbance is one of the most common comorbidities associated with tinnitus [11–13]. The prevalence of sleep disorders in patients with tinnitus varies from 25 to 77%, with almost 50% reporting insomnia [6, 14–16]. Hébert and Carrier found that patients suffering from tinnitus reported greater sleep difficulties compared to controls,

specifically in sleep efficiency and sleep quality [17]. Using questionnaires, other studies have found a higher prevalence of sleep complaints in tinnitus sufferers compared to the general population [13, 18]. It has also been shown that sleep disturbance strongly predicts lower tinnitus tolerance, while successful treatment of tinnitus results in fewer sleep complaints [11, 17, 19–21].

There is no definitive explanation of how tinnitus may lead to sleep disturbance. It has been postulated that when environmental noise wanes at night, tinnitus awareness may rise with the initiation of unhelpful thoughts, mood changes, and physical reactions, thereby initiating a cycle of anxiety, arousal, and distress [22]. Whatever the mechanism, it is important to note that insomnia is associated with functional impairment and decreased quality of life, especially among subjects with tinnitus who are older than 50 years of age [2, 11, 14, 23].

There are currently more than 20 million US veterans, a predominantly male, aging population with a history of noise exposure that is served by the Veterans Health Administration [24]. This cohort is especially prone to developing tinnitus, which has an increasing prevalence with age, and affects men more commonly than women [4, 25–27].

With the aid of the Epworth Sleepiness Scale (ESS), Tinnitus Handicap Inventory (THI), Tinnitus and Hearing Survey (THS), and Tinnitus Problem Checklist (TPC), we sought to address the following questions: can the ESS be used in the initial assessment of sleep disturbance in veterans with tinnitus? If so, among veterans with different degrees of tinnitus handicap severity, is there a difference in sleep disturbance? Are there any differences in demographics, hearing profiles, or psychiatric comorbidities that can distinguish veterans with different degrees of tinnitus? Can any characteristics of veterans with tinnitus help predict sleep disturbance?

2. Materials and Methods

2.1. Data Gathering. A retrospective chart review was conducted at the Veterans Affairs Medical Center (VAMC) in Loma Linda, CA, on patients with tinnitus complaints. The Loma Linda VAMC serves about 67,000 veterans living in the San Bernardino and Riverside Counties. Audiologic, otologic, and psychiatric data were retrieved from the computerized patient record system (CPRS). Charts for 117 patients were reviewed and 94 patients who had at least a completed Tinnitus Handicap Inventory and pure-tone audiometry data were included in the final analyses. These charts were from patients who visited the Loma Linda VAMC audiology clinic between 2010 and 2013. The data collected from CPRS included ICD-9 codes along with qualitative (e.g., type, severity, and degree) and quantitative (e.g., parametric results from diagnostic and screening tests) data when available. All procedures were reviewed and approved by the Institutional Review Board at the Loma Linda VAMC.

2.2. Epworth Sleepiness Scale (ESS). The ESS is a standardized tool used to measure daytime sleepiness. It contains 8 questions, each scoring 0–3 with increasing number signifying higher chance of "dozing" while engaged in specific activities of daily life. A score of less than 10 is generally considered clinically normal [28–30]. The ESS was developed in 1991, was modified in 1997, and has become the most frequently used method worldwide for assessing daytime sleepiness due to its reliability, consistency, and ease of use [28, 31, 32].

2.3. Tinnitus Handicap Inventory (THI). The THI is a survey containing 25 questions. Each question is worth up to 4 points, with 4 for "yes," 2 for "sometimes," and 0 for "no," for a total of 100 points. A score of 0–16 denotes no handicap from tinnitus, 18–36 denotes mild handicap, and 38–56 denotes moderate handicap, and higher scores denote severe handicap. The questions can be divided into three categories which contribute to three subscales: functional (11 questions, 48 points), emotional (9 questions, 32 points), and catastrophic (5 questions, 20 points). The functional score reflects the effect of tinnitus on mental, social, occupational, and physical functioning. The emotional score reflects affective response to

tinnitus. The catastrophic score reflects desperation, inability to escape, perception of having a terrible disease, lack of control, and inability to cope with tinnitus. The THI has been validated for being a robust tool for measuring the effect of tinnitus on daily life, with a score of 38 or higher suggesting significant tinnitus requiring intervention [33–36].

2.4. Tinnitus and Hearing Survey (THS). The THS contains 10 questions; each scored 0–4 for increasing tinnitus, hearing, and/or sound intolerance severity. Four questions are for tinnitus, 4 questions are for hearing loss, and 1 question is for hyperacusis. A final, unscored question is answered yes or no regarding severity of hyperacusis. The THS is a nonvalidated instrument that is used to rapidly determine how much of a reported problem is due to tinnitus, hearing, and/or hyperacusis. This measurement is often necessary because tinnitus patients tend to confuse hearing problems with tinnitus problem. Therefore, the THS is an efficient screening tool that allows clinicians to differentiate which of the three problems (tinnitus, hearing, and/or hyperacusis) is most troublesome to the patient [37, 38]. A total score of 3 or more on the tinnitus portion of the survey may suggest a need for clinical intervention [38–41].

2.5. Tinnitus Problem Checklist (TPC). The TPC is used to identify bothersome tinnitus situations [38]. The patient is instructed to select a situation where tinnitus is most bothersome. The patient then chooses the first, second, and third most bothersome tinnitus situations. The selections include falling asleep at night, staying asleep at night, waking up in the morning, reading, working on the computer, relaxing in my recliner, napping during the day, planning activities, driving, and others (where the patient can report a situation that is not listed among the choices).

2.6. Statistics. Analyses of continuous variables were performed using 2-tailed, unequal variance, Student's t-test, while analyses of nominal and ordinal variables were performed using Fisher's exact test. Fisher's exact test was chosen in place of Pearson's *chi*-squared test in order to eliminate limitations dealing with low counts of "yes" or "no" for some variables. Analysis of variance (ANOVA) was used to compare more than 2 groups of continuous variables. Linear regression was performed using Minitab 17. Odds ratios calculated from coefficients of the linear regression model are reported with 95% confidence intervals (CI). Other analyses were performed using Microsoft Excel 2010. Means are reported with ± standard deviations (SD). For all variables, a P value < 0.05 was considered to be statistically significant.

3. Results

Demographic, otologic, audiologic, and psychiatric profiles are presented in Table 1. Of 94 veterans, 93 (99% patients) were male and 1 was female. The mean age was 62 years. Veterans from the Army, Navy, and Air Force were represented. Military noise was the predominant source of noise

Table 1: Demographic, otologic, audiologic, and psychiatric profiles. SD: standard deviation, normal ear: tympanic membrane and external auditory canal, 3F-PTA: 3-frequency-pure-tone average (500, 1,000, and 2,000 Hz), SRT: speech reception threshold, WDS: word discrimination score, and PTSD: posttraumatic stress disorder.

Total of 94 patients	Patients	% (mean ± SD, median, min–max)	Unknown
Sex			
Male	93	99	0
Female	1	1	0
Age		(62 ± 10.3, 64, 31–84)	
Service			
Army	35		
Navy	13		41
Air force	5		
Noise exposure			
Military	67		24
Occupational	36		25
Recreational	21		39
All	69		21
Previous hearing aids use	18		7
Vertigo	23		20
Middle ear symptoms	14		9
Ear surgery	7		2
Ear injury	9		23
Ear infection	10		45
Ear pain	16		36
Aural fullness or pressure	18		32
Normal ear			
Left	91	97	0
Right	90	96	0
Left hearing loss			
Sensorineural	87	93	2
Mixed	2	2	
Right hearing loss			
Sensorineural	86	91	2
Mixed	2	2	
3F-PTA			
Left	94	(28 ± 14.3, 25, 6.7–83.3)	0
Right	94	(27 ± 15.3, 25, 5–93)	0
SRT			
Left	92	(25 ± 13.5, 25, 0–80)	2
Right	91	(24 ± 15.1, 20, 0–100)	3
WDS			
Left	92	(91 ± 12.7, 95, 0–100)	2
Right	92	(90 ± 15.1, 96, 20–100)	2
Sleep disorder	37	39	3
PTSD	77	82	4
Anxiety	75	80	2
Depression	57	61	1
Claustrophobia	9		48

exposure, affecting 67 (71%) patients. Vertigo was the most common otologic symptom, affecting 23 (24%) patients. The majority of veterans (90, 96%) had some degree of hearing loss in one ear or the other, and most of them (88, 94%) were diagnosed with sensorineural hearing loss. Sleep disorder, based on ICD-9 diagnoses by Behavioral Health Medicine, was found in 37 (39%) veterans. Furthermore, posttraumatic stress disorder (PTSD) was found in 77 (82%) patients,

TABLE 2: Tinnitus characteristics.

Total of 94 patients	Patients	% (mean ± SD, median, min−max)	Unknown
Tinnitus quality			
Bilateral	74		13
Unilateral	7		
Constant	56		14
Intermittent	24		
Tinnitus duration			
≤1 year	3		
2–10 years	20		
11–20 years	4		
21–30 years	17		37
31–40 years	5		
41–50 years	7		
>50 years	1		
Tinnitus Handicap Inventory			
Total score	94	(57 ± 23.5, 59, 4–96)	0
Functional score	94	(29 ± 11.4, 31, 0–44)	0
Emotional score	94	(17 ± 9.1, 18, 0–32)	0
Catastrophic score	94	(11 ± 4.8, 10, 2–20)	0
Tinnitus and Hearing Survey			
Tinnitus score	94	(10 ± 4.0, 10.5, 0–16)	0
Hearing score	94	(11 ± 4.5, 11.5, 0–16)	0
Hyperacusis score	94	(1.9 ± 1.6, 2, 0–4)	0
Tinnitus Problem Checklist: most bothersome situation			
Falling asleep at night	44		20
Staying sleep	5		
Waking up in the morning	2		
Napping during the day	0		
Epworth Sleepiness Scale score	91	(10 ± 5.4, 9, 1–22)	3

anxiety in 75 (80%) patients, and depression in 57 (61%) patients.

3.1. *Tinnitus Characteristics.* Features specific to tinnitus are presented in Table 2. Most veterans (74, 79%) had bilateral rather than monaural tinnitus, which was predominantly constant (versus intermittent) in 56 (60%) patients. More patients (20, 21%) began suffering from tinnitus within the last 1 to 10 years compared to any other time point. The most bothersome tinnitus situation was falling asleep at night (44 patients, 47%), followed by staying asleep at night (5 patients, 5%) and waking up in the morning (2 patients, 2%).

The average total THI score was 57 ± 23.5 (median 59, range 4–96), suggesting that this population of veterans fell within the severe level (score > 56) of tinnitus handicap and should undergo clinical intervention. The mean score on the tinnitus portion of the THS was 10 ± 4.0 (median 10.5, range 0–16), also indicating that this population had clinically significant tinnitus. The mean THS hearing score was 11 ± 4.5 (median 11.5, range 0–16), signifying the presence of concurrent hearing loss. The mean THS hyperacusis score was 1.9 ± 1.6 (median 2, range 0–4), implying a moderate problem with hyperacusis as well. The mean ESS score was 10 ± 5.4 (median 9, range 1–22), lying at the border of normal

and abnormal daytime sleepiness. Thirty-eight (42%) patients had an ESS score of 10 or more.

3.2. *The Epworth Sleepiness Scale as a Measure of Sleep Disturbance.* Of those veterans with sleep disorder, the average ESS score was 15.4 ± 3.6, compared to 6.0 ± 2.2 for those without sleep disorder ($P < 0.001$). Using an ESS score of 10 as a cutoff for clinical significance, all patients were divided into 2 groups: ESS score < 10 and ESS score ≥ 10. Sleep disorder was found in 0 of 53 patients in the former group and 37 of 38 (97%) patients in the latter ($P < 0.001$). The positive predictive value (PPV) of the ESS for sleep disorder given the above cutoff was 97%, and the negative predictive value (NPV) was 100%. Thus, we elected to use the ESS score as a measure of sleep disturbance in the subsequent analyses.

3.3. *Differences in Sleep Disturbance and Other Characteristics among Tinnitus Severity Groups.* Based on the THI total score, veterans were divided into 4 tinnitus handicap severity groups: no tinnitus handicap (0–16), mild (18–36), moderate (38–56), and severe (>56). The no tinnitus handicap group had a mean ESS of 5.8 ± 2.9, the mild group 7.8 ± 1.6, the moderate group 10.1 ± 4.3, and the severe group 10.7 ± 6.3. ANOVA testing was performed to assess whether

TABLE 3: Significant differences between tinnitus severity groups. THI: Tinnitus Handicap Inventory, SD: standard deviation, PTSD: posttraumatic stress disorder, R WDS: right ear word discrimination score, and THS: Tinnitus and Hearing Survey.

Factor	THI < 38		THI ≥ 38		P value
	Incidence	Mean ± SD	Incidence	Mean ± SD	
PTSD	58.80%		91.80%		0.002
Anxiety	41.20%		90.70%		<0.001
Sleep disorder	11.80%		47.30%		0.007
R WDS		96.0 ± 4.2		89.2 ± 16.5	0.002
THS score					
Tinnitus		4.5 ± 3.1		11.3 ± 3.0	<0.001
Hearing		6.5 ± 5.2		11.7 ± 3.7	0.001
Hyperacusis		0.9 ± 1.0		2.2 ± 1.6	<0.001

TABLE 4: Correlation coefficients for Tinnitus Handicap Inventory (THI) total score and Epworth Sleepiness Scale score.

Group	R^2
All patients	0.046
THI ≤ 46	0.332
THI > 46 and ESS ≥ 10	0.271
THI > 46 and ESS < 10	0.213

there was a difference in mean ESS score among the groups and no significant difference was found ($P = 0.071$). We proceeded with the analysis by aggregating the patients into fewer tinnitus handicap severity groups.

Since a THI total score of 38 was suggested as the cutoff for clinical significance, we divided the patients into 2 groups: THI total score <38 and ≥38. The former group had a mean ESS score of 6.8 and the latter a mean of 9.6 ($P = 0.006$). This is shown in Figure 1. Subsequently, we searched for a difference between the 2 tinnitus groups with respect to each variable listed in Tables 1 and 2. The group with THI total score <38 was found to have a significantly lower incidence of PTSD, anxiety, and sleep disorder, higher average right ear word discrimination score, and lower THS tinnitus, hearing, and hyperacusis scores. Notably, there was no difference in other measures of hearing loss, and there was a near-significant difference in rate of depression (39% in THI <38 group, 67% in THI ≥ 38 group, $P = 0.057$). Table 3 summarizes these significant factors.

A scatterplot was constructed to evaluate the global association between tinnitus (total THI score) and sleep disturbance (ESS score), as shown in Figure 2. On visual inspection, a portion of the data appeared to drift upwards while a portion appeared to plateau or drift slightly downwards at around an ESS score of 10. Taking this observation into account, the data was partitioned into 3 groups to more clearly define correlational attributes between these variables: patients with THI scores ≤46, designated as "normal"; patients with THI scores >46 and ESS scores ≥ 10, designated as "high-high"; and patients with THI scores >46 and ESS scores < 10, designated as "high-normal." Table 4 provides a summary of correlation coefficients (R^2). Comparing the

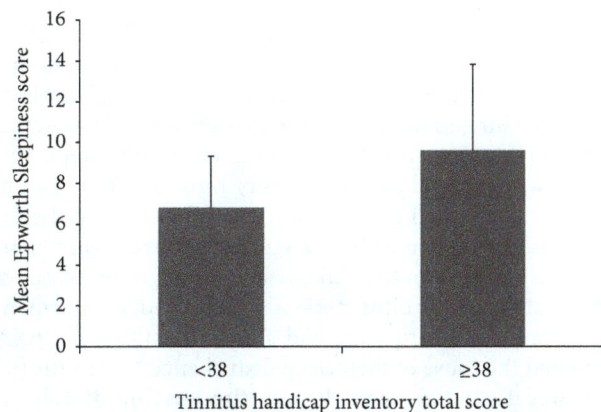

FIGURE 1: Mean Epworth Sleepiness Scale (ESS) score for Tinnitus Handicap Inventory (THI) total score <38 and ≥38. Vertical bars with caps indicate standard deviations.

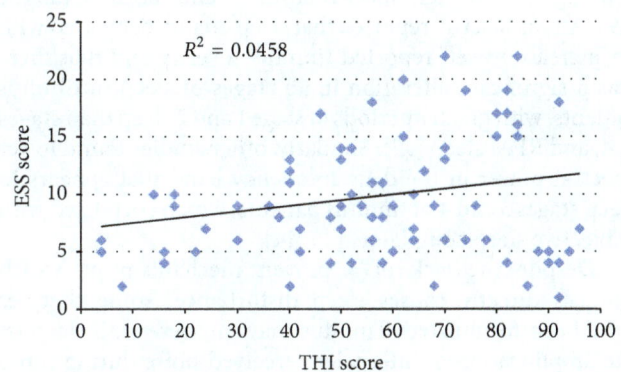

FIGURE 2: Scatterplot of Tinnitus Handicap Inventory (THI) score versus Epworth Sleepiness Scale (ESS) score.

high-high group and the high-normal group in terms of characteristics listed in Tables 1 and 2, the former had a higher percentage of bilateral tinnitus (100% versus 80%, $P = 0.025$), lower left ear word discrimination score (89.8 versus 93.8, $P = 0.049$), and higher THS hearing score (13.1 versus 11.4, $P = 0.028$).

3.4. Predictors of Sleep Disturbance among Tinnitus Patients. To reveal which demographic, otologic, audiologic, or psychiatric variables are associated with sleep disturbance in tinnitus patients, we performed linear regression using all factors listed in Tables 1 and 2 (except sleep disorder) as independent variables to predict sleep disturbance in terms of ESS score < 10 or ≥10. Three variables were found to be significantly associated with an ESS score of ≥10: bilateral tinnitus ($P = 0.006$), vertigo ($P = 0.036$), and anxiety ($P = 0.007$). The odds ratios were 1.80 (95% CI 1.20, 2.70), 1.30 (95% CI 1.02, 1.66), and 1.62 (95% CI 1.15, 2.27), respectively. The adjusted correlation coefficient (R^2) was 0.223.

4. Discussion

Noise, or a perception thereof, can be a natural obstacle to resting and initiating sleep. Many studies have examined the relationship between tinnitus and sleep. An Italian group found that 54% of study patients had sleep disorders and that maintaining sleep was the predominant complaint [22]. Lasisi and Gureje studied 1302 elderly subjects and found that 11.4% had tinnitus, with 51.9% of those with tinnitus reporting insomnia, compared to only 33.8% of those without tinnitus ($P = 0.002$) [16]. In the same study, it was found that difficulty falling asleep and morning wakefulness were significantly associated with tinnitus. Likewise, a large cross-sectional survey of 4,705 tinnitus patients conducted in Germany discovered that nearly 77% had sleep difficulty and 46.4% attributed the cause of their sleep disturbance to tinnitus [6].

Clinical studies have linked tinnitus specifically to decreased sleep quality [6, 15, 19, 20]. Alster et al. used the Mini Sleep Questionnaire to compare 80 tinnitus patients and a control group (both groups representing military personnel without major psychiatric comorbidities), to find that 77% of the tinnitus group had worse scores, particularly in prolonged sleep latency, microarousals, and morning fatigue [19]. Attanasio et al. reported that sleep quality decreased with an increase in self-reported tinnitus severity and that there was a significant alteration in all stages of sleep in tinnitus patients, with greater periods of stage 1 and 2 sleep than stages 3, 4, and REM sleep [42]. Similarly, other studies found lower spectral power in the delta frequency band that appears in sleep stages 3 and 4 of tinnitus patients, which correlated with subjective sleep complaints [43, 44].

Despite the lack of a proven mechanism by which tinnitus directly causes sleep disturbance, some theories have been formulated. Tinnitus may interfere with sleep by the amplification of internally perceived noise during times of low environmental noise. Also, increased awareness of tinnitus before falling asleep may lead to increased focus on tinnitus and undue anxiety which may lengthen sleep onset latency [6, 22]. On a physiological level, tinnitus has been suggested to lead to sleep disturbance through cortical pathways involving the auditory cortex as well as other nuclei. In the gerbil animal model, tinnitus was induced by salicylate injection or loud noise exposure, and c-fos, a marker of neuronal activity, was screened for and found to be consistently expressed in the auditory cortex, the frontal cortex, areas responsible for behavioral and physiological

stress reactions, and areas controlling autonomic function [45]. A similar pattern of c-fos expression was found in the brains of rats that were exposed to a stressor which led to increased sleep latency, decreased nonrapid eye movement (NREM) and REM sleep, and increased sleep fragmentation [46]. These and other animal studies have led to the notion that auditory information enters the amygdala from either the auditory cortex or the thalamic auditory relay nucleus and is thought to be enhanced in people with tinnitus. In doing so, areas of the amygdala are activated depending on the emotional significance of the stimuli, thereby eliciting a defensive response associated with fear [6].

Patients treated at Veterans Affairs (VA) Hospitals are particularly susceptible to tinnitus and its consequences. Veterans are exposed to high level of occupational noise, with increasing duration of military service correlating with lower hearing sensitivity [47]. Increased noise exposure is the most common cause of tinnitus [48]. As such, it was estimated in 2004 that 3 to 4 million American veterans were suffering from tinnitus and that tinnitus is regarded as one of the most disabling conditions caused by military service [49]. Its predominantly male sex and increased age make the VA population more vulnerable to tinnitus [24]. When the VA population is divided into 5-year age intervals, the greatest number of veterans lies between the ages of 65 and 69 [24]. Subjective tinnitus annoyance seems to increase in men with age, though this may partially be attributed to increased hearing problems with age [50]. For those older than 50 years, the likelihood of problems with sleep maintenance doubles [6].

Thirty-nine percent of our veteran population had an ICD-9 diagnosis of sleep disorder. This is within the range reported in the literature, as discussed previously (about 25–77%). An ESS score of 10 or above has been used as a cutoff for clinically abnormal daytime sleepiness. We found that, with this cutoff, the ESS was able to predict the presence of sleep disorder with a positive predictive value of 97% and negative predictive value of 100%. Therefore, the ESS can be an accurate tool for assessing the presence of sleep disturbance in veterans with tinnitus.

When veterans were divided into 4 tinnitus handicap severity groups, from no tinnitus handicap to severe, we did not find a significant difference in mean ESS score among the groups. However, the no tinnitus handicap and mild tinnitus groups had "normal" range (<10) (mean ESS scores 5.8 and 7.8, resp.), while the moderate and severe groups showed "abnormal" range (≥10) (ESS scores 10.1 and 10.7, resp.). Given the positive trend, there were possibly an insufficient number of subjects to detect a small difference in ESS scores. However, we were able to find a significant difference in ESS scores when patients were divided into 2 larger tinnitus handicap severity groups: THI < 38 and THI ≥ 38. We explored significant differences between these 2 groups and found that the THI < 38 group had a lower incidence of PTSD (59% versus 92%), anxiety (41% versus 91%), and sleep disorder (12% versus 47%). Fagelson found that the incidence of PTSD was 34% in a veteran population suffering from tinnitus, compared to our finding of 82% overall [51]. In primary care clinics, 5–13% of veterans have been found to have PTSD [52]. The general veteran population has been reported to have a lifetime PTSD prevalence of 31% in males and 27% in females [53]. Not only did our veteran population have a much higher rate of PTSD, but we also encountered a dramatic increase in PTSD with an increase in tinnitus handicap severity. This suggests that there is a positive linear or perhaps even exponential relationship between PTSD and tinnitus. Furthermore, there may be a synergistic effect involving tinnitus, PTSD, and sleep disorder in which the disease entities worsen one another's impact. Anxiety, which is closely related to PTSD, likely has a similar influence. Of note was the lower incidence of depression in the THI < 38 group compared to the THI ≥ 38 group (39% versus 67%). We suspect that depression also influences tinnitus, but perhaps our population was not large enough to capture the effect.

Interestingly, we discovered three distinct groups of patients as a function of THI and ESS scores. The group with THI total score ≤46 shared approximately 33% of the variance between THI and ESS scores. Above a score of 46, there was a group with increasing tinnitus handicap as well as increasing daytime sleepiness and a group with increasing tinnitus handicap and steady or decreasing daytime sleepiness. Coincidentally, the ESS cutoff score between the 2 groups approximately corresponds to the borderline of where sleepiness becomes clinically significant [28]. Previous documentation of this phenomenon was not found in the literature. The high-high group (THI > 46 and ESS ≥ 10) had a significantly higher percentage of bilateral tinnitus, lower left ear word discrimination score, and higher THS hearing score. No specific evidence relating tinnitus laterality to sleep disturbance was found in the literature. One can only speculate that unilateral tinnitus can be partially offset by head positioning on the pillow during sleep initiation. The low left ear word discrimination score combined with high THS hearing score might suggest retrocochlear involvement, but, in the absence of specific site-of-lesion assessments, such notions remain speculative.

Finally, we wanted to determine which factors may be used to predict sleep disturbance in a veteran population suffering from tinnitus. We found that bilateral tinnitus, vertigo, and anxiety were associated with ESS score ≥ 10. There is some evidence that lack of sleep may trigger migraines and migrainous vertigo, but no literature was found on a direct relationship between vertigo and sleep disturbance in tinnitus patients [54]. Anxiety has been well documented as a contributor to sleep disturbance [55, 56]. It has also been reported to correlate with tinnitus handicap severity [57].

It appears that PTSD, anxiety, and depression all exacerbate, to some degree, sleep disturbance and tinnitus in the veteran population. There are likely other psychiatric comorbidities that also play a role but were not studied in this paper. This underscores the importance of treatment for these disorders for patients with tinnitus. Antidepressants, such as selective serotonin reuptake inhibitors (SSRIs), have been shown to be effective in psychiatric disorders such as PTSD and depression [58, 59]. There is also evidence for sleep improvement when they are effectively used [60]. However, a 2006 Cochrane Review showed insufficient evidence that antidepressants improve tinnitus [61]. Perhaps future

prospective studies can focus on the efficacy of antidepressants in veterans who are prone to, and present with, both psychiatric disorders and tinnitus, along with sleep disorder. Another avenue for research would be to compare the efficacy of psychotherapy versus antidepressants. What is the cause and effect relationship among tinnitus, sleep, and psychiatric comorbidities? The fact that many patients present with these disorders simultaneously, the lack of objective measurements for severity, and overlapping disease mechanisms all contribute to the complexity of this question. Future physiological studies using more objective tools such as polysomnography, brain MRI, and other imaging modalities, and molecular markers may better elucidate the relationship.

5. Conclusions

The ESS can be used as a tool in the initial assessment of sleep disorders in veterans with tinnitus, with a PPV of 97% and NPV of 100%. There is a positive correlation between tinnitus and sleep disturbance in veterans, as has been shown in the general populations. However, we discovered a higher rate of PTSD (82%) in veterans with tinnitus than previously reported in the literature and found that veterans may suffer from comorbidities such as PTSD, anxiety, and depression which appear to act synergistically to worsen sleep disturbance and/or tinnitus. There appears to be a distinct population of veterans who have high tinnitus handicap severity, yet no sleep disturbance. Unlike this group, those with high tinnitus handicap severity and abnormal sleep perceive increased hearing loss despite a lack of audiometric evidence, the reason for which is unclear. Furthermore, vertigo and bilateral tinnitus seem to contribute to sleep disturbance in tinnitus patients, the mechanism of which has not been explored. Our study supports a need for multifaceted management of tinnitus in veterans, including treatment for psychiatric comorbidities and sleep disturbance, in order to achieve an improvement in tinnitus handicap severity.

Conflict of Interests

The authors declare that there is no conflict of interests regarding the publication of this paper.

Disclosure

The first author had full access to all of the data in the study and takes responsibility for the integrity of the data and the accuracy of the data analysis.

Acknowledgment

The authors would like to acknowledge and thank Dr. Najeeb A. Shirwany for his critical evaluation of this paper.

References

[1] R. R. Coles, "Epidemiology of tinnitus: (1) prevalence," The Journal of Lryngology and Otology, vol. 98, supplement S9, pp. 7–15, 1984.

[2] A. Axelsson and A. Ringdahl, "Tinnitus—a study of its prevalence and characteristics," *British Journal of Audiology*, vol. 23, no. 1, pp. 53–62, 1989.

[3] J. A. Henry, K. C. Dennis, and M. A. Schechter, "General review of tinnitus: prevalence, mechanisms, effects, and management," *Journal of Speech, Language, and Hearing Research*, vol. 48, no. 5, pp. 1204–1235, 2005.

[4] S. J. Veterans, *Tinnitus: Theory and Management*, BC Decker, Lewiston, NY, USA, 2008.

[5] J. Shargorodsky, G. C. Curhan, and W. R. Farwell, "Prevalence and characteristics of tinnitus among US adults," *The American Journal of Medicine*, vol. 123, no. 8, pp. 711–718, 2010.

[6] E. Wallhäusser-Franke, M. Schredl, and W. Delb, "Tinnitus and insomnia: is hyperarousal the common denominator?" *Sleep Medicine Reviews*, vol. 17, no. 1, pp. 65–74, 2013.

[7] R. F. F. Cima, J. W. S. Vlaeyen, I. H. L. Maes, M. A. Joore, and L. J. C. Anteunis, "Tinnitus interferes with daily life activities: a psychometric examination of the tinnitus disability index," *Ear and Hearing*, vol. 32, no. 5, pp. 623–633, 2011.

[8] B. Langguth, "A review of tinnitus symptoms beyond 'ringing in the ears': a call to action," *Current Medical Research & Opinion*, vol. 27, no. 8, pp. 1635–1643, 2011.

[9] J. M. Malouff, N. S. Schutte, and L. A. Zucker, "Tinnitus-related distress: a review of recent findings," *Current Psychiatry Reports*, vol. 13, no. 1, pp. 31–36, 2011.

[10] S. Rossiter, C. Stevens, and G. Walker, "Tinnitus and its effect on working memory and attention," *Journal of Speech, Language, and Hearing Research*, vol. 49, no. 1, pp. 150–160, 2006.

[11] R. S. Tyler and L. J. Baker, "Difficulties experienced by tinnitus sufferers," *The Journal of Speech and Hearing Disorders*, vol. 48, no. 2, pp. 150–154, 1983.

[12] L. Sanchez and D. Stephens, "A tinnitus problem questionnaire in a clinic population," *Ear and Hearing*, vol. 18, no. 3, pp. 210–217, 1997.

[13] R. Asplund, "Sleepiness and sleep in elderly persons with tinnitus," *Archives of Gerontology and Geriatrics*, vol. 37, no. 2, pp. 139–145, 2003.

[14] R. L. Folmer and S. E. Griest, "Tinnitus and insomnia," *American Journal of Otolaryngology*, vol. 21, no. 5, pp. 287–293, 2000.

[15] E. Marciano, L. Carrabba, P. Giannini et al., "Psychiatric comorbidity in a population of outpatients affected by tinnitus," *International Journal of Audiology*, vol. 42, no. 1, pp. 4–9, 2003.

[16] A. O. Lasisi and O. Gureje, "Prevalence of insomnia and impact on quality of life among community elderly subjects with tinnitus," *Annals of Otology, Rhinology & Laryngology*, vol. 120, no. 4, pp. 226–230, 2011.

[17] S. Hébert and J. Carrier, "Sleep complaints in elderly tinnitus patients: a controlled study," *Ear and Hearing*, vol. 28, no. 5, pp. 649–655, 2007.

[18] R. S. Hallam, "Correlates of sleep disturbance in chronic distressing tinnitus," *Scandinavian Audiology*, vol. 25, no. 4, pp. 263–266, 1996.

[19] J. Alster, Z. Shemesh, M. Ornan, and J. Attias, "Sleep disturbance associated with chronic tinnitus," *Biological Psychiatry*, vol. 34, no. 1-2, pp. 84–90, 1993.

[20] K. Eysel-Gosepath and O. Selivanova, "Characterization of sleep disturbance in patients with tinnitus," *Laryngo- Rhino- Otologie*, vol. 84, no. 5, pp. 323–327, 2005.

[21] T. Crönlein, B. Langguth, P. Geisler, and G. Hajak, "Tinnitus and insomnia," *Progress in Brain Research*, vol. 166, pp. 227–233, 2007.

[22] A. B. Fioretti, M. Fusetti, and A. Eibenstein, "Association between sleep disorders, hyperacusis and tinnitus: evaluation with tinnitus questionnaires," *Noise and Health*, vol. 15, no. 63, pp. 91–95, 2013.

[23] S. C. Jakes, R. S. Hallam, C. Chambers, and R. Hinchcliffe, "A factor analytical study of tinnitus complaint behaviour," *Audiology*, vol. 24, no. 3, pp. 195–206, 1985.

[24] US Department of Veterans Affairs, "Veteran Population," Veteran Population Statistics, 2013, http://www.va.gov/vetdata/Veteran_Population.asp.

[25] C. S. Hankin, A. Spiro III, D. R. Miller, and L. Kazis, "Mental disorders and mental health treatment among U.S. Department of Veterans Affairs outpatients: the Veterans Health Study," *The American Journal of Psychiatry*, vol. 156, no. 12, pp. 1924–1930, 1999.

[26] N. Ahmad and M. Seidman, "Tinnitus in the older adult: epidemiology, pathophysiology and treatment options," *Drugs & Aging*, vol. 21, no. 5, pp. 297–305, 2004.

[27] D. M. Nondahl, K. J. Cruickshanks, G.-H. Huang et al., "Tinnitus and its risk factors in the Beaver Dam offspring study," *International Journal of Audiology*, vol. 50, no. 5, pp. 313–320, 2011.

[28] M. W. Johns, "A new method for measuring daytime sleepiness: the Epworth sleepiness scale," *Sleep*, vol. 14, no. 6, pp. 540–545, 1991.

[29] M. W. Johns, "Reliability and factor analysis of the Epworth Sleepiness Scale," *Sleep*, vol. 15, no. 4, pp. 376–381, 1992.

[30] T. B. Kendzerska, P. M. Smith, R. Brignardello-Petersen, R. S. Leung, and G. A. Tomlinson, "Evaluation of the measurement properties of the Epworth sleepiness scale: a systematic review," *Sleep Medicine Reviews*, vol. 18, no. 4, pp. 321–331, 2014.

[31] M. W. Johns, "Sensitivity and specificity of the multiple sleep latency test (MSLT), the maintenance of wakefulness test and the epworth sleepiness scale: failure of the MSLT as a gold standard," *Journal of Sleep Research*, vol. 9, no. 1, pp. 5–11, 2000.

[32] D. J. Buysse, M. L. Hall, P. J. Strollo et al., "Relationships between the Pittsburgh Sleep Quality Index (PSQI), Epworth Sleepiness Scale (ESS), and clinical/polysomnographic measures in a community sample," *Journal of Clinical Sleep Medicine*, vol. 4, no. 6, pp. 563–571, 2008.

[33] C. W. Newman, G. P. Jacobson, and J. B. Spitzer, "Development of the tinnitus handicap inventory," *Archives of Otolaryngology—Head and Neck Surgery*, vol. 122, no. 2, pp. 143–148, 1996.

[34] A. McCombe, D. Baguley, R. Coles, L. McKenna, C. McKinney, and P. Windle-Taylor, "Guidelines for the grading of tinnitus severity: the results of a working group commissioned by the British Association of Otolaryngologists, Head and Neck Surgeons, 1999," *Clinical Otolaryngology and Allied Sciences*, vol. 26, no. 5, pp. 388–393, 2001.

[35] F. Zeman, M. Koller, R. Figueiredo et al., "Tinnitus handicap inventory for evaluating treatment effects: which changes are clinically relevant?" *Otolaryngology: Head and Neck Surgery*, vol. 145, no. 2, pp. 282–287, 2011.

[36] F. Zeman, M. Koller, M. Schecklmann et al., "Tinnitus assessment by means of standardized self-report questionnaires: psychometric properties of the Tinnitus Questionnaire (TQ), the Tinnitus Handicap Inventory (THI), and their short versions in an international and multi-lingual sample," *Health and Quality of Life Outcomes*, vol. 10, article 128, 2012.

[37] J. A. Henry, T. L. Zaugg, and M. A. Schechter, "Clinical guide for audiologic tinnitus management I: assessment," *American Journal of Audiology*, vol. 14, no. 1, pp. 21–48, 2005.

[38] J. A. Henry, T. L. Zaugg, M. A. Schechter et al., *How to Manage Your Tinnitus: A Step-by-Step Workbook*, VA National Center for Rehabilitative Auditory Research, Portland, Ore, USA, 2008.

[39] J. A. Henry, T. L. Zaugg, P. J. Myers, and M. A. Schechter, "The role of audiologic evaluation in progressive audiologic tinnitus management," *Trends in Amplification*, vol. 12, no. 3, pp. 170–187, 2008.

[40] J. A. Henry, T. L. Zaugg, P. J. Myers et al., "Pilot study to develop telehealth tinnitus management for persons with and without traumatic brain injury," *Journal of Rehabilitation Research and Development*, vol. 49, no. 7, pp. 1025–1042, 2012.

[41] T. Zaugg, M. Schechter, S. Fausti et al., "Difficulties caused by patients' misconceptions that hearing problems are due to tinnitus," in *Proceedings of the 7th International Tinnitus Seminar*, Perth, Australia, 2002.

[42] G. Attanasio, F. Y. Russo, R. Roukos, E. Covelli, G. Cartocci, and M. Saponara, "Sleep architecture variation in chronic tinnitus patients," *Ear and Hearing*, vol. 34, no. 4, pp. 503–507, 2013.

[43] I. de Andrés, M. Garzón, and F. Reinoso-Suárez, "Functional anatomy of non-REM sleep," *Frontiers in Neurology*, vol. 2, article 70, 2011.

[44] S. Hébert, S. Fullum, and J. Carrier, "Polysomnographic and quantitative electroencephalographic correlates of subjective sleep complaints in chronic tinnitus," *Journal of Sleep Research*, vol. 20, no. 1, part 1, pp. 38–44, 2011.

[45] C. B. Saper, G. Cano, and T. E. Scammell, "Homeostatic, circadian, and emotional regulation of sleep," *Journal of Comparative Neurology*, vol. 493, no. 1, pp. 92–98, 2005.

[46] G. Cano, T. Mochizuki, and C. B. Saper, "Neural circuitry of stress-induced insomnia in rats," *The Journal of Neuroscience*, vol. 28, no. 40, pp. 10167–10184, 2008.

[47] L. W. Henselman, D. Henderson, J. Shadoan, M. Subramaniam, S. Saunders, and D. Ohlin, "Effects of noise exposure, race, and years of service on hearing in U.S. army soldiers," *Ear and Hearing*, vol. 16, no. 4, pp. 382–391, 1995.

[48] A. Axelsson and D. Prasher, "Tinnitus induced by occupational and leisure noise," *Noise Health*, vol. 2, no. 8, pp. 47–54, 2000.

[49] J. A. Henry, C. Loovis, M. Montero et al., "Randomized clinical trial: group counseling based on tinnitus retraining therapy," *Journal of Rehabilitation Research & Development*, vol. 44, no. 1, pp. 21–32, 2007.

[50] C. Seydel, H. Haupt, H. Olze, A. J. Szczepek, and B. Mazurek, "Gender and chronic tinnitus: differences in tinnitus-related distress depend on age and duration of tinnitus," *Ear and Hearing*, vol. 34, no. 5, pp. 661–672, 2013.

[51] M. A. Fagelson, "The association between tinnitus and posttraumatic stress disorder," *American Journal of Audiology*, vol. 16, no. 2, pp. 107–117, 2007.

[52] The Management of MDD Working Group, "VA/ DoD Clinical Practice Guideline for Management of Major Depressive Disorder (MDD)," 2009, http://www.healthquality.va.gov/guidelines/MH/mdd/MDDFULL053013.pdf.

[53] F. H. Norris and L. B. Slone, "Understanding research on the epidemiology of trauma and PTSD," *PTSD Research Quarterly*, vol. 24, no. 2-3, p. 1, 2013.

[54] S. Salhofer, D. Lieba-Samal, E. Freydl, S. Bartl, G. Wiest, and C. Wöber, "Migraine and vertigo—a prospective diary study," *Cephalalgia*, vol. 30, no. 7, pp. 821–828, 2010.

[55] R. R. Rosa, M. H. Bonnet, and M. Kramer, "The relationship of sleep and anxiety in anxious subjects," *Biological Psychology*, vol. 16, no. 1-2, pp. 119–126, 1983.

[56] T. W. Uhde, B. M. Cortese, and A. Vedeniapin, "Anxiety and sleep problems: emerging concepts and theoretical treatment implications," *Current Psychiatry Reports*, vol. 11, no. 4, pp. 269–276, 2009.

[57] J. B. S. Halford and S. D. Anderson, "Anxiety and depression in tinnitus sufferers," *Journal of Psychosomatic Research*, vol. 35, no. 4-5, pp. 383–390, 1991.

[58] D. J. Stein, N. Zungu-Dirwayi, G. J. van der Linden, and S. Seedat, "Pharmacotherapy for posttraumatic stress disorder," *Cochrane Database of Systematic Reviews*, no. 4, Article ID CD002795, 2000.

[59] B. Arroll, C. R. Elley, T. Fishman et al., "Antidepressants versus placebo for depression in primary care," *Cochrane Database of Systematic Reviews*, no. 3, Article ID CD007954, 2009.

[60] S. Wilson and S. Argyropoulos, "Antidepressants and sleep: a qualitative review of the literature," *Drugs*, vol. 65, no. 7, pp. 927–947, 2005.

[61] P. Baldo, C. Doree, and P. Molin, "Antidepressants for patients with tinnitus," *Cochrane Database of Systematic Reviews*, vol. 9, p. CD003853, 2012.

28

Inferior Turbinate Size and CPAP Titration Based Treatment Pressures: No Association Found among Patients Who Have Not Had Nasal Surgery

Macario Camacho,[1,2] Soroush Zaghi,[3] Daniel Tran,[1] Sungjin A. Song,[1] Edward T. Chang,[1] and Victor Certal[4,5]

[1]*Otolaryngology-Head and Neck Surgery, Division of Sleep Surgery and Medicine, Tripler Army Medical Center, 1 Jarrett White Road, Honolulu, HI 96859, USA*
[2]*Department of Psychiatry and Behavioral Sciences, Sleep Medicine Division, Stanford Hospital and Clinics, Stanford, CA 94304, USA*
[3]*Otolaryngology-Head and Neck Surgery, Division of Sleep Surgery and Medicine, Stanford Hospitals and Clinics, Stanford, CA 94304, USA*
[4]*Department of Otorhinolaryngology, Sleep Medicine Centre, Hospital CUF, 4100-180 Porto, Portugal*
[5]*Centre for Research in Health Technologies and Information Systems (CINTESIS), University of Porto, 4200-450 Porto, Portugal*

Correspondence should be addressed to Macario Camacho; drcamachoent@yahoo.com

Academic Editor: Gerd J. Ridder

Objective. To evaluate the effect of turbinate sizes on the titrated continuous positive airway pressure (CPAP) therapeutic treatment pressures for patients with obstructive sleep apnea (OSA) who have not had nasal surgery. *Study Design*. Retrospective case series. *Methods*. A chart review was performed for 250 consecutive patients. *Results*. 45 patients met inclusion criteria. The mean ± standard deviation (M ± SD) for age was 54.6 ± 22.4 years and for body mass index was 28.5 ± 5.9 kg/m². The Spearman's rank correlation coefficient (r_s) between CPAP therapeutic treatment pressures and several variables were calculated and were weakly correlated (age r_s = 0.29, nasal obstruction r_s = −0.30), moderately correlated (body mass index r_s = 0.42 and lowest oxygen saturation r_s = −0.47), or strongly correlated (apnea-hypopnea index r_s = 0.60 and oxygen desaturation index (r_s = 0.62)). No statistical significance was found with one-way analysis of variance (ANOVA) between CPAP therapeutic treatment pressures and inferior turbinate size (right turbinates p value = 0.2012, left turbinate p value = 0.3064), nasal septal deviation (p value = 0.4979), or mask type (p value = 0.5136). *Conclusion*. In this study, CPAP titration based therapeutic treatment pressures were not found to be associated with inferior turbinate sizes; however, the CPAP therapeutic treatment pressures were strongly correlated with apnea-hypopnea index and oxygen desaturation index.

1. Introduction

There are several medical [1] and surgical [2, 3] treatment options for obstructive sleep apnea (OSA). Patients who use continuous positive airway pressure (CPAP) devices have been shown to have nasal obstruction as a common complaint (estimated prevalence: 25–45%) [4–6]. As described by Poiseuille's Law, airflow resistance is proportional to the length and is inversely proportion to the radius to the fourth power [7]. Because the radius is such an important variable, small changes, such as a 10% increase in the cross-sectional area of the nasal cavity airway, can result in a 21% increase in airflow [8]. Although surgery on the nose has not been shown to dramatically improve OSA [9], it can improve CPAP device use [10].

A recent systematic review and meta-analysis also demonstrated that isolated nasal surgery reduces CPAP device therapeutic treatment pressures by 2-3 centimeters of water pressure (cwp) [10]. Therefore, surgically increasing the size of the nasal airway decreases nasal resistance and reduces CPAP device pressure requirements [10]. However, to our knowledge, for patients who have not undergone nasal surgery it is unknown whether patients with smaller turbinates have lower CPAP therapeutic treatment pressure requirements when compared to patients with larger turbinates. A recently published systematic review did not identify any study in the international literature that used inferior turbinate size as a variable in mathematical equations to predict CPAP [11]. For this study we hypothesized that, in patients who have not had nasal surgery, large turbinates would require higher CPAP therapeutic treatment pressures than small inferior turbinates. Because it has previously been shown that nasal surgery can reduce CPAP therapeutic treatment pressures [12], we planned to exclude patients with prior nasal surgery in order to remove this confounding variable. The objective of this study is to evaluate the effect of turbinate sizes on the CPAP titration based therapeutic treatment pressures (in centimeters of water pressure) for patients with OSA who have not previously undergone nasal surgery.

2. Materials and Methods

The Stanford Hospital and Clinics Institutional Review Board was contacted and written approval was granted prior to commencing this study. The study design is a retrospective case series evaluating 250 consecutive patients. Inclusion criteria are as follows: (1) Stanford Sleep Medicine Clinic patients who had a nasal examination and underwent an attended in-lab CPAP titration study and (2) the nasal examination needed to include nasal septal deviation severity and inferior turbinate grades for the left and right sides separately. Exclusion criteria are as follows: (1) patients who have undergone nasal surgery. The CPAP titration pressures were obtained based on overnight, in-lab polysomnography. The American Academy of Sleep Medicine (AASM) Manual for the Scoring of Sleep and Associated Events was used by Stanford and outside institutions. The Stanford hypopnea scoring criteria included ≥10 seconds with ≥30% reduction in airflow measured by the nasal flow transducer associated with a 3% desaturation and/or an electroencephalogram arousal as described in the AASM scoring manual 2013, version 2.0.2 [13].

In order to fully evaluate the effect of inferior turbinate size, a tool ("Inferior Turbinate Classification System, Grades 1 to 4") [12] was utilized. This Inferior Turbinate Classification System provides a method for grading the amount of airway space that the anterior aspect of the inferior turbinate occupies relative to the total available airway space and is summarized as follows: grade 1 is 0–25% of the total airway space, grade 2 is 26–50% of the total airway space, grade 3 is 51–75% of the total airway space, and grade 4 is 76–100% of the total airway space [12]; see Figure 1. The Nasal Obstruction Symptom Evaluation (NOSE) scale was used to evaluate nasal obstruction and a patient with a score >40 was considered to have nasal obstruction [14].

3. Statistical Analysis

The data was cataloged using Microsoft Excel 2013 (Redmond, WA, USA). The IBM Statistical Package for Social Sciences (SPSS) software version 20 (Armonk, New York, USA) was used for statistical analyses. The patient data was analyzed by calculating the means, standard deviations (M ± SD), and 95% confidence intervals [95% CI]. One-way analysis of variance (ANOVA) was used to evaluate ordinal and nominal data; Spearman's rank correlation coefficient (r_s) was used for continuous data measures. The r_s was selected for correlating variables because it is less sensitive to strong outliers and it can also be used for calculating correlation coefficients for both continuous and discrete variables. The standard recommendations for r_s strengths were used [15]: 0.0–0.19 = very weak, 0.20–0.39 = weak, 0.40–0.59 = moderate, 0.60–0.79 = strong, and 0.80–1.0 = very strong. Variables evaluated included the CPAP titration data, age, and body mass index (BMI) in kilograms per meter squared (kg/m^2), race/ethnicity, apnea-hypopnea index (AHI), oxygen desaturation index (ODI), lowest oxygen saturation (LSAT), inferior turbinate size, nasal septal deviation severity, and other physical exam findings. For CPAP titration pressures, if a fixed pressure was prescribed, that value was used and if pressure ranges were prescribed, then the average of the pressure range was calculated and used as the CPAP therapeutic treatment pressure for analysis purposes. Multivariate analysis was performed using Standard Least Squares Linear Regression. A two-tailed p value < 0.05 was considered statistically significant.

4. Results

A total of 45 patients met study inclusion criteria. The mean ± standard deviation (M ± SD) for age was 54.6 ± 22.4 years and for body mass index was 28.5 ± 5.9 kg/m^2. Table 1 provides demographic information for the patients to include age, AHI, BMI, ODI, LSAT, NOSE Scale scores, race information, nasal septal deviation severity, inferior turbinate size, and mask type. The Spearman's rank correlation coefficient (r_s) between CPAP therapeutic treatment pressures and several variables were calculated and were weakly correlated (age r_s = 0.29, nasal obstruction r_s = −0.30), moderately correlated (body mass index r_s = 0.42 and lowest oxygen saturation r_s = −0.47), or strongly correlated (apnea-hypopnea index r_s = 0.60 and oxygen desaturation index (r_s = 0.62)). No statistical significance was found with one-way analysis of variance (ANOVA) between CPAP therapeutic treatment pressures and inferior turbinate size (right turbinates p value = 0.2012, left turbinate p value = 0.3064), nasal septal deviation (p value = 0.4979), or mask type (p value = 0.5136); see Table 2. The M ± SD for therapeutic CPAP for grade 1 (five patients): 12.8 ± 2.5 cwp, grades >1 to 2 (eleven patients): 11.5 ± 1.6 cwp, grades >2 to 3 (twenty-one patients): 11.3 ± 1.8 cwp, and grades >3 to 4 (eight patients): 12.2 ± 2.9 cwp, with a one-way ANOVA p value of 0.4599; see Table 3. Mean diagnostic CPAP titration based treatment pressure by inferior turbinate size (grades 1–4) was evaluated with multivariate analysis with the Standard Least Squares Linear Regression Model with an R^2 = 0.08, p value = 0.9953 consistent with no association to very weak association; see Figure 2.

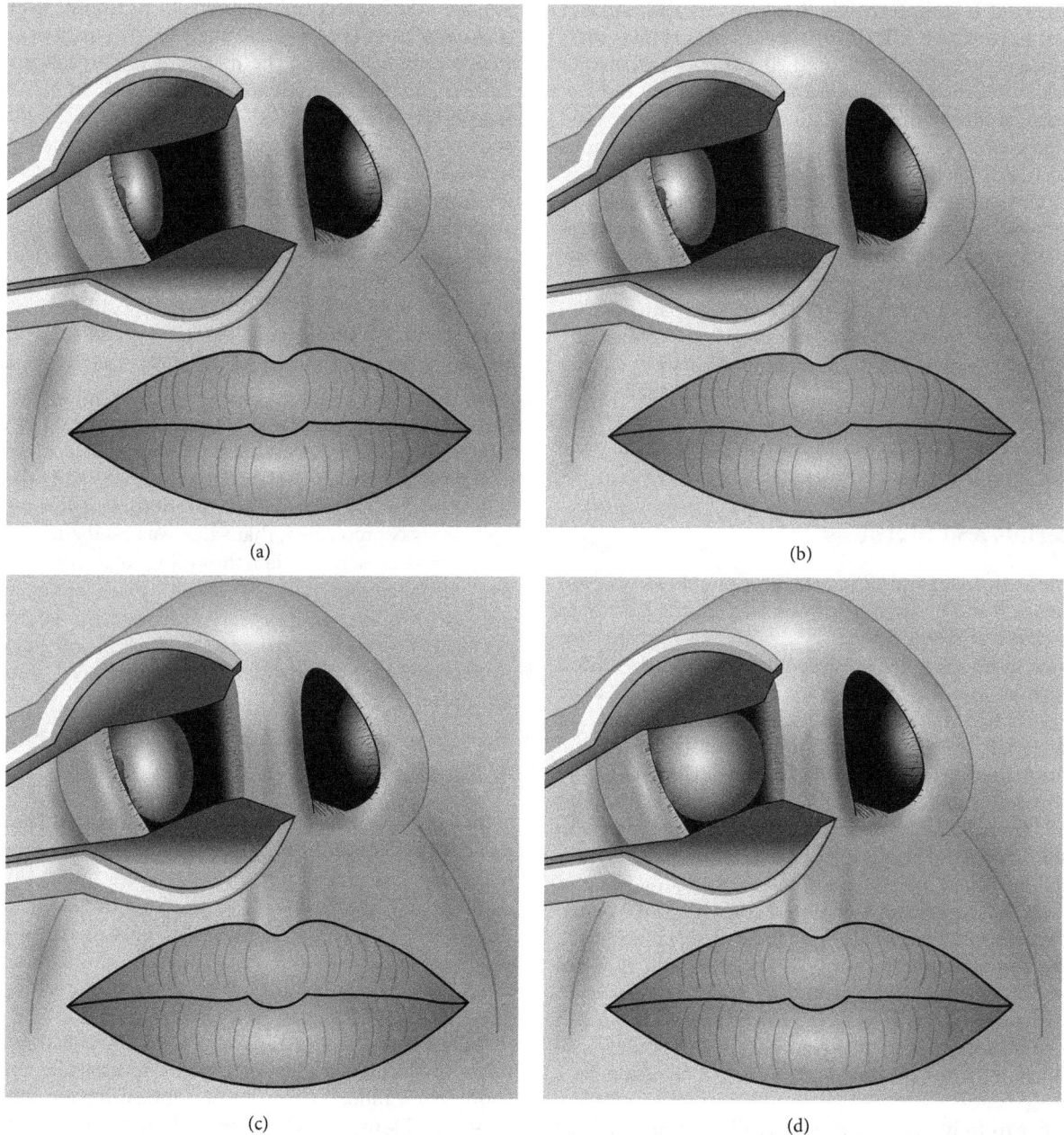

FIGURE 1: (a) Grade 1 (0%–25% of total airway space). (b) Grade 2 (26%–50% of total airway space). (c) Grade 3 (51%–75% of total airway space). (d) Grade 4 (76%–100% of total airway space). Reproduced with permission [12].

4.1. Sub-Analyses

4.1.1. Nasal Obstruction versus No Nasal Obstruction. Among a subgroup analysis of patients without nasal obstruction (as evaluated by a NOSE Scale Score [14] of 40 out of 100 or less, n = 34 patients) the M ± SD for age was 56.0 ± 23.8 years, for body mass index was 28.4 ± 6.6 kg/m^2, and for inferior turbinate size was 2.47 ± 0.80. The M ± SD for CPAP therapeutic treatment pressures for all 34 patients was 11.8 ± 2.2 cwp, for grade 1 (four patients): 13.3 ± 2.7 cwp, grades >1 to 2 (seven patients): 11.6 ± 1.7 cwp, grades >2 to 3 (eighteen): 11.5±1.8 cwp, and grades >3 to 4 (five patients) 12.1±3.5 cwp, with a one-way ANOVA p value of 0.5213; see Table 3. For

patients with complaints of nasal obstruction (11 patients) the M ± SD for age was 62.5 ± 15.4 years, for body mass index was 29.2 ± 3.5 kg/m^2, and for inferior turbinate size was 2.3 ± 0.9. The M ± SD for CPAP therapeutic treatment pressures for all 11 patients was 11.1±1.3 cwp, for grade 1 (one patient): 11 cwp, grades >1 to 2 (four patients): 11.3 ± 1.5 cwp, grades >2 to 3 (three patients): 10.0 ± 0.0 cwp, and grades >3 to 4 (three patients) 12.5 ± 0.7 cwp, with a one-way ANOVA p value of 0.4722; see Table 3.

4.1.2. Nasal Mask Type. There were three categories in the subanalysis for mask type: unknown mask types (7 patients), nasal masks (27 patients), and oronasal masks (11 patients).

TABLE 1: Variables for the patients included in the study.

Variables	N	M ± SD
All patients		
Age (years)	45	54.6 ± 22.4
AHI (events/hr)	44	34.7 ± 29.4
BMI (kg/m²)	45	28.5 ± 5.9
ODI (events/hr)	20	27.3 ± 32.7
LSAT (percent)	42	85.9 ± 6.2
NOSE Score (scaled 0–100)	45	28.9 ± 22.5
		CPAP
All patients	45	11.6 ± 2.0 cwp
Asian	6	12.0 ± 1.4 cwp
Black	3	13.3 ± 3.5 cwp
Caucasian	29	11.6 ± 2.0 cwp
Indian	4	11.4 ± 2.1 cwp
Latino	3	9.8 ± 0.8 cwp
Nasal deviation severity	40	
Grade 1 (0–25%)	24	12.0 ± 2.3 cwp
Grade 2 (26–50%)	11	11.0 ± 1.6 cwp
Grade 3 (51–75%)	3	10.8 ± 1.0 cwp
Grade 4 (76–100%)	2	11.0 ± 1.4 cwp
Inferior turbinate size: right		
Grade 1 (0–25%)	8	12.9 ± 2.0 cwp
Grade 2 (26–50%)	12	11.3 ± 1.5 cwp
Grade 3 (51–75%)	16	11.1 ± 1.7 cwp
Grade 4 (76–100%)	9	11.8 ± 2.8 cwp
Inferior turbinate size: left		
Grade 1 (0–25%)	10	11.9 ± 2.1 cwp
Grade 2 (26–50%)	11	11.3 ± 1.8 cwp
Grade 3 (51–75%)	17	11.1 ± 2.0 cwp
Grade 4 (76–100%)	7	12.8 ± 2.2 cwp
Mask type		
Unknown	7	11.3 ± 1.7 cwp
Nasal mask	27	11.8 ± 2.3 cwp
Oronasal mask	11	11.2 ± 1.5 cwp

AHI = apnea-hypopnea index; CPAP = continuous positive airway pressure; LSAT = lowest oxygen saturation; N = number of patients in the study with data available; NOSE Score = Nasal Obstruction Symptom Evaluation Scale score; and ODI = oxygen desaturation index.

The M ± SD for CPAP therapeutic treatment pressures for the seven patients with an unknown mask type was 11.3±1.7 cwp; the M ± SD turbinate sizes were 2.66 ± 0.30. The M ± SD for CPAP therapeutic treatment pressures for twenty-seven patients with nasal masks was 11.8 ± 2.3 cwp; the M ± SD turbinate sizes were 2.41 ± 0.96. For nasal masks, the one-way ANOVA p value of 0.9217, see Table 3. The M ± SD for CPAP therapeutic treatment pressures for eleven patients with oronasal masks was 11.2 ± 1.5 cwp; the M ± SD for turbinate sizes was 2.45 ± 0.82. For oronasal masks, the one-way ANOVA p value of 0.2732, see Table 3.

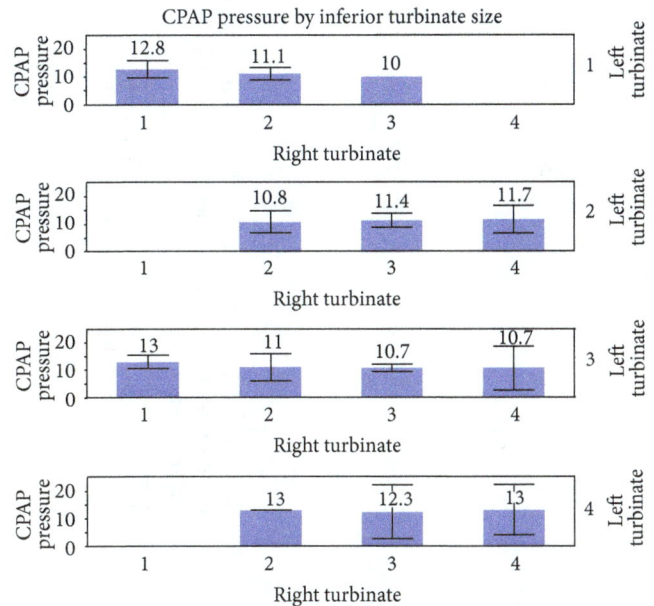

FIGURE 2: Mean diagnostic CPAP by inferior turbinate size (grades 1–4). Each error bar is constructed using a 95% confidence interval of the mean. Multivariate analysis with Standard Least Squares Linear Regression Model shows $R^2 = 0.08$, p value = 0.9953 consistent with no association to very weak association between CPAP and inferior turbinate size.

5. Discussion

There are two main findings to this study. First, CPAP therapeutic treatment pressures do not seem to be influenced by inferior turbinate sizes in patients who have not undergone nasal surgery. It has been shown that patients who have undergone nasal surgery will have a decrease in CPAP therapeutic treatment pressures by approximately 2-3 centimeters of water pressure [10]; therefore, patients with prior nasal surgery were intentionally excluded from the study in order to eliminate this variable as a confounder. The mean diagnostic CPAP and inferior turbinate sizes (grades 1–4) were evaluated with multivariate analysis with the Standard Least Squares Linear Regression Model with an $R^2 = 0.08$, p value = 0.9953 consistent with no association to very weak association.

Second, other variables were better correlated with CPAP therapeutic treatment pressures. There was a weak correlation between CPAP therapeutic treatment pressures and nasal obstruction using the NOSE Scale questionnaire (r_s was −0.21, two-tailed p value 0.57, not statistically significant) and a very weak correlation for patients without nasal obstruction using the NOSE Scale questionnaire (r_s was −0.05, two-tailed p value 0.78, not statistically significant). Given the lack of an association of the inferior turbinate sizes, nasal septal deviation severity, and nasal obstruction overall, these findings suggest that simply observing nasal abnormalities in a patient may not warrant surgery if they do not have complaints of nasal obstruction. Another finding was that lowest oxygen saturation r_s = −0.47 and body mass index

TABLE 2: Results of statistical tests for patient variables versus CPAP prescription pressures. Spearman's rank correlation coefficient (r_s) was used for continuous data measures; one-way ANOVA was used to evaluate ordinal and nominal data. A multivariate model was developed with Standard Least Squares Linear Regression using factors identified as significant on univariate analysis: AHI, BMI, LSAT, NOSE, and ODI ($n = 21$ observations, $R^2 = 0.56$, $p = 0.0030$); parameter estimates and standard errors are shown.

Variables versus CPAP	N	Correlation coefficient r_s	Univariate statistical test, p value: Spearman's rank correlation	Multivariate analysis: Standard Least Squares Linear Regression Model β estimate	Standard error	p value
Age (years)	45	0.29	0.058	Not included		
AHI (events/hr)	44	0.60	0.000005*	0.10	0.04	0.0131*
BMI (kg/m²)	45	0.42	0.0036*	0.13	0.05	0.0233*
LSAT (percent)	42	−0.47	0.0017*	−0.05	0.06	0.3804
NOSE Score (scaled 0–100)	45	−0.30	0.048*	−0.006	0.018	0.7449
ODI (events/hr)	20	0.62	0.0038*	−0.085279	0.036548	0.0340*
			One-way ANOVA			
Inferior turbinate size (1–4)	45	N/A	Right turbinate: 0.2012 / Left turbinate: 0.3064		Not included / Not included	
Nasal septal deviation (1–4)	40	N/A	0.4979		Not included	
Mask type: nasal versus oronasal	38	N/A	0.5136		Not included	

*Statistically significant (p value < 0.05). AHI = apnea-hypopnea index; BMI = body mass index; CPAP = continuous positive airway pressure; LSAT = lowest oxygen saturation; NOSE Score = Nasal Obstruction Symptom Evaluation Scale score; and ODI = oxygen desaturation index.

TABLE 3: Therapeutic continuous positive airway pressures, body mass index, and NOSE scale scores stratified by median inferior turbinate sizes. p values from statistical testing with one-way ANOVA are shown.

Variables	Median inferior turbinate size: right and left				p value
	Grade 1	Grade >1 to 2	Grade >2 to 3	Grade >3 to 4	
All patients ($N = 45$)	$N = 5$	$N = 11$	$N = 21$	$N = 8$	
BMI	28.1 ± 4.4	29.1 ± 6.1	27.7 ± 4.9	30.6 ± 9.7	0.8222
CPAP	12.8 ± 2.5	11.5 ± 1.6	11.3 ± 1.8	12.2 ± 2.9	0.4599
NOSE Score	33.0 ± 25.1	30.0 ± 18.1	26.0 ± 25.7	30.4 ± 20.7	0.8602
Patients w/o nasal obstruction ($N = 34$)	$N = 4$	$N = 7$	$N = 18$	$N = 5$	
BMI	26.8 ± 3.9	28.8 ± 7.5	28.0 ± 5.2	30.3 ± 11.7	0.8744
CPAP	13.3 ± 2.7	11.6 ± 1.7	11.5 ± 1.8	12.1 ± 3.6	0.5213
NOSE Score	23.8 ± 16.5	18.9 ± 11.2	16.8 ± 12.1	19.5 ± 11.2	0.7766
Patients with nasal obstruction ($N = 11$)	$N = 1$	$N = 4$	$N = 3$	$N = 3$	
BMI	33.0	29.7 ± 3.3	25.6 ± 1.9	31.3 ± 3.2	0.2911
CPAP	11.0	11.3 ± 1.5	10.0 ± 0.0	12.5 ± 0.7	0.4722
NOSE Score	70	49.4 ± 7.7	80.8 ± 8.0	57.5 ± 3.5	0.1125
Patients using nasal mask ($N = 27$)	$N = 4$	$N = 7$	$N = 12$	$N = 4$	
BMI	29.1 ± 4.3	28.1 ± 5.8	27.9 ± 4.2	30.5 ± 13.5	0.9122
CPAP	12.3 ± 2.5	11.9 ± 1.5	11.4 ± 1.7	11.9 ± 4.1	0.9217
NOSE Score	31.3 ± 28.7	25.7 ± 16.3	22.7 ± 20.4	21.8 ± 11.4	0.8826
Patients using oronasal mask ($N = 11$)	$N = 1$	$N = 4$	$N = 4$	$N = 2$	
BMI	23.9	31.1 ± 7.0	23.2 ± 5.4	26.8 ± 3.2	0.3645
CPAP	15.0	10.8 ± 1.5	10.9 ± 2.2	11.0 ± 1.4	0.2732
NOSE Score	40	37.5 ± 21.0	33.8 ± 39	55.0 ± 7.1	0.8611

BMI = body mass index in kg/m^2; CPAP = continuous positive airway pressure; N = number of patients; NOSE Score = Nasal Obstruction Symptom Evaluation questionnaire [14].

(r_s = 0.42) were moderately correlated. The moderate correlation with BMI is not unexpected as it is logical that a larger person would require more pressure than a thin person given the additional mass in the upper airway and in the abdomen. Two variables, apnea-hypopnea index (r_s = 0.60) and oxygen desaturation index (r_s = 0.62), were strongly correlated, which is a logical finding given that a CPAP titration is intended to reduce arousals and to improve oxygenation.

Additional research is needed in order to evaluate whether CPAP therapeutic treatment pressures are truly independent of inferior turbinate sizes. As a retrospective case series utilizing chart review, this study provides level 4 evidence. We would like to encourage researchers to incorporate and use the "Inferior Turbinate Classification System, Grades 1–4" as it is a tool which has high intra- and interrater reliability. By using the classification system, the influence that the inferior turbinate sizes have as related to nasal obstruction and CPAP can be more accurately ascertained. Furthermore, despite the lack of an association between CPAP therapeutic treatment pressures and inferior turbinate sizes in patients without nasal surgery we would still recommend that patients with nasal obstruction and large turbinates undergo turbinoplasties as several studies have demonstrated a quality of life benefit and improvement in CPAP use and decreased CPAP in patients who have undergone nasal surgery [10]. Additionally, to our knowledge, this study is the first to evaluate the association between

inferior turbinate sizes and therapeutic CPAP; therefore, we caution against making generalizations. In order to increase the level of evidence, we would also encourage prospective case series, case-control, cohort, and even randomized controlled trials. Once several studies have been published, a systematic review and meta-analysis would more accurately answer the question using statistical analysis with random effects modeling.

6. Limitations

There are limitations to this study. First, we are limited to the constraints which are shared by all retrospective studies in that only the previously collected data could be utilized and analyzed; therefore, if there are missing data, then patients may have had to be excluded solely based on the lack of documentation. Second, in this study we did not review CPAP device pressures for patients who had previous nasal surgery; however, this was done intentionally given that a meta-analysis of eighteen studies demonstrated a reduction by 2-3 centimeters of water pressure after isolated nasal surgeries [10]. Third, given that we did not have rhinomanometry nor acoustic rhinometry, we were not able to evaluate the relationship between the data from these tools and the inferior turbinate sizes and nasal function as it relates to CPAP; future studies could evaluate these relationships. Lastly, there was no rigid or flexible endoscopy performed in the assessment of these patients as the sleep medicine clinics do not have them available; however, each patient underwent a nasal examination by the first author who is a board-certified otolaryngologist.

7. Conclusion

In this study, CPAP titration based therapeutic treatment pressures were not found to be associated with inferior turbinate sizes; however, the CPAP therapeutic treatment pressures were strongly correlated with apnea-hypopnea index and oxygen desaturation index.

Disclosure

(i) There is no financial and no material support for this research and work. (ii) The authors have no financial interests in any companies or other entities that have an interest in the information in Authors' Contribution (e.g., grants, advisory boards, employment, consultancies, contracts, honoraria, royalties, expert testimony, partnerships, or stock ownership in medically related fields).

Disclaimer

The views herein are the private views of the authors and do not reflect the official views of the Department of the Army or the Department of Defense.

Conflict of Interests

The authors declare that they have no conflict of interests.

Authors' Contribution

All authors met the criteria for authorship established by the International Committee of Medical Journal Editors, specifically: Macario Camacho and Soroush Zaghi were responsible for substantial contribution to the conception, design, and statistical analysis and drafting the work, revising the work, and reviewing the paper. Daniel Tran, Sungjin A. Song, Edward T. Chang, and Victor Certal had substantial contributions to the analysis and interpretation of data for the work and revising the work critically for important intellectual content. Additionally, all authors provided final approval of the version to be published and agreed to be accountable for all aspects of the work including that each author ensures the accuracy and/or integrity of the work.

Acknowledgment

Institution where the work was primarily performed is Stanford Hospital.

References

[1] M. Camacho, V. Certal, J. Abdullatif et al., "Myofunctional therapy to treat obstructive sleep apnea: a systematic review and meta-analysis," *SLEEP*, vol. 38, pp. 669–675, 2015.

[2] V. Certal, N. Nishino, M. Camacho, and R. Capasso, "Reviewing the systematic reviews in OSA surgery," *Otolaryngology—Head and Neck Surgery*, vol. 149, no. 6, pp. 817–829, 2013.

[3] M. Camacho, S. Y. Liu, V. Certal, R. Capasso, N. B. Powell, and R. W. Riley, "Large maxillomandibular advancements for obstructive sleep apnea: an operative technique evolved over 30 years," *Journal of Cranio-Maxillofacial Surgery*, vol. 43, no. 7, pp. 1113–1118, 2015.

[4] V. Hoffstein, S. Viner, S. Mateika, and J. Conway, "Treatment of obstructive sleep apnea with nasal continuous positive airway pressure: patient compliance, perception of benefits, and side effects," *The American Review of Respiratory Disease*, vol. 145, no. 4 I, pp. 841–845, 1992.

[5] P. E. Brander, M. Soirinsuo, and P. Lohela, "Nasopharyngeal symptoms in patients with obstructive sleep apnea syndrome. Effect of nasal CPAP treatment," *Respiration*, vol. 66, no. 2, pp. 128–135, 1999.

[6] J. L. Pepin, P. Leger, D. Veale, B. Langevin, D. Robert, and P. Levy, "Side effects of nasal continuous positive airway pressure in sleep apnea syndrome: study of 193 patients in two French sleep centers," *Chest*, vol. 107, no. 2, pp. 375–381, 1995.

[7] S. M. Susarla, R. J. Thomas, Z. R. Abramson, and L. B. Kaban, "Biomechanics of the upper airway: changing concepts in the pathogenesis of obstructive sleep apnea," *International Journal of Oral and Maxillofacial Surgery*, vol. 39, no. 12, pp. 1149–1159, 2010.

[8] N. B. Powell, A. I. Zonato, E. M. Weaver et al., "Radiofrequency treatment of turbinate hypertrophy in subjects using continuous positive airway pressure: a randomized, double-blind, placebo-controlled clinical pilot trial," *The Laryngoscope*, vol. 111, no. 10, pp. 1783–1790, 2001.

[9] H.-Y. Li, P.-C. Wang, Y.-P. Chen, L.-A. Lee, T.-J. Fang, and H.-C. Lin, "Critical appraisal and meta-analysis of nasal surgery for obstructive sleep apnea," *American Journal of Rhinology & Allergy*, vol. 25, no. 1, pp. 45–49, 2011.

[10] M. Camacho, M. Riaz, R. Capasso et al., "The effect of nasal surgery on continuous positive airway pressure device use and therapeutic treatment pressures: a systematic review and meta-analysis," *SLEEP*, vol. 38, no. 2, pp. 279–286, 2015.

[11] M. Camacho, M. Riaz, A. Tahoori, V. Certal, and C. A. Kushida, "Mathematical equations to predict positive airway pressures for obstructive sleep apnea: a systematic review," *Sleep Disorders*, vol. 2015, Article ID 293868, 11 pages, 2015.

[12] M. Camacho, S. Zaghi, V. Certal et al., "Inferior turbinate classification system, grades 1 to 4: development and validation study," *The Laryngoscope*, vol. 125, no. 2, pp. 296–302, 2015.

[13] R. B. Berry, R. Brooks, C. E. Gamaldo et al., *The AASM Manual for the Scoring of Sleep and Associated Events: Rules, Terminology and Technical Specifications, Version 2.0.2*, American Academy of Sleep Medicine, Darien, Ill, USA, 2013, http://www.aasmnet.org/.

[14] M. G. Stewart, D. L. Witsell, T. L. Smith, E. M. Weaver, B. Yueh, and M. T. Hannley, "Development and validation of the Nasal Obstruction Symptom Evaluation (NOSE) scale," *Otolaryngology—Head and Neck Surgery*, vol. 130, no. 2, pp. 157–163, 2004.

[15] T. D. V. Swinscow and M. J. Campbell, *Correlation and Regression*, BMJ Publishing Group, Southampton, UK, 1997.

29

Patient Satisfaction with Postaural Incision Site

George Barrett, Susanne Koecher, Natalie Ronan, and David Whinney

Department ENT Head and Neck Surgery, Royal Cornwall Hospital, Truro TR1 3LJ, UK

Correspondence should be addressed to George Barrett; gwbarrett@hotmail.com

Academic Editor: Leonard P. Rybak

Introduction. Controversy exists over the optimum incision placement when performing ear surgery via the postauricular approach. Little is known about the impact of incision placement on future comfort in wearing audio or visual aids or the effect on the minor auricular muscles cut in the approach. *Objective.* (1) To establish patient satisfaction with their postauricular surgical incision, and to establish the impact on comfort wearing hearing or visual aids. (2) To establish whether patients' voluntary ear movements were affected by surgery. *Materials and Methods.* In January 2014, questionnaires were sent to 81 patients who underwent mastoid surgery requiring a postauricular incision between January 2004 and December 2012. The incision placement was broadly the same for all patients as they were operated on by the same surgeon (or under his supervision). The incision is sited far posteriorly at the hairline. *Results.* 42 (52%) of the patients contacted responded. 80% of patients wearing glasses reported no discomfort or problems associated with their incision. 82% of patients who wear hearing aids were comfortable. Only 1 of the 5 patients who could move their ears preoperatively noticed a change afterwards. *Conclusion.* A hairline incision is well tolerated by most of the patients.

1. Introduction

Postaural incisions are well established in middle ear surgery and are used as an approach to combined approach tympanoplasty and cortical mastoidectomy. Due to the cosmetic advantage from their concealed position and direct access to the mastoid air cells, they also play an increasing role in cochlear implant surgery [1, 2]. They are also used in other fields of head and neck surgery, including resection of benign parotid gland tumours [3] and robotic-assisted neck dissection [4].

There are two main surgical approaches for postaural incisions in the context of middle ear surgery. A curved incision can be made either in the postauricular sulcus (sulcus incision or in the groove incision) or along the hairline posterior to the sulcus (hairline incision or behind the groove incision), as shown in Figure 1.

There may be specific local factors such as skin lesions or previous scarring which dictate the precise site of surgery, but largely the incision location is based on surgeon preference and can vary considerably. After cutting through skin and subcutaneous tissue, the auricular muscles auricularis superior and posterior are generally divided to access and incise the periosteum overlying the mastoid bone. Depending on the surgery being performed a small amount of temporalis fascia may be harvested, but the underlying muscle is left intact.

Little is known about the role of these minor auricular muscles in humans. Infant mammals are believed to instinctively retract their auricles to comfortably position the head when nursing [5]. The postauricular reflex also appears to be triggered by seeing a happy expression on a female face [6]. In higher primates the auricular muscles are vestigial but seem to have a role in movements of the pinna. Some humans are able to voluntarily control the movements of their pinnae, and we aim to assess whether damage to this muscle group through postauricular incisions has an impact on this rudimentary function.

Some of the potential complications of postaural incisions have been investigated previously. Investigating cutaneous sensory deficit, Kang et al. [7] found that the sensation of the pinna returned to baseline within three months for sulcus incisions. However, a questionnaire-based study where the type of incision was not specified found that 26% of patients had persisting numbness beyond eight months [8]. Cosmetic outcomes have also been investigated. Retroauricular skin scars had an excellent aesthetic outcome in cochlear implant surgery [2]; and in a small follow up study, Hong et al. [9]

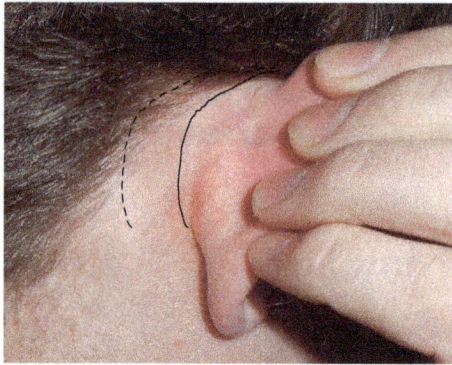

FIGURE 1: Photograph showing the locations of sulcal (solid line) and hairline (dashed line) postauricular incision for access to the mastoid.

noted that in 19 children a postauricular approach did not significantly affect pinna position. Shekhar and Bhavana [10] concluded that "behind the groove" incisions are better at preserving the conchomastoid angle than "in the groove" incisions and therefore give a better overall cosmetic result.

Little is known about the functional impact that a postauricular incision might have on the patient in daily life. Almost all patients will wear either sun glasses or vision correcting glasses at some stage during their postoperative lifetime, and the importance of a functional postauricular sulcus for eyeglass wearer has been highlighted [11, 12]. After ear surgery there is often an increased likelihood of needing to wear a hearing aid, and as behind the ear devices remain the most commonly used, there is a surprising lack of reports in the literature to examine patient comfort with this. In our study, we aimed to find out if patients perceived their "hairline scars" to affect comfort in wearing glasses and hearing aids.

2. Materials and Methods

2.1. Ethical Consideration. No ethics approval was required for this study. Approval was granted from the local Research and Development Department to carry out this questionnaire.

2.2. Study Design. The local Information services department provided the identities of all patients who underwent either "mastoidectomy," "combined approach tympanoplasty," or "cortical mastoidectomy" surgery between January 2004 and December 2012. These procedures all require drilling of the mastoid bone and therefore have the same incision site. Only procedures performed by or under direct supervision of one surgeon (DJW) were included. This information was derived from electronic theatre and admission records. No age restrictions were applied.

A printed paper questionnaire was designed to address the aims of the project, and the questions asked were as follows.

(1) Do you experience any pain or difficulty wearing glasses?

(2) Do you experience any pain or difficulty wearing a hearing aid?

(3) As part of the operation a small group of muscles behind the ear are cut. The function of these muscles is not clear, but they may have a role in moving the external ear as seen in other animals. Were you able to move or "wiggle" your ears before the operation?

(4) If so, has this movement been affected by the surgery?

Patients were asked to respond to each by highlighting "yes," "no," or "not applicable". Additional space was provided after each question, and participants (including those who did not wear audiovisual aids regularly) were encouraged to provide their comments.

Contact details were acquired from the hospital database, and questionnaires were then posted to participants in January 2014 complete with a stamped and addressed envelope for return. The results were collated over a 4-week period after which no further questionnaires were returned.

3. Results

3.1. Participants. A total of 100 operations were identified in the initial search as meeting the inclusion criteria. The search criteria excluded "tympanoplasties" and "myringoplasties." Whilst these can be performed through postaural incisions the authors favour an endaural incision for these procedures, and additionally the mastoid bone is usually preserved. Within the included operations, 5 patients had undergone bilateral surgery, 4 had a second look combined approach tympanoplasty, and further 4 patients had revision surgery or a conversion procedure (e.g., canal wall up converted to canal wall down). One patient was excluded at this stage as his operation was performed for acute mastoiditis and the incision site would therefore not be consistent with the other procedures.

A further 5 patients were excluded from questionnaires; 2 who had moved from the area but had not provided a forwarding address and 3 who were reported deceased on the hospital database.

In total, therefore, 81 questionnaires were posted. Completed responses were analysed for 42 patients (52%).

3.2. Wearing Glasses. In response to the first question relating to pain or difficulty wearing glasses 9 (21%) participants replied with "not applicable." Of the 33 responders who wear glasses, 26 (79%) denied any pain or difficulty, whilst 7 (21%) reported that they did experience some degree of pain or difficulty. One patient commented as follows: "irritated of wearing sunglasses/3D glasses/safety glasses after prolonged use more so on scar," whilst another replied as follows: "a little discomfort sometimes. Optician has to realign glasses on left due to indent in bone." There were others who complimented the outcome including "no pain at all to do with the incisions."

3.3. Wearing Hearing Aids. 20 responders indicated that this question was not applicable. Of the 22 patients wearing hearing aids, 18 (82%) reported no pain or difficulty associated with their use. One responded as follows: "I am very certain that if I did wear an aid my scar would not be of any problem either. Super job done, thank you." Four (18%) however did report problems including "still sore on the scar and finding it painful to keep hearing aid in longer than a couple of hours".

3.4. Voluntary Pinna Movement. 18 (43%) of participants did not know if they were able to voluntarily move their pinnae preoperatively. The majority (19, 45%) reported that they were unable to perform this function, whilst 5 (12%) reported that they were able to. Only one patient felt that the degree of movement was affected by the surgery, responding "I could "wiggle" both ears, but the ear operated on has lost a tiny bit of movement, approx. 15–20%."

4. Discussion

Key Results.

(i) 79% of glasses wearers reported no pain or discomfort.

(ii) 82% of hearing aid users reported no pain or discomfort.

Limitations. Inevitably with patient satisfaction questionnaires, several factors may bias the results. We tried to eliminate selection bias by contacting all patients who underwent surgery and fitted the time and operating consultant criteria. Response bias influences which patients respond to a questionnaire, and it is possible that we only had responses from patients who perceived their surgical episode to be either particularly good or particularly poor. Whilst a response rate of 50% is reasonable from a questionnaire we have to be cautious in speculating on the experiences of those who did not participate. We also acknowledge that racial demographics of the local population are quite different to some other areas of the country being almost exclusively Caucasian in this study, and therefore keloid scarring is unusual.

It would be useful to compare the patient satisfaction of this cohort with a group who have had a more anterior, sulcal incision. This would help establish which approach is more comfortable for patients.

Whilst all procedures were performed under the supervision of one consultant, the operating surgeon, particularly at the point of wound closure, will have varied from patient to patient. However in each case the same technique is used (interrupted deep sutures followed by continuous subcutaneous wound closure with 4-0 absorbable synthetic polyfilament).

Finally it is acknowledged that at the time of participation in the questionnaire many patients were not regular glasses or hearing aid users, but with time they may become so. It is not possible to comment on whether they will have problems with their scars in the future.

4.1. Wearing Glasses. The position of the pinna can be affected by incisions used to access the mastoid [13], but the effect of

this and the scar site itself are rarely considered. Our results suggest that generally a far posterior incision is compatible with comfort in wearing glasses. One patient commented on the change of alignment required as a result of the "indent." Irrespective of the surgical approach, a mastoidectomy will leave this deficit, and it is worth considering this when consenting patients particularly those who are regular glasses wearers.

4.2. Wearing Hearing Aids. After mastoid surgery it is reasonable to expect a higher incidence of hearing aid use than that of the general population. Although there is a range of aids available, the most commonly worn are behind the ear aids. Most of these rely on the natural support of the pinna and sit close to the retroauricular sulcus so may cause more irritation to a scar in this area.

4.3. Voluntary Pinna Movement. The movements of the ear in humans cannot be isolated to the postauricular muscles alone as there are contributions from temporalis and frontalis. Whilst in humans the postauricular reflex is vestigial, it is possible to measure the contractions in these muscles using EMG. The fact that only one of the patients who could voluntarily move his pinnae preoperatively noticed a change in function after surgery would also imply that this muscle group is of limited importance, but the response rate and low study numbers mean that no robust conclusions can be drawn from this. It is possible that some muscle contractions are feasible with healing postoperatively, but no active attempt is made to close the muscle layers as functional units. It is more likely in this isolated case that the fibrosis and scarring affected the degree of fixation of the pinna onto surrounding tissues.

5. Conclusions

This survey has provided evidence that most patients who wear glasses and hearing aids can do so without discomfort from the far posterior postauricular incision. It would be interesting to compare these results with patients who have incisions closer to the retroauricular groove. Whilst infrequent but serious complications of middle ears surgery such as facial nerve injury are usually discussed as part of the preoperative consent process, we feel that patients should also be informed of the far more frequent problems they may face with wearing audio and visual aids as a result of the operation.

Disclosure

The authors accept responsibility for authorship and review of the paper.

Conflict of Interests

The authors declare that there is no conflict of interests regarding the publication of this paper.

References

[1] W. P. R. Gibson, H. C. Harrison, and C. Prowse, "A new incision for placement of cochlear implants," *Journal of Laryngology and Otology*, vol. 109, no. 9, pp. 821–825, 1995.

[2] T. Braun, T. Langhagen, A. Berghaus, and E. Krause, "Evaluation of skin scars following cochlear implant surgery," *The Journal of International Advanced Otology*, vol. 10, no. 1, pp. 30–32, 2014.

[3] D.-Y. Kim, G. C. Park, Y.-W. Cho, and S.-H. Choi, "Partial superficial parotidectomy via retroauricular hairline incision," *Clinical and Experimental Otorhinolaryngology*, vol. 7, no. 2, pp. 119–122, 2014.

[4] R. G. F. Blanco, P. K. Ha, J. A. Califano, C. Fakry, J. Richmon, and J. M. Saunders, "Robotic-assisted neck dissection through a pre- and post-auricular hairline incision: preclinical study," *Journal of Laparoendoscopic and Advanced Surgical Techniques*, vol. 22, no. 8, pp. 791–796, 2012.

[5] G. M. Johnson, F. Valle-Inclán, D. C. Geary, and S. A. Hackley, "The nursing hypothesis: an evolutionary account of emotional modulation of the postauricular reflex," *Psychophysiology*, vol. 49, no. 2, pp. 178–185, 2012.

[6] U. Hess, G. Sabourin, and R. E. Kleck, "Postauricular and eye-blink startle responses to facial expressions," *Psychophysiology*, vol. 44, no. 3, pp. 431–435, 2007.

[7] H.-S. Kang, S.-K. Ahn, S.-Y. Jeon et al., "Sensation recovery of auricle following chronic ear surgery by retroauricular incision," *European Archives of Oto-Rhino-Laryngology*, vol. 269, no. 1, pp. 101–106, 2012.

[8] S. J. Frampton and M. Pringle, "Cutaneous sensory deficit following post-auricular incision," *The Journal of Laryngology and Otology*, vol. 125, no. 10, pp. 1014–1019, 2011.

[9] P. Hong, T. Arseneault, and F. Makki, "A long-term analysis of auricular position in pediatric patients who underwent post-auricular approaches," *International Journal of Pediatric Otorhinolaryngology*, vol. 78, no. 3, pp. 471–473, 2014.

[10] C. Shekhar and K. Bhavana, "Aesthetics in ear surgery: a comparative study of different post auricular incisions and their cosmetic relevance," *Indian Journal of Otolaryngology and Head and Neck Surgery*, vol. 59, no. 2, pp. 187–190, 2007.

[11] G. Datta and S. Carlucci, "Reconstruction of the retroauricular fold by "nonpedicled" superficial mastoid fascia: details of anatomy and surgical technique," *Journal of Plastic, Reconstructive and Aesthetic Surgery*, vol. 61, no. 1, pp. S92–S97, 2008.

[12] R. D. Eavey, "Microtia repair: creation of a functional postauricular sulcus," *Otolaryngology—Head and Neck Surgery*, vol. 120, no. 6, pp. 789–793, 1999.

[13] M. S. Ali, "Unilateral secondary (acquired) postmastoidectomy low-set ear: postoperative complication with potential functional and cosmetic implications," *Journal of Otolaryngology—Head and Neck Surgery*, vol. 38, no. 2, pp. 240–245, 2009.

30

Bolus Residue Scale: An Easy-to-Use and Reliable Videofluoroscopic Analysis Tool to Score Bolus Residue in Patients with Dysphagia

Nathalie Rommel,[1,2,3] **Charlotte Borgers,**[1] **Dirk Van Beckevoort,**[4] **Ann Goeleven,**[1,5] **Eddy Dejaeger,**[6] **and Taher I. Omari**[1,7,8]

[1]*Neurosciences, ExpORL, KU Leuven, 3000 Leuven, Belgium*
[2]*Gastroenterology, Neurogastroenterology and Motility, University Hospitals Leuven, 3000 Leuven, Belgium*
[3]*Translational Research Center for Gastrointestinal Diseases (TARGID), KU Leuven, 3000 Leuven, Belgium*
[4]*Radiology, University Hospitals Leuven, Leuven, Belgium*
[5]*ENT, Head & Neck Surgery, MUCLA, University Hospitals Leuven, Leuven, Belgium*
[6]*Geriatric Medicine, University Hospitals Leuven, Leuven, Belgium*
[7]*School of Medicine, Flinders University, Bedford Park, Australia*
[8]*The Robinson Research Institute, University of Adelaide, Adelaide, Australia*

Correspondence should be addressed to Nathalie Rommel; nathalie.rommel@med.kuleuven.be

Academic Editor: Gerd J. Ridder

Background. We aimed to validate an easy-to-use videofluoroscopic analysis tool, the bolus residue scale (BRS), for detection and classification of pharyngeal retention in the valleculae, piriform sinuses, and/or the posterior pharyngeal wall. *Methods.* 50 randomly selected videofluoroscopic images of 10 mL swallows (recorded in 18 dysphagia patients and 8 controls) were analyzed by 4 experts and 6 nonexpert observers. A score from 1 to 6 was assigned according to the number of structures affected by residue. Inter- and intrarater reliabilities were assessed by calculation of intraclass correlation coefficients (ICCs) for expert and nonexpert observers. Sensitivity, specificity, and interrater agreement were analyzed for different BRS levels. *Results.* Intrarater reproducibility was almost perfect for experts (mean ICC 0.972) and ranged from substantial to almost perfect for nonexperts (mean ICC 0.835). Interjudge agreement of the experts ranged from substantial to almost perfect (mean ICC 0.780), but interrater reliability of nonexperts ranged from substantial to good (mean 0.719). BRS shows for experts a high specificity and sensitivity and for nonexperts a low sensitivity and high specificity. *Conclusions.* The BRS is a simple, easy-to-carry-out, and accessible rating scale to locate pharyngeal retention on videofluoroscopic images with a good specificity and reproducibility for observers of different expertise levels.

1. Introduction

In patients with dysphagia, pharyngeal bolus residue is a significant predictor of postswallow aspiration [1, 2]. Residue is the result of incomplete bolus clearance due to poor propulsion, weak pharyngeal vigor, and/or impaired upper esophageal sphincter (UES) relaxation [2, 3]. As a result, this bolus residual material poses an aspiration risk as it may enter the airway after swallowing. A higher risk for postswallow aspiration is expected with increased volume of the residue, because a larger amount of retention will overflow the boundaries of the available space [2]. In particular, pharyngeal bolus residue is most commonly located in the valleculae and/or the piriform sinuses [4].

To date, the gold standard to detect postswallow residue in a clinical setting is a videofluoroscopic swallow study

(VFS). In order to evaluate those VFS recordings, several qualitative and quantitative methods have been developed to evaluate pharyngeal retention.

First, on a VFS image, pharyngeal residue can be rated using qualitative, also called observational, methods. Dejaeger et al. classified pharyngeal residue into one of four categories based on residue presence and location: no residue, residue in valleculae, residue in piriform sinuses, and residue in both locations (diffuse) [5]. This approach is limited due to the lack of information about the amount of residual material [6]. Hence, an alternative manner to rate pharyngeal residue is to use an ordinal scale. An example of such a scale is Hind's three-point ordinal scale. This scale estimates the amount of residue (with 0 = no residue; 1 = coating of residue; 2 = pooling of residue) at various locations such as the oral cavity, valleculae, posterior pharyngeal wall, piriform sinuses, and the upper esophageal sphincter (UES) [7]. Also, Rosenbek et al. described an equivalent scale with 0 = no residue, 1 = minimal residue, and 2 = moderate-to-substantial residue [8]. Yet, these ordinal rating scales are limited by lack of specific cut-off score for minimal or moderate-to-substantial residue or pooling [6]. An example of a semiquantitative method is the scale of Han et al. (2001). They rated pharyngeal residue as a percent-filled space by assigning four grades based on perception of the amount of residue in comparison to the width of the valleculae [6, 9]. A "0" grade represents no residue, "1" refers to <10% filling of the width of the valleculae, "2" refers to 10–50%, and "3" refers to >50%. In addition, Eisenhuber et al. developed a 1–3 grading scale to score the amount of residue in the valleculae or the piriform sinuses [2]. Grade "1" is mild bolus residue and corresponds to <25% of the height of the valleculae or the piriform sinuses filled with residue. Grades "2" and "3" represent moderate (25–50% of the height) and severe (>50% of the height) pharyngeal retention in the valleculae or piriform sinuses.

Apart from observational methods, a few quantitative analysis methods for the measurement of the area of residue on radiographic images have been suggested. Two recently published methods are the Vallecular Residue Ratio Scale (VRRS) [10] and the Normalized Residue Ratio Scale (NRRS) [6].

This paper presents an easy-to-use observational method developed to rate the presence or absence of bolus residue. The aim of the current paper was to describe inter- and intrarater reliability as well as sensitivity and specificity of this simple method to measure pharyngeal residue on lateral videofluoroscopy images of swallowing.

2. Methods

2.1. Study Database Swallows and Selection. Fifty 10 mL bolus swallows were randomly selected from a master database of bolus swallows recorded in 30 patients and 10 control subjects who had undergone videofluoroscopy under the aegis of clinical research protocols approved by the Research Ethics Committee (S51993-B32220097615), University Hospitals Leuven, Belgium. The order of individual master database swallows was randomized and 50 were consecutively selected comprising 30 dysphagic patient swallows and 20 control

TABLE 1: Bolus residue scale (BRS) scores according to the number of structures affected by residue.

BRS score	Indication of residue
1	No residue
2	Residue in valleculae
3	Residue in posterior pharyngeal wall *or* piriform sinus
4	Residue in valleculae *and* posterior pharyngeal wall *or* piriform sinus
5	Residue in posterior pharyngeal wall *and* piriform sinus
6	Residue in valleculae *and* posterior pharyngeal wall *and* piriform sinus

swallows. The 30 randomly selected patient swallows were from 18 patients (12 male, mean 64 yrs, range 13–95 yrs) of whom twelve had a neurological history (7: stroke, 1: Parkinson's disease, 2: dementia, 1: postneurosurgery, and 1: neuromuscular disorder), 1 had postcervical surgery, and 5 had unknown etiologies at the time of study. The 20 randomly selected control swallows were from ten subjects (3 male, mean 37 yrs, range 24–47 yrs). The number of swallows selected for each patient/control ranged from one to four (11 with 1 swallow analyzed; 8 with 2 swallows; 4 with 3 swallows; 3 with 4 swallows).

Controls had no swallowing difficulties nor other symptoms suggestive of a motility disorder.

As per routine clinical fluoroscopy, test boluses were administered orally via syringe. Boluses were standardized across all patients and controls studied. A standard liquid contrast material (MicropaqueH) was given as liquid bolus and used with thickener (Thick & Easy) for semisolid bolus test conditions. A low osmotic hydrosoluble iodinated contrast agent (UltravistH) was used when aspiration was suspected. The corresponding videofluoroscopy files of all selected swallows were compiled into a study database for sequential analysis by observers.

2.2. Fluoroscopy Analysis. Video-loops of the fluoroscopic images of swallows were acquired at 25 frames per second. Each observer performed repeat BRS analyses of deidentified video-loops edited such that only one bolus swallow was displayed per video-loop.

The BRS scored for the presence or absence of postswallow residue in the valleculae, piriform sinuses, and/or posterior pharyngeal wall. A bolus residue scale (BRS) score between 1 and 6 according to the number of structures showing evidence of residue was assigned: no residue in any of these structures was assigned a BRS score of 1. If residue was present, then additional scores were weighted towards the anatomical regions in which residue posed an aspiration risk (Table 1). A higher BRS score is more severe and corresponds to a higher risk of aspiration because the location is closer to the airway. A BRS score of 4–6 was considered highly clinically significant as indicative of residue on at least two structures. Examples of videofluoroscopic images for different BRS levels are shown in Figure 1.

BRS 1
No residue

BRS 2
Valleculae

BRS 3
Posterior pharyngeal
wall/piriform sinus

BRS 4
Valleculae and
posterior pharyngeal
wall/piriform sinus

BRS 5
Posterior pharyngeal
wall and piriform
sinus

BRS 6
Valleculae and
posterior pharyngeal
wall and piriform
sinus

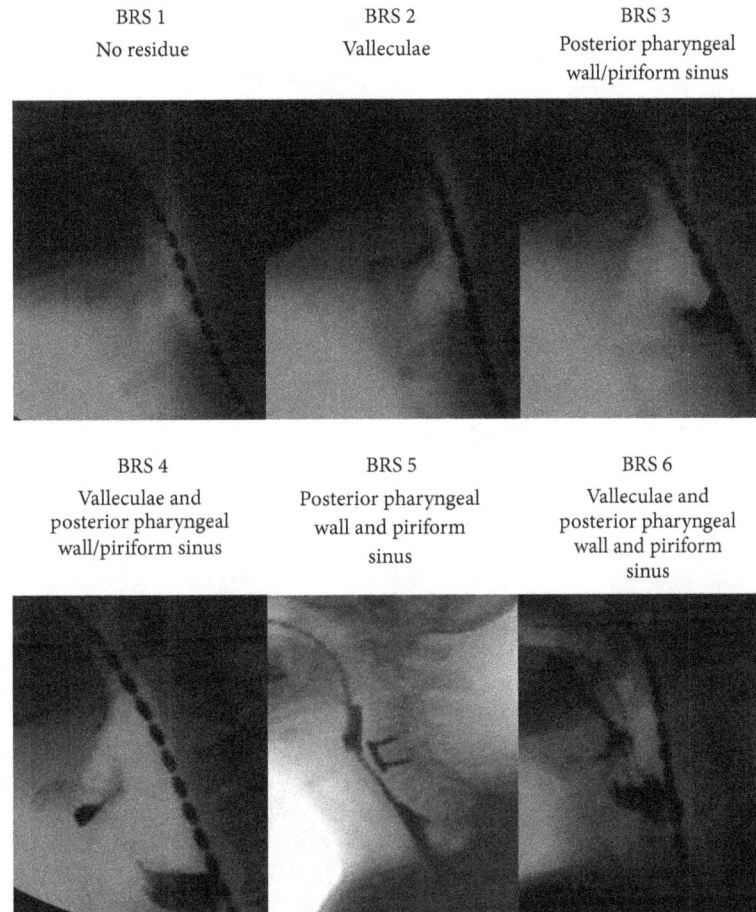

FIGURE 1: Videofluoroscopic image for each BRS score (1–6).

2.3. Observers. Ten observers with ranging experience were asked to participate in the study. Four observers were considered to be "experts" in fluoroscopy as they routinely reviewed fluoroscopy images (geriatrician, radiologist, and two speech pathologists); six were considered informed nonexperts (a medical student, a research assistant, two nurses, and two gastroenterology trainees). All observers received identical training in the BRS. Reference material, demonstration videos, and practice swallows were provided to allow the observers to develop competence in the BRS before proceeding to their formal analysis of the database swallows. Each observer performed repeat analyses of all swallows in their own time.

2.4. Statistical Analysis. Intrarater test/retest reproducibility and interrater reliability of the BRS were assessed by calculation of intraclass correlation coefficients (ICCs). For intrarater reproducibility, data derived during the first and second analyses were correlated for each observer. For interrater reliability, data derived from the first analysis were correlated for each combination of observers.

An expert consensus BRS score was determined for each swallow based upon the most frequently assigned BRS score for that swallow as determined by the experts (if two BRS scores were equally frequently assigned, the average was taken). The degree of agreement between the expert consensus score and individual experts/nonexperts was determined for the different levels of BRS (BRS 2+ to 6) by using Cohen's kappa statistic (κ), weighted kappa that corrects for the effect of chance and bias [11]. The interrater agreement between the expert consensus score and individual scorings of expert and nonexpert observers compares BRS scores greater than a specified cut-off consensus score. As a result, any observer scoring greater as the cut-off score agrees. For example, when a cut-off consensus of 3 (BRS 3+) is chosen, then all observer gradings higher than BRS 3 (BRS 4–6) agree with the consensus. The interpretation for ICC and κ values is as follows: 0.00 = no agreement, 0.00–0.2 = slight (poor), 0.21–0.40 = fair, 0.41–0.60 = moderate, 0.61–0.8 = substantial (good), and 0.81–1.00 = almost perfect (very good) [12]. Prognostic value was also assessed through calculation of sensitivity and specificity.

3. Results

Complete repeat scorings were returned by all observers. Inter- and intrarater ICCs for individual experts and non-experts as well as expert consensus scores are shown in

TABLE 2: Intra- and interrater test/retest reproducibility for expert and nonexpert observers assessed by calculation of intraclass correlation coefficients (ICC).

Observer	Intrarater ICC	Interrater ICC	Expert consensus
Expert 1	0.997		0.880
Expert 2	0.895	0.780	0.820
Expert 3	1.000		0.893
Expert 4	0.997		0.915
Nonexpert 1	0.789		0.834
Nonexpert 2	0.716		0.752
Nonexpert 3	0.796	—	0.639
Nonexpert 4	0.926		0.732
Nonexpert 5	0.797		0.533
Nonexpert 6	0.987		0.823
Average experts	0.972	—	0.877
Average nonexperts	0.835	—	0.719

TABLE 3: Cross-classifications of both gradings given by 4 experts are calculated for 50 swallows: the pattern of agreement (diagonal) and the total frequency of assigned scores for gradings 1 and 2 are shown.

	Grading 2						Total	%
	1	2	3	4	5	6		
Grading 1								
1	85	3	0	0	0	0	88	44
2	1	25	0	1	1	1	29	14.5
3	0	0	10	1	1	0	12	6
4	0	0	0	40	0	1	41	20.5
5	0	0	0	1	0	1	2	1
6	0	0	0	1	0	27	28	14
Total	86	28	10	44	2	30	200	100
%	43	14	5	22	1	15		

Table 2. The intrarater reproducibility of the BRS was almost perfect for both experts (mean ICC 0.972, range 0.895–1.000) and ranged from substantial to almost perfect for nonexperts (mean ICC 0.835, range 0.716–0.987). To evaluate the degree of agreement of nonexperts with experts, the ICC for expert consensus score versus nonexpert scoring of the BRS was calculated. Nonexperts seemed to be less reliable in detecting residue compared to experts with the ICC ranging from moderate to almost perfect (mean ICC 0.719, range 0.533–0.834). The interrater ICCs were as expected highly variable as presented in Table 2. Because of the less reliable intrarater reproducibility of the nonexperts, interrater ICCs between individual nonexperts were not computed. Interjudge agreement between expert observers ranged from substantial to almost perfect (mean ICC 0.780, range 0.716–0.880) (Table 2).

The cross-classifications of the scores given by the experts and the nonexperts are shown in Tables 3 and 4, respectively,

TABLE 4: Cross-classifications of both gradings given by 6 nonexperts are calculated for 50 swallows: the pattern of agreement (diagonal) and the total frequency of assigned scores for gradings 1 and 2 are shown.

	Grading 2						Total	%
	1	2	3	4	5	6		
Grading 1								
1	70	6	5	5	0	2	88	29.3
2	5	44	2	7	0	4	62	20.7
3	1	3	23	2	0	2	31	10.3
4	1	2	1	28	3	7	42	14
5	0	0	0	2	1	4	7	2.3
6	0	4	1	5	1	59	70	23.3
Total	77	59	32	49	5	78	300	100
%	25.7	19.7	10.7	16.3	1.7	26		

as well as the total frequencies of the assigned scale scores for the first and second grading by both experts and nonexperts. The diagonal in both tables represents the pattern of agreement (i.e., identical scores) between the first and second grading per judge. The experts gave an identical score in 187 of 200 replicate gradings, which corresponds to an agreement percentage of 94%. The nonexperts had an agreement percentage of 75% (225 of 300 replicates gradings). When both experts and nonexperts did not assign an identical score on both gradings, a score within 1 unit (3.5% and 9.7%, resp.) or 2 units (2% and 9%, resp.) was given as second score.

The sensitivity and specificity as well as the kappa-coefficients for every grading of bolus residue are shown in Figure 2 for expert and nonexpert observers. The kappa-coefficients compare the amount of agreement between a single observer (expert/nonexpert) and the expert consensus for different levels of the BRS score (i.e., a cut-off score). In the same way, sensitivity, specificity, and average kappa-coefficients on each BRS level are displayed in Table 5 for both experts and nonexperts. A substantial agreement was observed between expert scoring and expert consensus for different BRS levels. However, this agreement could be expected since expert observers showed good inter- and intrarater reliability. Expert scoring of any residue (2+) and clinically significant residue (4+) agreed substantially with the expert consensus (mean κ 0.737, sens. 0.88, spec. 0.89 and 0.731, sens. 0.79, and spec 0.98, resp.). In contrast, nonexpert scoring revealed higher variability on different BRS levels. In detecting the presence of any residue (BRS 2+), nonexpert scoring agreed moderately with the expert consensus score (mean κ 0.543, sens. 0.73, and spec. 0.92). With a view to determine the presence of clinically significant residue (BRS 4+), nonexpert scoring agreed substantially with the expert consensus score (mean κ 0.623, sens. 0.67, and spec. 0.96), although individual agreement ranged from κ 0.452 (moderate) to κ 0.847 (almost perfect). A low reliability was observed in detecting clinical significant residue in all structures (BRS 6) (mean κ 0.36, sens. 0.97, and spec. 0.33).

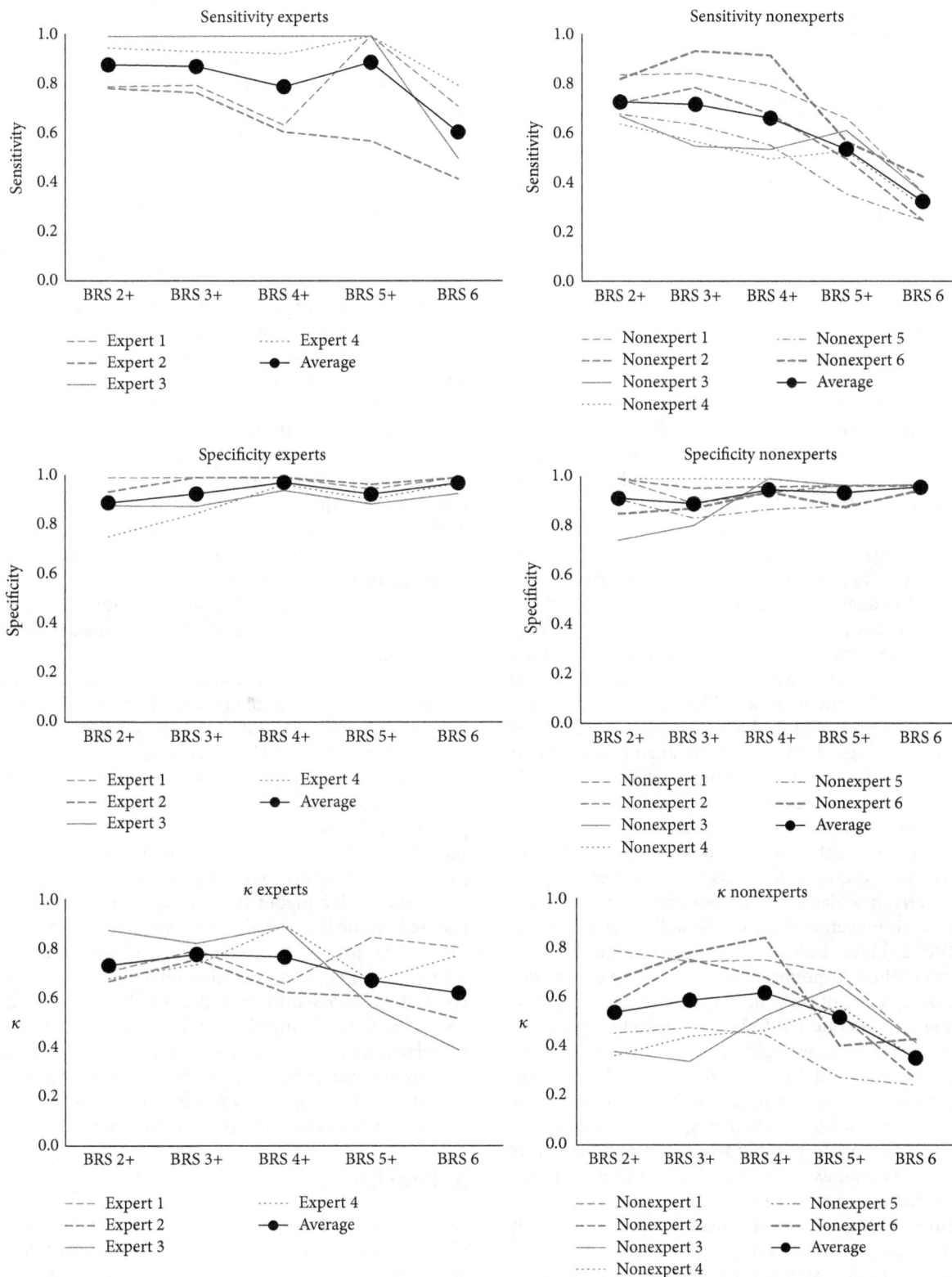

FIGURE 2: Specificity, sensitivity, and agreement (κ) of nonexperts and experts with the expert consensus score in relation to different bolus residue scale scores.

TABLE 5: Averaged intraclass kappa (κ), sensitivity, and specificity for experts and nonexperts by scale scores.

	BRS 2+	BRS 3+	BRS 4+	BRS 5+	BRS 6
Experts					
Intraclass κ	0.74	0.78	0.77	0.68	0.62
Specificity	0.90	0.93	0.98	0.93	0.98
Sensitivity	0.88	0.88	0.79	0.89	0.61
Nonexperts					
Intraclass κ	0.54	0.59	0.62	0.52	0.36
Specificity	0.92	0.90	0.96	0.94	0.97
Sensitivity	0.73	0.72	0.67	0.54	0.33

4. Discussion

The bolus residue scale (BRS) is an observational scale to determine the absence or presence of residue in the valleculae, the piriform sinuses, and/or the posterior pharyngeal wall. To evaluate whether this scale can be used as a reliable tool to grade residue, the reproducibility and reliability of this radiological-based method in both expert and nonexpert observers were assessed in this study. Fifty fluoroscopic images were repeatedly scored by four experts and six nonexperts by assigning a grade ranging from 1 to 6 according to the anatomic structures in which the residual material was located. The BRS appeared reproducible in the hands of different observers. The intra- and interrater reproducibility of experts were almost perfect. In fact, our experts were fairly unanimous, which makes the BRS a reliable instrument for clinical use. The less experienced observers in radiological assessment obtained poorer results compared to expert observers. Interrater reliability between nonexperts and experts was rather moderate, as there was a large variability between individual nonexperts. Additionally, the agreement on both gradings was more variable for nonexperts than experts (75% versus 94%). For both experts and nonexperts, nonidentical gradings differed by only one or two units. Moreover, experts agreed well in detecting any residue (BRS 2+) and clinically significant residue (BRS 4+) locating in 1 of the 3 locations. Nonexpert observers showed a substantial agreement with the expert consensus scoring in detecting any residue (BRS 2+) or clinically significant residue (BRS 4+). Interestingly, in both groups, a larger variability on BRS 5+ and BRS 6 was observed, indicating that it may be more difficult to rate residue which affects more than one anatomical site. Presumably, a related difficulty could be to differentiate pooling from coating. Pooling of bolus material is seen as any material that is present in the pharynx or larynx cavities before and/or after swallowing [13]. Coating is the condition where bolus residue only moistens the pharyngeal walls [14].

BRS scoring of nonexperts has a high specificity for both BRS 2+ score (any residue) and BRS 4+ score (clinically significant residue). However, both BRS 2+ and BRS 4+ showed low sensitivity (0.73 and 0.67, resp.), indicating that a large proportion of the population will potentially be undetected (false negative) or that residue severity will be underestimated. For experts, both sensitivity and specificity were higher for 2+ and 4+. These findings support the use of the BRS to screen for patients with pharyngeal retention by trained clinicians. Hereby, at-risk patients can be referred for further investigation and diagnosis, thereby preventing further pulmonary complications and chronic undetected dysphagia. Our data show however that nonexperts (such as nurses, researchers, and medical students) can but need to be trained to reliably judge fluoroscopic images with respect to pharyngeal residue grading.

Several quantitative and qualitative analysis methods have been developed to evaluate pharyngeal retention performed on videofluoroscopic recordings. Advantage of software-based techniques such as NRRS or VRRS is their quantitative nature and high interrater reliability, but a limitation of these methods for routine clinical practice is that they require extra handling of the VFS data for analysis [10]. As a result, those methods can be time consuming. Therefore, we believe an efficient and easy-to-use method like the BRS can be useful due to the low handling complexity of the scale.

Besides quantitative and observational methods, semiquantitative methods have been developed. Those methods take into account severity as well as the amount of residue. Although these semiquantitative ordinal scales were designed to improve the accuracy of residue detection, it is well accepted that they have limited precision and they showed poor reliability [15]. The BRS does not rate the volume of the residue as it may be inaccurate to estimate a 3D volume on a 2D VFS image.

It is important to emphasize that the BRS is a qualitative assessment. Counting this potential limitation, Omari et al. however reported a significant correlation between the BRS and an objective nonradiological marker of clinically relevant postswallow residue, called the integrated nadir impedance to impedance ratio. This metric is an objectively derived parameter for bolus residue using impedance manometry recordings [3]. Furthermore, it is assumed that increased postswallow residue, marked as a higher BRS score, will be associated with a higher risk for aspiration. This assumption is based on the fact that the areas covered with bolus residue (according to the BRS score) are closely located at the airway entrance. Omari et al. confirmed this suggestion by correlating BRS scores with the Swallow Risk Index (SRI). SRI is an objective metric correlating to aspiration which is calculated using four pharyngeal pressure flow parameters [16]. In summary, objective evidence is emerging that the BRS outcome is linked not only to detection of bolus residue but also to aspiration in patients with dysphagia.

5. Conclusion

In summary, this paper described the validation of a new observational scale, the bolus residue scale (BRS), to detect and classify bolus residue in the valleculae, piriform sinuses, and/or posterior wall of the pharynx. This study explored the reliability and reproducibility of this method as well as sensitivity and specificity for both expert and nonexpert observers. The bolus residue scale seems to have a good specificity and reproducibility for different types of observers.

The study shows that even nonexperts showed a good but a more variable agreement with lower sensitivity than experts. Hence, the BRS showed to be a reliable instrument that can be used in the clinical setting by professionals experienced in evaluating radiological swallow studies. The BRS is a simple, easy-to-carry-out, and accessible analysis method to rate and locate pharyngeal retention. In clinical practice, the BRS can be used to indicate the severity of pharyngeal residue as a quantifiable score.

Abbreviations

BRS: Bolus residue scale
UES: Upper esophageal sphincter.

Conflict of Interests

Professor Nathalie Rommel has AIM technology patent to disclose. Professor Taher I. Omari has AIM technology patent to disclose. Other authors have no conflict of interests to disclose.

Authors' Contribution

Nathalie Rommel was responsible for study concept and design, analysis, and interpretation of data; drafting and critical revision of the paper; statistical analysis; and study supervision. Charlotte Borgers was responsible for drafting of the paper and critical revision. Dirk Van Beckevoort was responsible for acquisition and analysis of data; critical revision of the paper for important intellectual content; and technical or material support. Ann Goeleven carried out analysis of data and critical revision of the paper for important intellectual content. Eddy Dejaeger carried out analysis of data and critical revision of the paper. Taher I. Omari was responsible for study concept and design; analysis and interpretation of data; drafting of the paper; critical revision; and study supervision.

Acknowledgments

The authors are very thankful to the wonderful nursing staff of the Department of Radiology, University Hospitals Leuven, Belgium.

References

[1] W. J. Dodds, J. A. Logemann, and E. T. Stewart, "Radiologic assessment of abnormal oral and pharyngeal phases of swallowing," *American Journal of Roentgenology*, vol. 154, no. 5, pp. 965–974, 1990.

[2] E. Eisenhuber, W. Schima, E. Schober et al., "Videofluoroscopic assessment of patients with dysphagia: pharyngeal retention is a predictive factor for aspiration," *American Journal of Roentgenology*, vol. 178, no. 2, pp. 393–398, 2002.

[3] T. I. Omari, E. Dejaeger, J. Tack, D. Vanbeckevoort, and N. Rommel, "An impedance-manometry based method for non-radiological detection of pharyngeal postswallow residue," *Neurogastroenterology & Motility*, vol. 24, no. 7, pp. e277–e284, 2012.

[4] J. A. Logemann, *Evaluation and Treatment of Swallowing Disorders*, PRO-ED, Austin, Tex, USA, 1998.

[5] E. Dejaeger, W. Pelemans, E. Ponette, and E. Joosten, "Mechanisms involved in postdeglutition retention in the elderly," *Dysphagia*, vol. 12, no. 2, pp. 63–67, 1997.

[6] W. G. Pearson Jr., S. M. Molfenter, Z. M. Smith, and C. M. Steele, "Image-based measurement of post-swallow residue: the normalized residue ratio scale," *Dysphagia*, vol. 28, no. 2, pp. 167–177, 2013.

[7] J. A. Hind, M. A. Nicosia, E. B. Roecker, M. L. Carnes, and J. Robbins, "Comparison of effortful and noneffortful swallows in healthy middle-aged and older adults," *Archives of Physical Medicine and Rehabilitation*, vol. 82, no. 12, pp. 1661–1665, 2001.

[8] J. C. Rosenbek, J. A. Robbins, E. B. Roecker, J. L. Coyle, and J. L. Wood, "A penetration-aspiration scale," *Dysphagia*, vol. 11, no. 2, pp. 93–98, 1996.

[9] T. R. Han, N.-J. Paik, and J. W. Park, "Quantifying swallowing function after stroke: a functional dysphagia scale based on videofluoroscopic studies," *Archives of Physical Medicine and Rehabilitation*, vol. 82, no. 5, pp. 677–682, 2001.

[10] J. C. Dyer, P. Leslie, and M. J. Drinnan, "Objective computer-based assessment of valleculae residue: is it useful?" *Dysphagia*, vol. 23, no. 1, pp. 7–15, 2008.

[11] J. Cohen, "A coefficient of agreement for nominal scales," *Educational and Psychological Measurement*, vol. 20, no. 1, pp. 37–46, 1960.

[12] J. R. Landis and G. G. Koch, "An application of hierarchical kappa-type statistics in the assessment of majority agreement among multiple observers," *Biometrics*, vol. 33, no. 2, pp. 363–374, 1977.

[13] D. Farneti, "Pooling score: an endoscopic model for evaluating severity of dysphagia," *Acta Otorhinolaryngologica Italica*, vol. 28, no. 3, pp. 135–140, 2008.

[14] J. Murray, S. E. Langmore, S. Ginsberg, and A. Dostie, "The significance of accumulated oropharyngeal secretions and swallowing frequency in predicting aspiration," *Dysphagia*, vol. 11, no. 2, pp. 99–103, 1996.

[15] S. J. Stoeckli, T. A. G. M. Huisman, B. Seifert, and B. J. W. Martin-Harris, "Interrater reliability of videofluoroscopic swallow evaluation," *Dysphagia*, vol. 18, no. 1, pp. 53–57, 2003.

[16] T. I. Omari, E. Dejaeger, D. Van Beckevoort et al., "A novel method for the nonradiological assessment of ineffective swallowing," *The American Journal of Gastroenterology*, vol. 106, no. 10, pp. 1796–1802, 2011.

The Importance of the Neutrophil-Lymphocyte Ratio in Patients with Idiopathic Peripheral Facial Palsy

M. Mustafa Kiliçkaya,[1] Mustafa Tuz,[1] Murat Yariktaş,[1] Hasan Yasan,[1] Giray Aynalı,[1] and Özkan Bagci[2]

[1]*Department of Otolaryngology, Medical Faculty of Suleyman Demirel University, 32100 Isparta, Turkey*
[2]*Department of Medical Genetics, Medical Faculty of Suleyman Demirel University, 32100 Isparta, Turkey*

Correspondence should be addressed to M. Mustafa Kiliçkaya; drmmkilic@gmail.com

Academic Editor: Jose Antonio Lopez-Escamez

Objective. The purpose of this study was to investigate whether or not there was a correlation between the neutrophil-to-lymphocyte ratio (NLR) value and the severity of idiopathic peripheral facial palsy (IPFP) and to determine whether or not NLR could be used as an early predictive parameter in the prognosis of IPFP patients. *Material and Method.* This retrospective study was conducted on 146 patients who were diagnosed with IPFP. The control group comprised 140 patients. Patients with IPFP were categorized according to the House-Brackmann grading system (HBS). The NLR value was obtained by dividing the neutrophil value by the lymphocyte value. *Results.* In the IPFP group, the mean NLR value was 3.63 ± 2.74 and, in the control group, 1.84 ± 0.78. The mean NLR value was significantly higher in IPFP patients than in the control subjects ($p < 0.0001$). The mean NLR value in group A (Grades I-II) was 2.61 ± 2.28, in group B (Grades III-IV) 3.22 ± 2.65, and in group C (Grades V-VI) 10.69 ± 6.30. *Conclusion.* We determined that as the severity of IPFP increased, the NLR value increased. The NLR value can be used as a prognostic factor in the early prediction of IPFP prognosis.

1. Introduction

Idiopathic peripheral facial palsy (IPFP) is a disease seen in 20–30 people per 100,000 per year [1]. IPFP, which generally affects a single side of the face, is an acute IPFP [2]. Although the pathology is not fully known, viral infections, vascular ischaemia, and inflammation are widely held responsible [2]. Of viruses, varicella-zoster virus (VZV) and herpes simplex virus (HSV) are most commonly blamed [3, 4]. There are several systems to evaluate the severity of IPFP, of which the most widely used is the House-Brackmann grading system (HBS). Grading is made from I to VI with Grade I as normal and Grade VI as total palsy. On the HBS scale, Grades I-II are stated as mild paralysis, Grades III-IV as moderate paralysis, and Grades V-VI as severe paralysis with a poor prognosis [5].

Some studies, if not all, recognize diabetes, hypertension, hypercholesterolemia, old age, and paralysis severity as factors associated with poor prognosis of IPFP [6, 7]. In the early stages of this disease, many tests are applied to predict prognosis, including stapes reflex (SR), electromyography (EMG), nerve excitability test (NET), and electroneuronography (ENoG) and blink reflex tests [8]. White blood cells (WBC) and the number of subtypes such as neutrophils in particular are accepted as classic inflammatory markers. Several studies have reported that the NLR could be used as a marker of inflammation. In addition, it has been used as an indicator of prognosis in some diseases such as cardiac diseases and neoplasia [9, 10].

Our aim was to investigate whether or not there was a correlation between the severity of IPFP, which is thought to be related to inflammation and a high level of the NLR value and to determine whether or not NLR could be used as an early predictive parameter of prognosis in patients with IPFP.

2. Materials and Methods

This retrospective study was performed on 146 patients (76 males, 70 females) who were diagnosed with IPFP in the Otorhinolaryngology Clinic of Suleyman Demirel University Faculty of Medicine Hospital between February 2009 and January 2015. Ethics board approval for this study was granted by the Suleyman Demirel University Medical Faculty, in accordance with the Declaration of Helsinki. Patients were excluded with diseases which could affect the NLR, such as active ear disease, acute inflammation or infection, acute or chronic renal failure, chronic liver disease, heart disease, chronic obstructive pulmonary disease, neurological disorders, or neoplasm. We included patients with diabetes, hypertension, and hypercholesterolemia in the study. The control group comprised 140 patients (70 males, 70 females) with no active ear disease or facial nerve pathology who were undergoing preoperative tests in the ENT polyclinic for septoplasty or myringoplasty operations. The study group and control group were retrospectively scanned for the neutrophil and lymphocyte values. More than half of the patients had their facial paralysis severity grades (on early referral and control examination) recorded in patient files based on the House-Brackmann grading system. Some patients' grades were not indicated. We provided detailed descriptions of their mimic muscle movements, and found their HBS grade based on such data. All patients included in the study referred to our clinic in the first three days of paralysis, and we measured, as a routine, their complete blood count on early referral. In the case of facial paralysis, instead of the grade measured on early referral, we took the grade that corresponded to the most advanced stage of paralysis as initial grade, for paralysis may grow worse in a couple of days. In the patient follow-up, those with facial motor deficit at the end of 1 year were accepted as patients with permanent motor deficit. Follow-up period for the patients included in the study varied between six months and six years. The group composed of twelve patients with permanent facial motor deficit had a minimum follow-up period of two years. We reinvited those patients with permanent facial motor deficit to a control examination in order to determine their paralysis grades based on the HBS. The IPFP patients were classified according to the HBS as follows: a diagnosis of Grades I-II paresis was made in 61 patients (41.78%), Grades III-IV in 72 (49.31%), and Grades V-VI in 13 (8.90%). Grades I-II patients were designated as group A, Grades III-IV patients as group B, and Grades V-VI as group C. The NLR values of groups A, B, and C were calculated and statistical analysis was applied. All the patients were treated with steroids or steroids+antiviral medication. After 15 days, additional physical therapy was applied to some patients in whom paralysis continued.

2.1. Hematological Analysis.
Blood samples were collected into tubes containing calcium EDTA and an automated blood cell counter was used for complete blood count (CBC) test measurements (Beckman Coulter LH 780 Hematology Analyzer, USA). The NLR value was obtained mathematically by dividing the neutrophil value by the lymphocyte value.

2.2. Statistical Analysis.
In the statistical analysis, the t-test was used to evaluate the mean NLR in the IPFP and control groups, Kruskal-Wallis analysis was applied to the differences

TABLE 1: The age distribution of groups A, B, and C.

Age	Group A	Group B	Group C
≤15	15 (24.59%)	18 (25.35%)	1 (7.69%)
16–45	16 (26.22%)	27 (38.02%)	5 (38.46%)
46≤	30 (49.18%)	26 (36.61%)	7 (53.84%)

TABLE 2: The average age of groups A, B, and C.

	Mean age ± Std. deviation
Group A	38.90 ± 22.77
Group B	36.04 ± 21.77
Group C	42.30 ± 17.43

TABLE 3: The distribution of patients with diabetes mellitus.

	The patients with diabetes mellitus
Group A ($n = 61$)	15 (24.59%)
Group B ($n = 72$)	10 (13.88%)
Group C ($n = 13$)	2 (15.38%)

between groups A, B, and C to determine from which group the difference originated, and Bonferroni correction was performed. Mann-Whitney U test was used to compare differences between the IPFP patients with complete recovery and those with permanent motor function deficit. A value of p smaller than 0.05 was considered significant.

2.3. Results.
The average age of the patients with IPFP was 41.62 ± 22.32 and that of the control group subjects was 43.64 ± 11.68 years. Tables 1 and 2 present the age distribution and average age figures for groups A, B, and C. It was shown that NLR was not affected by age in control groups (Figure 1). One-way ANOVA analysis revealed no statistically significant difference between the groups in terms of average age ($p = 0.560$). All patients had unilateral palsies: 72 cases were right-sided and 73 left-sided. The mean NLR value was 1.84 ± 0.78 in the control group and 3.63 ± 2.74 in the IPFP group. The average NLR value was found to be remarkably higher in patients with IPFP than in the control group ($p = 0.000$). No statistically remarkable difference was determined between IPFP patients with DM (26 patients, 17.80%) and IPFP patients without DM (122 patients, 83.56%) ($p = 0.547$). There was no statistically significant difference between the groups in terms of patients with DM ($p > 0.05$) (Table 3).

The mean NLR value in group A was determined as 2.61 ± 2.28, in group B as 3.22 ± 2.65, and in group C as 10.69 ± 6.30. According to the results of the Kruskal-Wallis analysis, the difference between the mean NLR values of the 3 groups was statistically highly significant ($p < 0.0001$). As the severity of the paralysis increased in the IPFP patients in this study, the NLR value increased (Figure 2). To determine from which group the difference originated, Bonferroni correction was applied and it was determined that the difference originated in group C ($p = 0.000$, $p = 0.000$, and $p = 0.136$, groups C-A, groups C-B, and groups A-B, resp.).

TABLE 4: The initial NLR values in the 12 patients with permanent facial motor function deficit.

Patients	Age	Initial grading of HBS	Final grading of HBS	Initial NLR value
Case 1	51	Grade II	Grade II	1,87
Case 2	67	Grade III	Grade II	1,05
Case 3	57	Grade IV	Grade II	**4,51**
Case 4	32	Grade IV	Grade II	**3,25**
Case 5	20	Grade IV	Grade II	**15,00**
Case 6	13	Grade IV	Grade II	0,96
Case 7	79	Grade IV	Grade II	**2,64**
Case 8	11	Grade IV	Grade II	**3,48**
Case 9	18	Grade IV	Grade II	1,78
Case 10	21	Grade V	Grade II	**11,22**
Case 11	13	Grade VI	Grade II	**17,00**
Case 12	47	Grade VI	Grade IV	**3,56**
Mean				**5.55 ± 4.41**

NLR: Neutrophil-to-lymphocyte ratio. HBS: House-Brackmann grading system.

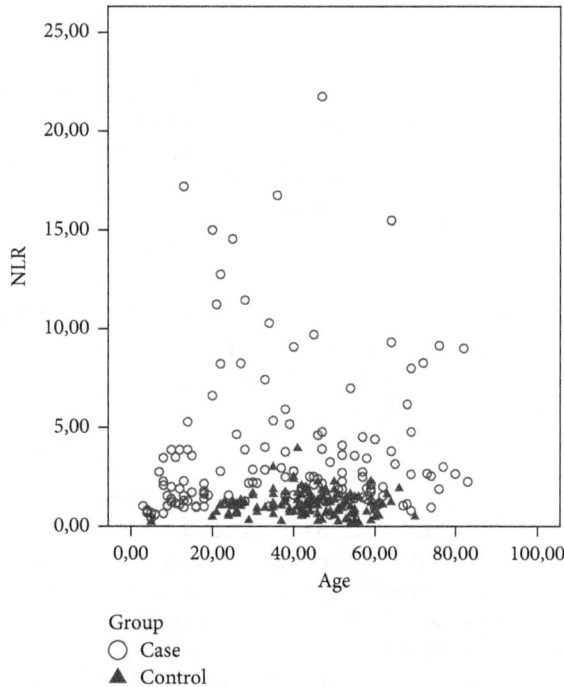

Group
○ Case
▲ Control

FIGURE 1: The distribution according to age of NLR in case and control groups.

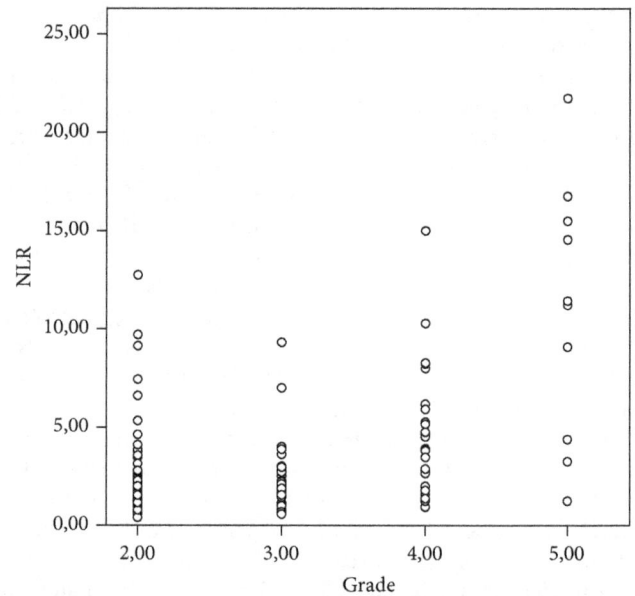

FIGURE 2: The distribution according to grade of NLR in IPFP.

At the end of the follow-up period, 12 of 146 patients were determined with permanent facial motor deficit. The mean NLR value of 8 (66.66%) of these 12 patients was found to be high compared to the control group (Table 4). The mean NLR of the IPFP patients with complete recovery was 3.44 ± 2.50 and in the 12 patients with permanent facial motor function deficit the mean NLR value was found to be 5.55 ± 4.41. According to the Mann-Whitney U analysis, there was no as statistical remarkable difference ($p = 0.11$).

3. Discussion

Rapid response to acute inflammation is provided by leukocytes and plasma proteins. The basic leukocytes in acute infection are neutrophils. Acute inflammation is triggered by events such as bacterial or viral infections, trauma, tissue necrosis, and immune reactions. In the response to viral infections of the body, the T-lymphocytes play a greater role [11]. In the current study, the mean NLR values of the patients with IPFP were significantly higher than those of the control group and it was also determined that as the severity of IPFP increased, the NLR value increased. In some studies, it has been reported that when there is an increase in the initial degree of IPFP the prognosis worsens [12]. Therefore, it can be considered that patients with a high NLR value could have a poor prognosis. In addition, generally the disease progresses within a few days from the initial symptoms to maximal paralysis [5]. Certain electrophysiological tests, such as EMG and ENoG, are employed to estimate IPFP prognosis. However, they are not very reliable in the first week of paralysis [13, 14]. The NLR value may be high in blood tests made on the first day. Therefore, the NLR value on the first day of presentation may be a significant indicator in the prediction of prognosis.

Some studies report increased NLR associated with age and smoking [15]. In our study, we found that NLR was not affected by age. As smoking status was not recorded for all patients in patient files, we could not examine possible impacts of smoking on NLR.

There are studies in literature which have stated that steroid use is the most effective treatment in the early stage for IPFP patients [12, 16]. Just as it has been advocated that there is no benefit from antiviral medications in IPFP treatment, some clinical studies have reported that the combination of steroids with antiviral drugs was more beneficial [17, 18]. Considering that the prognosis could be poor for patients with a high NLR value in the blood tests made on the first day, it may be useful to inform the patient and immediately start steroid+antiviral therapy and the importance of this therapy for the patient can also be suggested.

4. Conclusion

NLR is accepted as a new potential marker of inflammation. As the severity of the paralysis increased in the IPFP patients in this study, the NLR value increased and the majority of the patients with permanent facial motor function deficit were determined to have a high NLR value. Therefore, the NLR value can be used as an early predictive prognostic factor of IPFP.

Disclosure

The authors declare no financial support. The paper is not being considered or reviewed by any other publication. This paper describes original work and it has not been published elsewhere. The paper contains no libellous or unlawful statements; all authors approved the paper and this submission. All authors of the paper have participated sufficiently in the conception and design of the work and in writing the paper and take public responsibility for it.

Conflict of Interests

The authors declare that there is no conflict of interests regarding the publication of this paper.

References

[1] S. G. Yeo, Y. C. Lee, D. C. Park, and C. I. Cha, "Acyclovir plus steroid vs steroid alone in the treatment of Bell's palsy," *American Journal of Otolaryngology—Head and Neck Medicine and Surgery*, vol. 29, no. 3, pp. 163–166, 2008.

[2] K. P. Peng, Y. T. Chen, J. L. Fuh, C. H. Tang, and S. J. Wang, "Increased risk of Bell palsy in patients with migraine: a nationwide cohort study," *Neurology*, vol. 84, no. 2, pp. 116–124, 2015.

[3] L. Tolstunov and G. A. Belaga, "Bell's palsy and dental infection: a case report and possible etiology," *Journal of Oral and Maxillofacial Surgery*, vol. 68, no. 5, pp. 1173–1178, 2010.

[4] C. Bodénez, I. Bernat, J.-C. Willer, P. Barré, G. Lamas, and F. Tankéré, "Facial nerve decompression for idiopathic Bell's palsy: report of 13 cases and literature review," *Journal of Laryngology and Otology*, vol. 124, no. 3, pp. 272–278, 2010.

[5] A. Greco, A. Gallo, M. Fusconi, C. Marinelli, G. F. Macri, and M. de Vincentiis, "Bell's palsy and autoimmunity," *Autoimmunity Reviews*, vol. 12, no. 2, pp. 323–328, 2012.

[6] M. Riga, G. Kefalidis, and V. Danielides, "The role of diabetes mellitus in the clinical presentation and prognosis of bell palsy," *Journal of the American Board of Family Medicine*, vol. 25, no. 6, pp. 819–826, 2012.

[7] J. Finsterer, "Management of peripheral facial nerve palsy," *European Archives of Oto-Rhino-Laryngology*, vol. 265, no. 7, pp. 743–752, 2008.

[8] M. Ushio, K. Kondo, N. Takeuchi, H. Tojima, T. Yamaguchi, and K. Kaga, "Prediction of the prognosis of Bell's palsy using multivariate analyses," *Otology and Neurotology*, vol. 29, no. 1, pp. 69–72, 2008.

[9] A. Dirican, B. B. Kucukzeybek, A. Alacacioglu et al., "Do the derived neutrophil to lymphocyte ratio and the neutrophil to lymphocyte ratio predict prognosis in breast cancer?" *International Journal of Clinical Oncology*, vol. 20, no. 1, pp. 70–81, 2015.

[10] B. A. Williams and M. E. Merhige, "Association between neutrophil-lymphocyte ratio and impaired myocardial perfusion in patients with known or suspected coronary disease," *Heart & Lung: The Journal of Acute and Critical Care*, vol. 42, no. 6, pp. 436–441, 2013.

[11] V. Kumar, A. K. Abbas, and J. C. Aster, "General pathology of infectious diseases," in *Robbins Basic Pathology*, chapter 8, pp. 309–326.e1, Elsevier, 9th edition, 2013.

[12] S. Axelsson, T. Berg, L. Jonsson et al., "Prednisolone in Bell's palsy related to treatment start and age," *Otology and Neurotology*, vol. 32, no. 1, pp. 141–146, 2011.

[13] T. Fujiwara, N. Hato, K. Gyo, and N. Yanagihara, "Prognostic factors of Bell's palsy: prospective patient collected observational study," *European Archives of Oto-Rhino-Laryngology*, vol. 271, no. 7, pp. 1891–1895, 2014.

[14] N. Takemoto, A. Horii, Y. Sakata, and H. Inohara, "Prognostic factors of peripheral facial palsy: multivariate analysis followed by receiver operating characteristic and Kaplan-meier analyses," *Otology and Neurotology*, vol. 32, no. 6, pp. 1031–1036, 2011.

[15] N. Alkhouri, G. Morris-Stiff, C. Campbell et al., "Neutrophil to lymphocyte ratio: a new marker for predicting steatohepatitis and fibrosis in patients with nonalcoholic fatty liver disease," *Liver International*, vol. 32, no. 2, pp. 297–302, 2012.

[16] F. M. Sullivan, I. R. C. Swan, P. T. Donnan et al., "Early treatment with prednisolone or acyclovir in Bell's palsy," *The New England Journal of Medicine*, vol. 357, no. 16, pp. 1598–1607, 2007.

[17] H. Y. Lee, J. Y. Byun, M. S. Park, and S. G. Yeo, "Steroid-antiviral treatment improves the recovery rate in patients with severe Bell's palsy," *The American Journal of Medicine*, vol. 126, no. 4, pp. 336–341, 2013.

[18] N. Hato, H. Yamada, H. Kohno et al., "Valacyclovir and prednisolone treatment for Bell's palsy: a multicenter, randomized, placebo-controlled study," *Otology and Neurotology*, vol. 28, no. 3, pp. 408–413, 2007.

32

Antrochoanal Polyps: How Long Should Follow-Up Be after Surgery?

Saisawat Chaiyasate,[1] Kannika Roongrotwattanasiri,[1] Jayanton Patumanond,[2] and Supranee Fooanant[1]

[1]*Department of Otolaryngology, Faculty of Medicine, Chiang Mai University, Chiang Mai 50000, Thailand*
[2]*Clinical Research Center, Faculty of Medicine, Thammasat University, Pathum Thani 12120, Thailand*

Correspondence should be addressed to Saisawat Chaiyasate; saisawat.c@cmu.ac.th

Academic Editor: David W. Eisele

Objective. To investigate the length of follow-up needed to detect recurrence of antrochoanal polyps. *Methods*. A retrospective investigation was performed on patients who had been operated on with a preoperative diagnosis of antrochoanal polyps in Chiang Mai University hospital from 2006 to 2012. *Results and Discussion*. Of the 38 cases of choanal polyps, 27 were adults (71%). The median age was 23.5, ranging from 7 to 64 years old. Eighteen patients were male (47.4%). The origin of choanal polyps was the maxillary antrum in 32 patients. The most common symptom was nasal obstruction (97.4%). The surgical procedures were polypectomy in one child and combined endoscopic and transcanine fossa approach in two adults. The remainder of the patients underwent endoscopic removal of the polyps. The follow-up time ranged from 1 day to 8 years. There were 5 cases of recurrence of which four were in children. The time for recurrence was 1.2 ± 0.6 years (95% CI 0.51, 1.97). *Conclusion*. Antrochoanal polyps are more common in younger patients. Recurrence was significantly higher in children. Follow-up of patients should be for at least 2 years postoperatively in order to detect 95% of recurrence.

1. Introduction

The condition of antrochoanal polyps (Killian polyps) is a distinctive clinical disease. It is characterized by polyps originating from the maxillary antrum, which then extend through the natural or accessory ostium into the nasal cavity, choana, and nasopharynx. The maxillary portion is cystic though there are some reports of solid forms (polyps), while nasal and choanal portions are usually solid [1]. Choanal polyps may come from the sphenoid sinus, the nasal septum, and other parts of the nasal cavity [2–4]. Antrochoanal polyps occur as 4–6% of adult polyps [5] and 33% of childhood polyps [6]. The most common presenting symptom is nasal obstruction, either unilateral or bilateral. Other complaints are rhinorrhea, sinusitis, snoring, dysphagia, and so forth. Complete surgical removal of the nasal and antral portion of the polyp is the standard treatment to prevent recurrence. However, in some patients with a small maxillary sinus or in revision cases, the origin of the polyp could not be well

identified. This study is to investigate the length of follow-up needed to detect recurrence of polyps in patients. The authors also would like to discern if there are differences in recurrence between children and adults.

2. Materials and Methods

A retrospective investigation was carried out on patients who had been operated on with a preoperative diagnosis of antrochoanal polyps in Chiang Mai University hospital from 2006 to 2012. After excluding 6 cases of inverted papilloma and 1 case of maxillary mucopyocele, 38 cases of patients with choanal polyps were included in this study. Clinical data and operative findings were reviewed, and the latest follow-up data were collected. Delayed diagnosis was defined as treating patients with another diagnosis such as sinusitis or allergic rhinitis for more than 3 visits to the outpatient document without recording incidence of polyps. The treatment of antrochoanal polyps was complete surgical

TABLE 1: Patient characteristics according to age group.

	Total (38 patients)	Age <15 years (11 patients)	Age ≥15 years (27 patients)	p value
Age (year)	Median 23.5			
Mean ± SD	28.1 ± 16.3	10.7 ± 2.6	35 ± 14	
Range	7–64	7–14	15–64	
Sex				
Male : female		6 : 5	12 : 15	0.724
Symptoms				
Nasal obstruction	37 (97.4%)	11 (100%)	26 (96.3%)	1.000
Unilateral		7 (63.6%)	15 (55.6%)	
Bilateral		4 (36.4%)	11 (40.7%)	
None		0	1 (3.7%)	
Positional change	9 (23.7%)	3 (27.3%)	6 (22.2%)	1.000
Progression		10 (90.9%)	17 (63%)	0.124
Purulent rhinorrhea	27 (71.1%)	9 (81.8%)	18 (66.7%)	0.452
Epistaxis	5 (13.2%)	2 (18.2%)	3 (11.1%)	0.615
Pain	10 (26.3%)	2 (18.2%)	8 (29.6%)	0.690
Sore throat	3 (7.9%)	—	3 (11.1%)	0.542
Delayed diagnosis	9 (23.7%)	1 (9.1%)	8 (29.6%)	0.237
Follow-up				
Less than a month	7 (18.4%)	2 (18.2%)	5 (18.5%)	
Median (year)	1.22	1.24	1.20	0.721
Range	1 day–8 years	1 day–7 years	1 day–8 years	
Operation				
Endoscopic polypectomy		1	—	
Endoscopic removal		10	25	
Combined endoscopic and transcanine fossa		—	2	
Origin				
Maxillary sinus		11	21	
Sphenoethmoidal recess/superior turbinate		—	6	
Recurrence		4 (36.4%)	1 (3.7%)	0.019

removal with either an endoscopic approach alone or an endoscopic approach combined with the transcanine fossa approach.

The data were analyzed using the STATA program version 11.0 (STATA Corporation, Texas, USA). The exact probability test was used for the proportion of the investigative variables between the age groups, and survival analysis was used for evaluating the potential factors affecting recurrence.

The Research Ethics Committee of the Faculty of Medicine of Chiang Mai University approved the study protocol.

3. Results

Of the 38 cases of choanal polyps, 27 were adults (71%). The median age was 23.5, ranging from 7 to 64 years. Eighteen patients were male (47.4%). There was no statistical difference in the sex of the age groups (Table 1). The origin of choanal polyps was the maxillary antrum in 32 patients. The other polyps originated from the superior turbinate or

sphenoethmoidal recess, totaling 6 adult patients. The most common symptom was nasal obstruction (97.4%), either unilateral (57.9%) or bilateral (39.5%). Positional changing of the obstruction in the supine or lateral decubitus was found in 9 patients (23.7%). Other symptoms were purulent rhinorrhea (71%), pain (26.3%), epistaxis or bloody nasal discharge (13.2%), and sore throat (7.9%). One adult patient who presented with a sore throat and a mass in the oropharynx for 3 days had no nasal obstruction at all. The duration of symptoms ranged from 3 days to 4.5 years, with a median time of 1 year.

When comparing between age groups, the symptoms showed no significant difference. However, purulent rhinorrhea was more common in children (88.8% compared to 66.7%) and pain was more common in adults (29.6% compared to 18.2%). Delayed diagnosis was more common in adults (29.6%) than in children (9.1%).

The surgical procedures were polypectomy in one child and combined endoscopic and transcanine fossa approach in

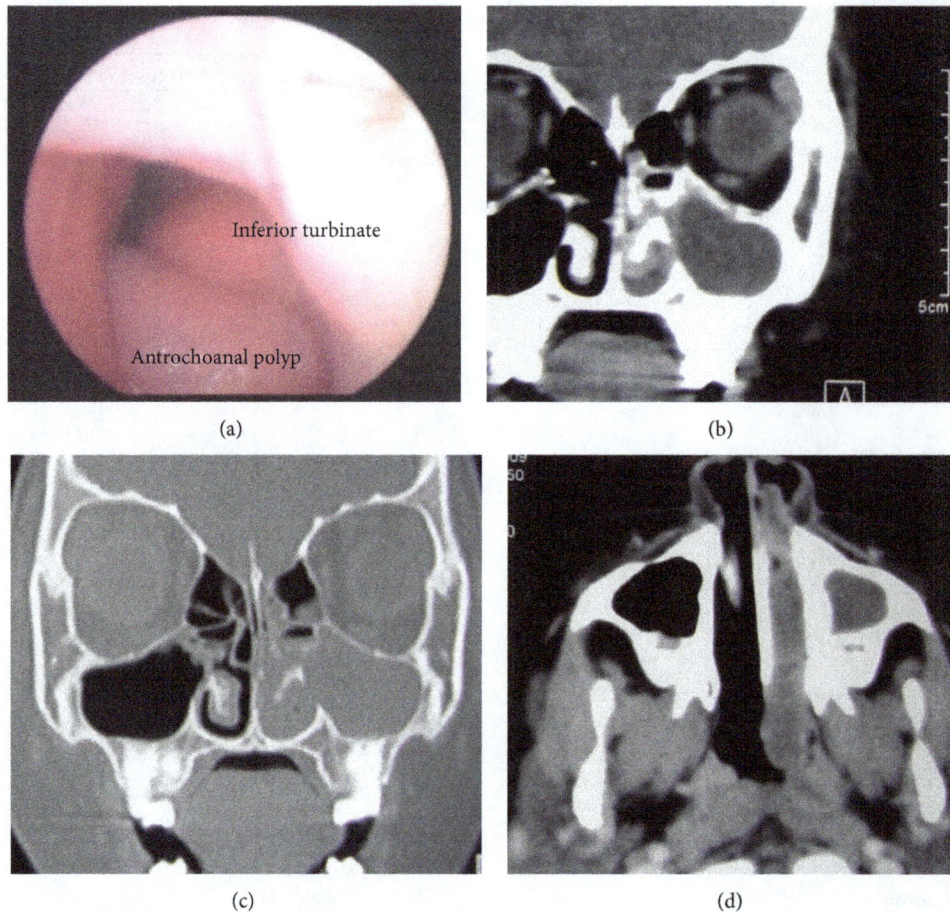

FIGURE 1: (a) Left nasal cavity endoscopic view showing antrochoanal polyp at inferior meatus CT scans. (b) Coronal view, soft tissue window showing cystic component in the maxillary antrum. (c) Coronal view, bone window showing defect of medial maxillary wall below the inferior turbinate. (d) Axial view, soft tissue window; polyp extending into the nasopharynx.

two adults. The remainder of the patients underwent endoscopic removal of the polyps by a middle meatus antrostomy with an operative note of incomplete removal of the maxillary part in the case of one child. All but one polyp extended into the nasal cavity through the middle meatus, via either natural or accessory ostium. Only one case differed in the children, where the polyp extended through the inferior meatus (Figure 1).

The follow-up time ranged from 1 day to 8 years, the median being 1.2 years. Two patients failed to keep appointments for the postoperative care that was scheduled. There were 5 cases of recurrence of which four were in children. The time for recurrence was 1.2 ± 0.6 years (95% CI 0.51, 1.97). The case of recurrence in an adult was where the surgery had been carried out in another hospital. After the recurrence a revision was carried out at CMU and no further recurrence occurred in the one-year follow-up period. The origin of the polyps from all recurrent cases was from the maxillary sinus, while none of sphenoethmoidal polyps recurred.

The sex, age group, and infection were tested as risk parameters for recurrence. The origin of polyps and type of surgical procedure were not tested because of the limited numbers of patients in each subgroup (Table 2). The polyps

TABLE 2: Multivariable odds ratios (OR) and 95% confidence interval (CI) of potential factors affecting recurrence of antrochoanal polyps.

Parameters	OR	95% CI		p value
Young age group	10.52	1.17	94.71	0.036
Sex	1.03	0.16	6.51	0.978
Infection	1.78	0.19	17.14	0.617

recurred significantly more in the group of children when compared to that of the adults ($p = 0.036$).

4. Discussion

Antrochoanal polyps have been known about for some time; for example, in 1691 a polyp from the antrum of Highmore was mentioned by Fredrik Ruysch. Antrochoanal polyps (ACP) are also known as Killian polyps after Gustav Killian, the doctor who stressed this special type of polyp from the maxillary antrum to choana in 1906 [1]. Though the pathogenesis is still unknown, Berg et al. studied the macro- and microarchitecture of ACPs and suggested that they develop from an expanding intramural cyst, protruding through the maxillary ostium into the nasal cavity [7]. Frosini et al., in the largest study of 200 cases, suggested that they occurred from the combination of an antral cyst and a maxillary ostium obstruction with an association with an anatomical abnormality such as a deviated nasal septum and a turbinate alteration [1]. Mostafa et al., on the other hand, studied 25 cases of ACPs in which only 5% of the antral parts were cystic [8]. They compared the transitional zone of an ACP with chronic sinusitis with nasal polyps and found a higher density of lymphatic markers on the ACP group (88% versus 16%). Mostaf et al. suggested that the lymphatic obstruction might be a process associated with ACP development.

Antrochoanal polyps were found in patients with a wide age range from 5 to 81 years [1, 3, 9]. The patients in this study ranged from 7 to 64 years of age. The median age of 21 years showed that this type of polyp was more common in the younger age group as was found in many previous studies [1, 10–12]. Other studies found that the ACP occurred more commonly in males, but this was not found to be the case in this study. When comparing the clinical presentations and the outcome of treatment in children and adults, there was no statistical significant difference in clinical presentations though infection was more common in the younger age group. The key of successful treatment is complete removal of the polyp from the maxillary origin. The inflammatory mucosa of sinusitis was mentioned as a possible risk of recurrence in some studies as it led to difficulty in identifying the origin in the antrum [9, 13]. The polyps originating from the lateral, anterior, and inferior walls of the maxillary antrum were difficult to view and remove with the transnasal endoscopic approach alone [9–11]. Special instruments or a combined transcanine fossa approach may be needed to complete surgical removal [9, 11, 14–16]. In children, the anatomically narrow sinuses, the nonerupted teeth, and concern of maxillary growth may effect surgeons' decision on the surgical approach, leading to recurrence.

The choanal polyps which originated from the superior turbinate or the sphenoethmoidal recess showed no recurrence. This type of polyp might be different from those developing from the maxillary antrum and is easier to locate and remove from its origin. No other types of choanal polyps in children were found, though several have been reported in other studies [17, 18].

This study found that the age group alone was significantly associated with recurrence (p value = 0.036). In other studies, the occasion of recurrence was found as early as 6 months in the cases of incomplete removal [10] to as long as 3 years [3]. Ten percent of our patients did not come back for postoperative evaluation as they lived very far away or came from neighboring countries. In this group of patients, the postoperative cleaning was carried out before discharge to ensure sinus drainage was adequate. The median follow-up time was 1.2 years, though the longest was up to 8 years. The overall time of recurrence in this study was 1.2 ± 0.6 years (95% CI 0.51, 1.97). We suggested monitoring ACP patients for at least 2 years in order to detect 95% of recurrence.

5. Conclusions

Antrochoanal polyps are more common in younger patients. Recurrence was significantly higher in children. Follow-up of patients should be for at least 2 years postoperatively in order to detect 95% of recurrence.

Conflict of Interests

The authors declare that there is no conflict of interests regarding the publication of this paper.

Acknowledgment

The authors would like to thank Ms. Chidchanok Ruengorn, Ph.D., for her expertise in the statistical review.

References

[1] P. Frosini, G. Picarella, and E. de Campora, "Antrochoanal polyp: analysis of 200 cases," Acta Otorhinolaryngologica Italica, vol. 29, no. 1, pp. 21–26, 2009.

[2] Ö. Aydin, G. Keskin, E. Üştündağ, M. Işeri, and H. Özkarakaş, "Choanal polyps: an evaluation of 53 cases," American Journal of Rhinology, vol. 21, no. 2, pp. 164–168, 2007.

[3] Y. Kizil, U. Aydil, A. Ceylan, S. Uslu, V. Batürk, and F. Leri, "Analysis of choanal polyps," Journal of Craniofacial Surgery, vol. 25, no. 3, pp. 1082–1084, 2014.

[4] M. M. Lessa, R. L. Voegels, F. Pádua, C. Wiikmann, F. R. Romano, and O. Butugan, "Sphenochoanal polyp: diagnose and treatment," Rhinology, vol. 40, no. 4, pp. 215–216, 2002.

[5] J. M. Chen, M. D. Schloss, and M. E. Azouz, "Antro-choanal polyp: a 10-year retrospective study in the pediatric population with a review of the literature," Journal of Otolaryngology, vol. 18, no. 4, pp. 168–172, 1989.

[6] V. L. Schramm Jr. and M. Z. Effron, "Nasal polyps in children," Laryngoscope, vol. 90, no. 9, pp. 1488–1495, 1980.

[7] O. Berg, C. Silfversward, and A. Sobin, "Origin of the choanal polyp," Archives of Otolaryngology—Head & Neck Surgery, vol. 114, no. 11, pp. 1270–1271, 1988.

[8] H. S. Mostafa, T. O. Fawzy, W. R. Jabri, and E. Ayad, "Lymphatic obstruction: a novel etiologic factor in the formation of antrochoanal polyps," Annals of Otology, Rhinology and Laryngology, vol. 123, no. 6, pp. 381–386, 2014.

[9] T.-J. Lee and S.-F. Huang, "Endoscopic sinus surgery for antrochoanal polyps in children," Otolaryngology—Head and Neck Surgery, vol. 135, no. 5, pp. 688–692, 2006.

[10] C. Bozzo, R. Garrel, F. Meloni, F. Stomeo, and L. Crampette, "Endoscopic treatment of antrochoanal polyps," European Archives of Oto-Rhino-Laryngology, vol. 264, no. 2, pp. 145–150, 2007.

[11] N. Choudhury, A. Hariri, and H. Saleh, "Endoscopic management of antrochoanal polyps: a single UK centre's experience," European Archives of Oto-Rhino-Laryngology, 2014.

[12] B. S. Gendeh, Y.-T. Long, and K. Misiran, "Antrochoanal polyps: clinical presentation and the role of powered endoscopic polypectomy," Asian Journal of Surgery, vol. 27, no. 1, pp. 22–25, 2004.

[13] A. L. Woolley, R. A. Clary, and R. P. Lusk, "Antrochoanal polyps in children," The American Journal of Otolaryngology—Head & Neck Medicine & Surgery, vol. 17, no. 6, pp. 368–373, 1996.

[14] R. Kamel, "Endoscopic transnasal surgery in antrochoanal polyp," *Archives of Otolaryngology—Head and Neck Surgery*, vol. 116, no. 7, pp. 841–843, 1990.

[15] A. El-Guindy and M. H. Mansour, "The role of transcanine surgery in antrochoanal polyps," *The Journal of Laryngology & Otology*, vol. 108, no. 12, pp. 1055–1057, 1994.

[16] S. K. Hong, Y.-G. Min, C. N. Kim, and S. W. Byun, "Endoscopic removal of the antral portion of antrochoanal polyp by powered instrumentation," *Laryngoscope*, vol. 111, no. 10, pp. 1774–1778, 2001.

[17] W.-K. Lim and T. Sdralis, "Regression of a sphenochoanal polyp in a child," *Laryngoscope*, vol. 114, no. 5, pp. 903–905, 2004.

[18] F. Tosun, S. Yetiser, T. Akcam, and Y. Özkaptan, "Sphenochoanal polyp: endoscopic surgery," *International Journal of Pediatric Otorhinolaryngology*, vol. 58, no. 1, pp. 87–90, 2001.

33

Vestibular Disorders after Stapedial Surgery in Patients with Otosclerosis

Ditza de Vilhena, Inês Gambôa, Delfim Duarte, and Gustavo Lopes

Department of Otolaryngology and Head & Neck Surgery, Hospital Pedro Hispano, Matosinhos, 4150-800 Porto, Portugal

Correspondence should be addressed to Ditza de Vilhena; ditzadevilhena@gmail.com

Academic Editor: Wouter A. Dreschler

Introduction and Objectives. Vertigo is a described complication of stapedial surgery. Many studies have been conducted to assess the improvement of hearing loss, but there are few studies that assess vestibular function after stapedial surgery. The aim of this study was to evaluate the presence and characterize the vertigo after stapedial surgery. *Methods.* We conducted a prospective observational study. Patients undergoing stapedial surgery in our hospital between October 2013 and December 2014 were invited to participate. The vertigo was assessed before and 4 months after surgery, using the Dizziness Handicap Inventory. *Results.* We included 140 patients in the study. 12 patients (8.6%) reported vertigo before surgery, and all of them denied vertigo after surgery. 36 patients (25.7%) reported vertigo four months after surgery, and none of them had vertigo before surgery. Postoperative total scores in patients with vertigo ranged between 2 and 18 points. *Conclusion.* The study shows that vestibular disorders may remain after the immediate postoperative period and reinforces the need for clarification of the patient in the informed consent act.

1. Introduction

Otosclerosis was first described in 1741 by Valsalva, who noted ankylosis of the stapes in an autopsy on a deaf patient and in 1894 Politzer defined otosclerosis as a clinical condition. It is an illness that affects the optic capsule, which forms part of the group of osteodystrophies, caused by changes in bone metabolism. It is characterised by the presence of several spots of reabsorption and bone repositioning. Despite significant research having been undertaken on the topic, the cause of otosclerosis remains unknown, although most authors consider it a multifactorial disease. There would appear to be a genetic predisposition with autosomal dominant inheritance, although it may occur sporadically.

Caucasians are most typically affected, although the prevalence rate of clinical otosclerosis is lower than 1% [1–3]. It is most common amongst the middle aged, with women most commonly affected [4–7]. Otosclerosis is a bilateral condition in approximately 60 to 80% of cases[6].

It is one of the most common causes of conductive hearing loss and tends to be progressive in nature.

Treatment tends to be medical or surgical, with surgery being the preferred option, namely, a stapedotomy or stapedectomy. Although uncommon, in certain circumstances, some health professionals treat the condition medically with bisphosphonates or fluorine compounds, normally during the initial stages of the illness [8], either separate from or in combination with calcium and vitamin D [9]. The use of glucocorticoids has also been proposed when there is an associated sensorineural component [9, 10], and even the use of calcitonin has been suggested [11].

Dizziness is a complication of stapedial surgery mentioned in the literature, as it poses a significant risk of vestibular damage, perilymphatic fistula and prosthesis displacement, in addition to other complications [12, 13].

Various studies have been carried out to assess the improvement in conductive hearing loss or sensorineural loss after stapedial surgery; however, little research has been undertaken to assess vestibular functions after surgery.

Symptoms related to vestibular function disorders in patients with otosclerosis have also been documented prior to surgery [14, 15], with clinical evidence demonstrating the presence of dizziness in almost 17 to 23% of otosclerosis patients [15, 16]. The purpose of this study is to assess this presence and distinguish between dizziness before and dizziness after surgery in patients with otosclerosis.

2. Methods

We have designed a prospective and observational study, which was approved by the ethics committee at our hospital. All patients on whom stapedial surgery was carried out at our hospital between October 2013 and December 2014 were invited to participate.

As part of the service, partial posterior stapedotomy/ stapedectomy are carried out under general anesthetic by employing a transcanal approach. By means of a horizontal incision in the skin of the outer ear canal's posterior superior wall, 5-6 mm from the annulus, a tympanomeatal flap is created that makes it possible to access the tympanic cavity. To guarantee better control of the oval window, curettage or drilling is performed several times in the canal's posterior superior wall, sparing the tympanic chord. After confirming the security of the stapes, the platinotomy, incudostapedial joint disarticulation, sectioning of the stapes muscle tendon, fracturing of the stapes superstructure, lengthening of the platinotomy/platinectomy, and installation of the Causse-type polytetrafluoroethylene prosthesis (Teflon) are carried out. For stapedial surgery, we accepted the recommendation of an air-bone gap equal to or greater than 30 dB.

The presence of dizziness was assessed before and 4 months after surgery. For instances of dizziness, the Portuguese version of the Dizziness Handicap Inventory questionnaire was used. The questionnaire comprises 25 simple questions, grouped into three categories: physical, emotional, and functional, with a variable score of between 0 and 100. Furthermore, the following data was collected: age, gender, and laterality. Patients submitted to revision surgery and those that failed to attend follow-ups were excluded. For the purposes of statistical analysis, the SPSS program was used and a level of statistical significance of $P < 0.05$ was allocated.

3. Results

140 patients were included in the study, 96 of whom (68.6%) were women. Age varied between 23 and 66, with an average age of 42. In regard to the ear operated on, right ear was for 91 patients (65%) and left ear was for 49 patients (35%). 11 patients (7.9%) showed signs of a bilateral illness.

48 patients (34.3%) mentioned dizziness in one of the two study periods. Before surgery, when questioned on the presence of any kind of vestibular disorder, 12 patients (8.6%) mentioned dizziness.

4 months after surgery, none of these patients mentioned any dizziness. 36 patients (25.7%) mentioned dizziness 4 months after surgery, of whom none had mentioned dizziness before surgery. 28.1% of the patients, without dizziness before surgery, developed vestibular complains after surgery. 92 patients (65.7%) did not mention any dizziness before or after surgery. These numbers are resumed at Tables 1 and 2. The total postoperation scores of the questionnaire on patients

TABLE 1: Number and percentage of patients with and without dizziness, before and after surgery.

	Before surgery (n (%))	4 months after surgery (n (%))
Dizziness	12 (8.6%)	36 (25.7%)
No dizziness	128 (91.4%)	104 (74.3%)

TABLE 2: Evolution of the two groups of patients (with and without dizziness before surgery), after the surgery.

Before surgery	4 months after surgery
Group of patients with dizziness (n = 12)	(i) All without dizziness
Group of patients without dizziness (n = 128)	(ii) 36 with dizziness (28.1%)
	(iii) 92 without dizziness (71.9%)

with dizziness varied between 2 and 18 points, with an average of 10 points. The most affected categories were physical and functional. There was no significant statistical difference between gender and age and the presence or seriousness of dizziness, whether in the presurgical period or in the 4 months after surgery.

4. Discussion

Women suffer otosclerosis more frequently than men, with a variable ratio of women to men of up to 2 : 1 [3]. Amongst patients subject to stapedial surgery at our hospital, during the study period, 96 (68.4%) were women and 44 (31.4%) were men. This data is similar to the figures obtained by other authors: 68.4% women in a study carried out in Spain [17] and 67% women in a French study [18]. We obtained a ratio of women to men of 2 : 1, which is also consistent with the literature [3, 17, 18].

Age varied between 23 and 66, with an average age of 42. The most affected age range was between 40 and 49 years of age (56%). In a study carried out on 475 Spanish patients, the most affected age range was between 15 and 45 years of age (62.2%) [17] whereas, as part of a study carried out in England on 65 English patients, the most affected age range was between 40 and 49 years of age [19]. Therefore, our results with regard to the most affected age range align with the results of publications released by other authors in the literature.

The condition was bilateral for 11 patients (7.9%) as part of our study, somewhat lower than in most of the studies published. As part of a study carried out in India, the condition was bilateral for 70% of study patients [20], whereas in an Iranian study this figure stood at just 18.2% [21]. The cause of a lower value having been recorded may be attributable to the fact that patients with previous stapedial surgery were excluded from the study.

As part of this study, when asked regarding the presence of any kind of vestibular disorder before surgery, 12 patients (8.6%) mentioned dizziness. This amount is lower than what is provided in the literature, with most studies returning dizziness rates of ranges between 17% and 23% [15, 16], for patients with otosclerosis. Amongst these patients, dizziness reduced after surgery, a phenomenon also identified by other authors [22]. The likely mechanism suggested by other authors is the fact that the quick recession is attributable to the sudden ruptures in the membranous labyrinth that cause changes in intralabyrinthine pressure due to changes in the volume of inner ear fluids. After stapedial surgery, as a result of movement in the ossicles and due to the prosthesis, a compensatory mechanism is established that prevents changes in pressure, which could explain the disappearance of dizziness.

As part of this study, in the 4th month following surgery, 36 patients (25.7%) reported dizziness. Dizziness is a common case in the days following surgery on the stapes [23, 24]; however, it rarely lasts longer than a week. Generally speaking, patients affected develop a permanent vestibular hypofunction, and over time they get used to the condition and are asymptomatic [25]. Birch and Elbrond reported a rate of dizziness lasting longer than one week of 4% [25], and Plaza Mayor recently reported a rate of persistent vertigo lasting 12 months of 2.6% [26]. The results obtained from this study were higher than those reported by the above authors, but very few studies assessing the presence of dizziness in the months following stapedial surgery have been carried out. Amongst these patients, as part of our study, all denied experiencing dizziness before surgery, which has made it possible to conclude that stapedial surgery could cause new vestibular disorders that are not related to the condition as such, which would remain in place after a 4-month period.

As part of this study, the total questionnaire scores in the postoperating period for patients with dizziness varied between 2 and 18 points, with an average score of 10 points; thus, dizziness can be considered light (whenever the result of the questionnaire is <30), with no significant effect on day-to-day activities.

5. Conclusion

Our study demonstrates that vestibular disorders may persist after the immediate postoperating period and highlights the need for patient clarifications at the time of providing informed consent.

Conflict of Interests

The authors declare that there is no conflict of interests regarding the publication of this paper.

References

[1] M. Ealy and R. J. H. Smith, "Otosclerosis," *Advances in Oto-Rhino-Laryngology*, vol. 70, pp. 122–129, 2011.

[2] T. Karosi and I. Sziklai, "Etiopathogenesis of otosclerosis," *European Archives of Oto-Rhino-Laryngology*, vol. 267, no. 9, pp. 1337–1349, 2010.

[3] B. Bouaity, M. Chihani, M. Touati, Y. Darouassi, K. Nadour, and H. Ammar, "Otosclerosis: retrospective study of 36 cases," *The Pan African Medical Journal*, vol. 18, article 242, 2014.

[4] W. Arnold, R. Busch, A. Arnold, B. Ritscher, A. Neiss, and H. P. Niedermeyer, "The influence of measles vaccination on the incidence of otosclerosis in Germany," *European Archives of Oto-Rhino-Laryngology*, vol. 264, no. 7, pp. 741–748, 2007.

[5] Y. D. Redfors and C. Möller, "Otosclerosis: thirty-year's follow-up after surgery," *Annals of Otology, Rhinology & Laryngology*, vol. 120, no. 9, pp. 608–614, 2011.

[6] J. W. House and C. D. Cunningham III, "Otosclerosis," in *Cummings Otolaryngology-Head and Neck Surgery*, P. W. Flint, B. H. Haughey, V. J. Lund, J. K. Niparko, M. A. Richardson, K. T. Robbins et al., Eds., pp. 2028–2035, Elsevier Mosby, Philadelphia, Pa, USA, 5th edition, 2010.

[7] S. Nemati, E. Naghavi, E. Kazemnejad, M. Aghajanpour, and O. Abdollahi, "Middle ear exploration results in suspected otosclerosis cases: are ossicular and footplate area anomalies rare?" *Iranian Journal of Otorhinolaryngology*, vol. 25, no. 72, pp. 155–159, 2013.

[8] S. Uppal, Y. Bajaj, and A. P. Coatesworth, "Otosclerosis 2: the medical management of otosclerosis," *International Journal of Clinical Practice*, vol. 64, no. 2, pp. 256–265, 2010.

[9] B. Liktor, Z. Szekanecz, T. J. Batta, I. Sziklai, and T. Karosi, "Perspectives of pharmacological treatment in otosclerosis," *European Archives of Oto-Rhino-Laryngology*, vol. 270, no. 3, pp. 793–804, 2013.

[10] Y. Imauchi, M. Lombès, P. Lainé, O. Sterkers, E. Ferrary, and A. B. Grayeli, "Glucocorticoids inhibit diastrophic dysplasia sulfate transporter activity in otosclerosis by interleukin-6," *Laryngoscope*, vol. 116, no. 9, pp. 1647–1650, 2006.

[11] J. L. Lacosta Nicolás, A. Sánchez del Hoyo, and J. García Cano, "Posible benefits of calcitonin in the treatment of otosclerosis," *Acta Otorrinolaringologica Espanola*, vol. 54, no. 3, pp. 169–172, 2003.

[12] J. R. G. Testa, I. Millas, I. M. De Vuono, M. E. L. R. B. V. Neto, and M. F. Lobato, "Otosclerose-resultados de estapedotomias," *Revista Brasileira de Otorrinolaringologia*, vol. 68, pp. 251–253, 2002.

[13] H. Kojima, M. Komori, S. Chikazawa et al., "Comparison between endoscopic and microscopic stapes surgery," *Laryngoscope*, vol. 124, no. 1, pp. 266–271, 2014.

[14] P. Eza-Nuñez, M. Manrique-Rodriguez, and N. Perez-Fernandez, "Otosclerosis amoung patients with dizziness," *Revue de Laryngologie Otologie Rhinologie*, vol. 131, no. 3, pp. 199–206, 2010.

[15] S. V. Morozova, V. E. Dobrotin, L. A. Kulakova, G. R. Kaspranskaia, and I. M. Ovchinnikov, "Vestibular disorders in patients with otosclerosis: prevalence, diagnostic and therapeutic options," *Vestnik Otorinolaringologii*, no. 2, pp. 20–22, 2009.

[16] M. S. Vartanian and T. V. Banashek-Meshchiarkova, "The incidence of vestibular disorders among the patients suffering from otosclerosis," *Vestnik Otorinolaringologii*, vol. 2, no. 2, pp. 23–26, 2013.

[17] J. J. Pérez-Lázaro, R. Urquiza, A. Cabrera, C. Guerrero, and E. Navarro, "Effectiveness assessment of otosclerosis surgery," *Acta Oto-Laryngologica*, vol. 125, no. 9, pp. 935–945, 2005.

[18] R. Vincent, N. M. Sperling, J. Oates, and M. Jindal, "Surgical findings and long-term hearing results in 3,050 stapedotomies for primary otosclerosis: a prospective study with the otology-neurotology database," *Otology and Neurotology*, vol. 27, no. 8, pp. S25–S47, 2006.

[19] C. H. Bulman, "Audit of stapedectomy in the north west of England for 1996 and an analysis of the criteria used to describe

success," *Clinical Otolaryngology & Allied Sciences*, vol. 25, no. 6, pp. 542–546, 2000.

[20] S. Ahmed, N. Raza, L. Ali, S. Ullah, and S. Iqbal, "Hearing improvement after stapedotomy using Teflon loop prosthesis," *Journal of the College of Physicians and Surgeons Pakistan*, vol. 16, no. 10, pp. 659–661, 2006.

[21] N. Saki, S. Nikakhlagh, M. Hekmatshoar, and N. M. Booshehri, "Evaluation of hearing results in otosclerotic patients after stapedectomy," *Iranian Journal of Otorhinolaryngology*, vol. 23, no. 65, pp. 127–132, 2011.

[22] N. K. Panda, A. K. Saha, A. K. Gupta, and S. B. S. Mann, "Evaluation of vestibular functions in otosclerosis before and after small fenestra stapedotomy," *Indian Journal of Otolaryngology and Head and Neck Surgery*, vol. 53, no. 1, pp. 23–27, 2001.

[23] J. Kuczkowski, W. Sierszeń, T. Przewoźny, and D. Paradowska, "Treatment results of otosclerosis regarding different types of prosthesis," *Otolaryngologia Polska*, vol. 66, no. 4, supplement, pp. 25–29, 2012.

[24] T. P. Hirvonen and H. Aalto, "Immediate postoperative nystagmus and vestibular symptoms after stapes surgery," *Acta Oto-Laryngologica*, vol. 133, no. 8, pp. 842–845, 2013.

[25] L. Birch and O. Elbrond, "Stapedectomy and vertigo," *Clinical Otolaryngology & Allied Sciences*, vol. 10, no. 4, pp. 217–223, 1985.

[26] G. Plaza Mayor, C. Herraiz Puchol, B. Martínez Rodríguez, and G. de los Santos Granados, "Delayed vertigo after stapedotomy with good hearing results," *Anales Otorrinolaringológicos Ibero-Americanos*, vol. 34, no. 5, pp. 447–457, 2007.

Permissions

List of Contributors

Anila Narayanan and Bini Faizal
Department of ENT, Amrita Institute of Medical Sciences, Amrita Vishwa Vidyapeetham, Kochi, Kerala 682041, India

Kei Nakajima
Division of Clinical Nutrition, Department of Medical Dietetics, Faculty of Pharmaceutical Sciences, Josai University, 1-1 Keyakidai, Sakado, Saitama 350-0295, Japan

Eiichiro Kanda
Department of Nephrology, Tokyo Kyosai Hospital, Nakameguro 2-3-8, Meguroku, Tokyo 153-8934, Japan

Ami Hosobuchi
Division of Clinical Nutrition, Department of Medical Dietetics, Faculty of Pharmaceutical Sciences, Josai University, 1-1 Keyakidai, Sakado, Saitama 350-0295, Japan

Kaname Suwa
Saitama Health Promotion Corporation, 519 Kamiookubo, Saitama, Saitama 338-0824, Japan

M. Sayma, R. Hyne, M. Sharma, L. Kyle, M. Abo Khatwa, I. MacKay-Davies, A. Poulios and H. S. Khalil
Plymouth Hospitals NHS Trust and Peninsula College of Medicine and Dentistry, Plymouth, UK

Mehmet Metin
Hendek State Hospital, 54300 Sakarya, Turkey

Zeynep Kizilkaya Kaptan
Ankara Research and Training Hospital, Ministry of Health, 06340 Ankara, Turkey

Sedat Dogan
Faculty of Medicine, Adiyaman University, Ear Nose Throat Clinic, 02200 Adiyaman, Turkey

Hasmet Yazici
Faculty of Medicine, Balikesir University, Ear Nose Throat Clinic, 10145 Balikesir, Turkey

Cem Bayraktar
Faculty of Medicine, Adiyaman University, Ear Nose Throat Clinic, 02200 Adiyaman, Turkey

Hakan Gocmen and Etem Erdal Samim
Ankara Research and Training Hospital, Ministry of Health, 06340 Ankara, Turkey

Rolf Haye and Liv Kari Døsen
The Department of Oto-Rhino-Laryngology, Lovisenberg Diakonale Hospital, Norway

Magnus Tarangen and Olga Shiryaeva
The Department of Quality, Lovisenberg Diakonale Hospital, Norway

Sohil Vadiya
Pramukhswami Medical College and Shree Krishna Hospital, Karamsad, Gujarat 388325, India

Abebe Bekele
Department of Surgery, School of Medicine, Addis Ababa University, Ethiopia

Ramesh Parajuli
Department of Otorhinolaryngology, Chitwan Medical College Teaching Hospital, P.O. Box 42, Chitwan, Nepal

Yousseria Elsayed Yousef
Department of Pediatric Nursing, Faculty of Nursing, Sohag University, Egypt

Essam A. Abo El-Magd
ENT, Faculty of Medicine, Aswan University, Egypt

Osama M. El-Asheer
Pediatrics, Faculty of Medicine, Assiut University, Egypt

Safaa Kotb
Public Health, Faculty of Nursing, Assiut University, Egypt

Ke Heng Chen and Susan A. Small
University of British Columbia, Vancouver, BC, Canada V6T 1Z3

Kerem Erkalp, M. Salih Sevdi, Hacer Yeter, SertuL Sinan Ege and Aysin Alagol
Istanbul Bagcilar Educational and Training Hospital, 34200 Istanbul, Turkey

Nuran Kalekoglu Erkalp
Ventigoo ENT and Balance Center, 34180 Istanbul, Turkey

A. Yasemin Korkut
Istanbul Sisli Etfal Training Hospital, 34360 Istanbul, Turkey

Veysel Erden
Istanbul Educational and Research Hospital, 34104 Istanbul, Turkey

Lara Ferris and Taher Omari
Gastroenterology Unit, Child, Youth & Women's Health Service, Adelaide, SA, Australia
School of Medicine, Flinders University, Adelaide, SA, Australia

Margot Selleslagh and Nathalie Rommel
Translational Research Center for Gastrointestinal Disorders, KU Leuven, Leuven, Belgium
ExpORL, Department of Neurosciences, KU Leuven, Leuven, Belgium

Eddy Dejaeger
Geriatric Medicine, University Hospital Leuven, Leuven, Belgium
Center for Swallowing Disorders, University Hospital Leuven, Leuven, Belgium

Jan Tack
Translational Research Center for Gastrointestinal Disorders, KU Leuven, Leuven, Belgium

Dirk Vanbeckevoort
Center for Swallowing Disorders, University Hospital Leuven, Leuven, Belgium
Radiology, University Hospital Leuven, Leuven, Belgium

Thomas S. Rau, Thomas Lenarz and Omid Majdani
Department of Otolaryngology, Hannover Medical School, Carl-Neuberg-Straße 1, 30625 Hannover, Germany

H. P. Barham
Department of Otolaryngology-Head and Neck Surgery, Louisiana State University Health Sciences Center, 533 Bolivar Street, Suite 566, New Orleans, LA 70112, USA

P. Collister, V. D. Eusterman and A.M. Terella
Department of Otolaryngology-Head and Neck Surgery, University of Colorado, Aurora, CO, USA

Hussein Walijee, Ali Al-Hussaini, Andrew Harris and David Owens
Department ofOtorhinolaryngology,Head and Neck Surgery, University Hospital of Wales, Cardiff CF14 4XW, UK

Vinaya Manchaiah
Department of Vision and Hearing Sciences, Anglia Ruskin University, Cambridge CB1 1PT, UK
Linnaeus Centre HEAD,The Swedish Institute for Disability Research, Department of Behavioral Science and Learning, Linköping University, 58183 Linköping, Sweden

Berth Danermark
The Swedish Institute for Disability Research, Örebro University, 702 81 Örebro, Sweden

Jerker Rönnberg
Linnaeus Centre HEAD,The Swedish Institute for Disability Research, Department of Behavioral Science and Learning, Linköping University, 58183 Linköping, Sweden

Thomas Lunner
Linnaeus Centre HEAD,The Swedish Institute for Disability Research, Department of Behavioral Science and Learning, Linköping University, 58183 Linköping, Sweden

Eriksholm Research Centre, Oticon A/S, 20 Rørtangvej, 3070 Snekkersten, Denmark

Sampath Chandra Prasad, Nikhil Dinaker Thada and Kishore Chandra Prasad
Department of Otolaryngology, Head and Neck Surgery, Srinivas Institute of Medical Sciences and Research, 5-7-712/3 ASRP Street, Dongerkery, Kodialbail, Mangalore, Karnataka 575001, India

Arun Azeez
Department of Otolaryngology, Head and Neck Surgery, Kasturba Medical College, Mangalore, Karnataka, India

Pallavi Rao
Department of Radiodiagnosis, Kasturba Medical College, Mangalore, Karnataka, India

Andrea Bacciu
Department of Clinical and Experimental Medicine, Otolaryngology Unit, University Hospital of Parma, Parma, Italy

Mahmoud El-Sayed Ali
Department of Otolaryngology, Mansoura University Hospital, Mansoura University, Egypt
Institute for Cell and Molecular Biosciences, Newcastle University, Faculty of Medical Sciences, Newcastle upon Tyne NE2 4HH, UK

DavidM. Bulmer and Jeffrey P. Pearson
Institute for Cell and Molecular Biosciences, Newcastle University, Faculty of Medical Sciences, Newcastle upon Tyne NE2 4HH, UK

PeterW. Dettmar
Castle Hill Hospital, Castle Road, Cottingham, East Yorkshire HU16 5JQ, UK

Jerome R. Lechien
Laboratory of Anatomy and Cell Biology, Faculty of Medicine, UMONS Research Institute for Health Sciences and Technology, University of Mons (UMons), Avenue du Champ de Mars 6, B7000 Mons, Belgium
Laboratory of Phonetics, Faculty of Psychology, Research Institute for Language Sciences and Technology,University ofMons (UMons), B7000 Mons, Belgium

Olivier Filleul and Pedro Costa de Araujo
Laboratory of Anatomy and Cell Biology, Faculty of Medicine, UMONS Research Institute for Health Sciences and Technology, University of Mons (UMons), Avenue du Champ de Mars 6, B7000 Mons, Belgium

Julien W. Hsieh
Laboratory of Neurogenetics and Behavior, Rockefeller University, 1230 York Avenue, New York City, NY 10065, USA

Gilbert Chantrain
Department of Otorhinolaryngology, Head, and Neck Surgery, CHU Saint-Pierre, Faculty of Medicine, Universit´e Libre de Bruxelles (ULB), B1000 Brussels, Belgium

Sven Saussez
Laboratory of Anatomy and Cell Biology, Faculty of Medicine, UMONS Research Institute for Health Sciences and Technology, University of Mons (UMons), Avenue du Champ de Mars 6, B7000 Mons, Belgium
Department of Otorhinolaryngology, Head, and Neck Surgery, CHU Saint-Pierre, Faculty of Medicine, Universit´e Libre de Bruxelles (ULB), B1000 Brussels, Belgium

Henri Traboulsi, Elie Alam and Usamah Hadi
Department of Otolaryngology-Head and Neck Surgery, American University of Beirut Medical Center, Phase I, 6th Floor, Room C-638, Bliss Street, P.O. Box 11-0236, Beirut, Lebanon

Mahmoud El-Sayed Ali
Department of Otolaryngology, Mansoura University Hospital, Mansoura University, Mansoura 35516, Egypt
Institute for Cell and Molecular Biosciences, Faculty of Medical Sciences, Newcastle University, Newcastle upon Tyne NE2 4HH, UK

Jeffrey P. Pearson
Institute for Cell and Molecular Biosciences, Faculty of Medical Sciences, Newcastle University, Newcastle upon Tyne NE2 4HH, UK

Holger A. Rambold
Department of Neurology, County Hospitals of Altötting and Burghausen, 84503 Altötting, Germany
Department of Neurology, University of Regensburg, 93053 Regensburg, Germany

Sushil Gaur, Sanjeev Kumar Awasthi, Sunil Kumar Singh Bhadouriya, Rohit Saxena,
Vivek Kumar Pathak and Mamta Bisht
Department of E.N.T. and Head & Neck Surgery, School of Medical Science & Research, Greater Noida 201306, India

Priscila Carvalho Miranda and Rafaela Aquino Fernandes Lopes
Brasília University Hospital, Hospital Universitário de Brasília-HUB, SGAN 605, Avenida L2 Norte, 70830-200 Brasília, DF, Brazil

André Luiz Lopes Sampaio, Alessandra Ramos Venosa and Carlos Augusto Costa Pires de Oliveira
Brasília University Hospital, Hospital Universitário de Brasília-HUB, SGAN 605, Avenida L2 Norte, 70830-200 Brasília, DF, Brazil
Universidade de Brasília (UnB), Campus Universitário Darcy Ribeiro, 70910-900 Brasília, DF, Brazil

Saisawat Chaiyasate, Supranee Fooanant, Niramon Navacharoen and Kannika Roongrotwattanasiri
Department of Otolaryngology, Faculty of Medicine, Chiang Mai University, Chiang Mai 50000,Thailand

Pongsakorn Tantilipikorn
Department of Otorhinolaryngology, Faculty of Medicine, Siriraj Hospital, Mahidol University, Bangkok 10700, Thailand

Jayanton Patumanond
Division of Clinical Epidemiology, Department of Community Medicine, Faculty of Medicine, Chiang Mai University, Chiang Mai 50000,Thailand
Clinical Research Center, Faculty of Medicine,Thammasat University, Pathum Thani 12120, Thailand

Jinwei Hu and Helen Xu
Department ofOtolaryngology and Head & Neck Surgery, Loma Linda University Medical Center, Loma Linda, CA, USA
Loma Linda Veterans Affairs Medical Center, Loma Linda, CA, USA

Jane Xu and Matthew Streelman
Loma Linda University Medical School, Loma Linda, CA, USA

O'neil Guthrie
Department ofOtolaryngology and Head & Neck Surgery, Loma Linda University Medical Center, Loma Linda, CA, USA
Loma Linda Veterans Affairs Medical Center, Loma Linda, CA, USA
Cell & Molecular Pathology Laboratory, Department of Communication Sciences and Disorders, Northern Arizona University, Flagstaff, AZ, USA

Yuan F. Liu and Jinwei Hu
Department of Otolaryngology-Head and Neck Surgery, Loma Linda University Medical Center, 11234 Anderson Street, Loma Linda, CA 92354, USA

Matthew Streelman
Loma Linda University School of Medicine, 11175 Campus Street, Loma Linda, CA 92350, USA

O'neilW. Guthrie
Department of Otolaryngology-Head and Neck Surgery, Loma Linda University Medical Center, 11234 Anderson Street, Loma Linda, CA 92354, USA
Loma Linda University School of Medicine, 11175 Campus Street, Loma Linda, CA 92350, USA
Loma Linda Veterans Affairs Medical Center, 11201 Benton Street, Loma Linda, CA 92357, USA

Macario Camacho
Otolaryngology-Head and Neck Surgery, Division of Sleep Surgery andMedicine, Tripler ArmyMedical Center, 1 JarrettWhite Road, Honolulu, HI 96859, USA
Department of Psychiatry and Behavioral Sciences, SleepMedicine Division, Stanford Hospital and Clinics, Stanford, CA 94304, USA

Soroush Zaghi
Otolaryngology-Head and Neck Surgery, Division of Sleep Surgery and Medicine, Stanford Hospitals and Clinics, Stanford, CA 94304, USA

Daniel Tran, Sungjin A. Song and Edward T. Chang
Otolaryngology-Head and Neck Surgery, Division of Sleep Surgery andMedicine, Tripler ArmyMedical Center, 1 JarrettWhite Road, Honolulu, HI 96859, USA

Victor Certal
Department of Otorhinolaryngology, Sleep Medicine Centre, Hospital CUF, 4100-180 Porto, Portugal
Centre for Research in Health Technologies and Information Systems (CINTESIS), University of Porto, 4200-450 Porto, Portugal

George Barrett, Susanne Koecher, Natalie Ronan and DavidWhinney
Department ENT Head andNeck Surgery, Royal Cornwall Hospital, Truro TR1 3LJ, UK

Nathalie Rommel
Neurosciences, ExpORL, KU Leuven, 3000 Leuven, Belgium
Gastroenterology, Neurogastroenterology and Motility, University Hospitals Leuven, 3000 Leuven, Belgium
Translational Research Center for Gastrointestinal Diseases (TARGID), KU Leuven, 3000 Leuven, Belgium

Charlotte Borgers
Neurosciences, ExpORL, KU Leuven, 3000 Leuven, Belgium

Dirk Van Beckevoort
Radiology, University Hospitals Leuven, Leuven, Belgium

Ann Goeleven
Neurosciences, ExpORL, KU Leuven, 3000 Leuven, Belgium
ENT,Head&Neck Surgery, MUCLA, University Hospitals Leuven, Leuven, Belgium

Eddy Dejaeger
Geriatric Medicine, University Hospitals Leuven, Leuven, Belgium

Taher I. Omari
Neurosciences, ExpORL, KU Leuven, 3000 Leuven, Belgium

School of Medicine, Flinders University, Bedford Park, Australia
The Robinson Research Institute, University of Adelaide, Adelaide, Australia

M. Mustafa Kiliçkaya, Mustafa Tuz, Murat YariktaG, Hasan Yasan and Giray AynalJ
Department of Otolaryngology, Medical Faculty of Suleyman Demirel University, 32100 Isparta, Turkey

Özkan Bagci
Department of Medical Genetics, Medical Faculty of Suleyman Demirel University, 32100 Isparta, Turkey

Saisawat Chaiyasate, Kannika Roongrotwattanasiri and Supranee Fooanant
Department of Otolaryngology, Faculty of Medicine, Chiang Mai University, Chiang Mai 50000, Thailand

Jayanton Patumanond
Clinical Research Center, Faculty of Medicine,Thammasat University, Pathum Thani 12120, Thailand

Ditza de Vilhena, Inês Gambôa, Delfim Duarte and Gustavo Lopes
Department of Otolaryngology and Head & Neck Surgery, Hospital Pedro Hispano, Matosinhos, 4150-800 Porto, Portugal